RADIOLOGY:
MGH Clinical Review

RADIOLOGY:
MGH Clinical Review

Daniel I. Rosenthal, M.D.
Associate Radiologist-in-Chief and Director
of Bone and Joint Radiology
Massachusetts General Hospital

Associate Professor of Radiology
Harvard Medical School
Boston, Massachusetts

William E. Palmer, M.D.
Assistant Radiologist
Massachusetts General Hospital

Assistant Professor of Radiology
Harvard Medical School
Boston, Massachusetts

Felix S. Chew, M.D.
Assistant Radiologist
Massachusetts General Hospital

Assistant Professor of Radiology
Harvard Medical School
Boston, Massachusetts

Daniel P. Barboriak, M.D.
Assistant in Neuroradiology
Massachusetts General Hospital

Clinical Assistant Instructor
Harvard Medical School
Brockton MRI Center
Boston, Massachusetts

Andrew E. Rosenberg, M.D.
Associate Pathologist and Director
of Musculoskeletal Pathology
Massachusetts General Hospital

Assistant Professor of Radiology
Harvard Medical School
Boston, Massachusetts

W.B. SAUNDERS COMPANY
A Division of Harcourt Brace & Company
Philadelphia   London   Toronto   Montreal   Sydney   Tokyo

W.B. Saunders Company
A Division of Harcourt Brace & Company

The Curtis Center
Independence Square West
Philadelphia, Pennsylvania 19106

Library of Congress Cataloging-in-Publication Data

Radiology : MGH clinical review / edited by Daniel I. Rosenthal . . .
  [et al.] ; contributors, Stephen M. Bloch . . . [et al.].—1st ed.
     p. cm.
   ISBN 0-7216-4609-3
     1. Radiography, Medical—Case studies.   I. Rosenthal, Daniel I.
(Daniel Ira).
    [DNLM: 1. Radiology—examination questions.   WN 18 R12972 1994]
  RC78.15.R28   1994
  616.07′57′076—dc20
  DNLM/DLC   93-20747

Credits

The American Roentgen Ray Society has granted permission to reproduce the
following material from the *American Journal of Roentgenology:*

AJR No.	Author	Case
159:756, 1992	Brown JH, Chew FS	Case 4
156:474, 1991	Chew FS, Smith PL, Barboriak DP	Case 82
156:724, 1991	Palmer WE, Gerard-McFarland EL, Chew FS	Case 9
156:1144, 1991	Palmer WE, Chew FS	Case 3
157:318, 1991	Brown JH, Chew FS	Case 53
157:468, 1991	Chew FS, Weissleder R	Case 98
157:792, 1991	Chew FS, Weissleder R	Case 39
157:950, 1991	Palmer WE, Rivitz SM, Chew FS	Case 94
157:1278, 1991	Prince MR, Chew FS	Case 74
158:62, 1992	Palmer WE, Bloch SM, Chew FS	Case 33
158:330,1992	Chew FS, Crenshaw WB	Case 32
158:570, 1992	Prince MR, Chew FS	Case 51

RADIOLOGY:MGH CLINICAL REVIEW   ISBN 0-7216-4609-3

Printed in the United States of America

Last digit is the print number: 9   8   7   6   5   4   3   2   1

Preparing a conference can be drudgery.
Cases must be selected, films found,
findings reviewed, entities researched.
We are indebted to the industrious residents
who helped collect and prepare this material
and dedicate this volume
to all radiology residents,
past, present, and future.

Preface

This volume is a collection of cases culled from the Radiologic-Pathologic Conferences of the Massachusetts General Hospital (MGH), a series of educational seminars that has been conducted continuously for two thirds of a century. Early workers in radiology realized the importance of correlating radiology with pathology. In the preface to their 1919 textbook, Drs. George W. Holmes* and Howard E. Ruggles wrote: "The necessity of a medical training as a prerequisite in [roentgenology] is, of course, recognized, but the particular importance of thorough grounding in pathology is not always sufficiently plain. In attempting to study gross changes by means of shadows, a knowledge of pathology is as essential to the roentgenologist as anatomy to the surgeon."[6]

During Dr. Holmes' tenure as chief, a weekly teaching seminar in roentgenology was organized in 1927 by Dr. John D. Camp†[9,10,12] for the purpose of correlating radiology with clinical and pathological findings. The following 1927 description of the conference remains accurate: "The staff of the department conducts a weekly seminar which has been well attended and at which the clinical, operative, or autopsy findings are compared with those of the x-ray."[1] In the 1940s the seminar was held on Wednesday afternoons from 4 to 6 PM, and the entire radiology department, at that time consisting of six staff and three residents (one in each year of training), attended, along with a pathologist and many visitors. The cases were presented by the residents and discussed extemporaneously by a staff member. The major emphasis at the time was on difficult cases in which the diagnosis had been prospectively missed or delayed. Afterwards, it was usual to repair to a nearby Irish pub—a small, dark place with checkered table cloths—on a site now occupied by a filling station. In general, every man paid for his own drinks, but sometimes the chief would buy beer for the three residents.[17]

Six "case reports from the weekly seminar, Department of Roentgenology, Massachusetts General Hospital" were published in the American Journal of Roentgenology (AJR) in 1938 and 1939 by Dr. James R. Lingley‡, beginning with a case of intestinal adenocarcinoma, discussed by Drs. Aubrey O. Hampton# and Benjamin Castleman[7] and

---

*Dr. Holmes (1876–1959) was roentgenologist-in-chief of the MGH from 1916 to 1941. Dr. Holmes established what is thought to be the first radiology residency in the United States at the MGH in 1916.[9,12]

†Dr. Camp (1889–1969) in 1927 was an assistant roentgenologist.[13] Dr. Camp left the MGH the following year and subsequently rose to national prominence as a neuroradiologist at the Mayo Clinic.[14] He was president of the Radiological Society of North America in 1937, and president of the American College of Radiology in 1952. Dr. Camp ended his career as Director of Radiology at Good Samaritan Hospital in Los Angeles.

‡Dr. Lingley (1903–1978) was a radiology resident at MGH from 1930 to 1931, and then an assistant roentgenologist beginning in 1931.[13] After service in World War II, he returned briefly to the MGH before entering private practice in Worcester, MA.[16]

#Drs. Hampton (1900–1955) and Castleman wrote the definitive paper on pulmonary embolism and infarction.[2,5] During the late 1930s they conducted a weekly lung-cutting session in the pathology department, during which they correlated the roentgenograms with the pathology. This conference expanded to consider other types of pathology and was ultimately merged with the weekly radiology seminar.[17] Dr. Hampton was roentgenologist-in-chief in 1941 and 1942, but his tenure was cut short by Army service, and he did not return to the MGH after the war. Dr. Castleman was pathologist-in-chief from 1953 to 1974.

ending with a case of follicular gastritis.[8] From 1961 to 1972, 123 cases were published in JAMA as a monthly feature called X-Ray Seminars, beginning with a case of gastric adenocarcinoma masquerading as varices[15] and ending with osteoblastic multiple myeloma.[4] A collection of the first 100 of these cases was published in 1971 as a book.[11] In 1989, beginning with a case of candidal splenic abscesses,[3] cases drawn from the weekly X-Ray Seminar, now called the Radiologic-Pathologic Conference, are again being published as a monthly feature in AJR.

Over the years, the number of teaching exercises in the Department of Radiology has increased so that the Radiologic-Pathologic Conference is only one of many formal department-wide teaching conferences. Currently conducted by Dr. Jack Wittenberg, these exercises consist of the presentation of four to six unknown cases, chosen primarily for their diagnostic difficulty and the correlation between the radiologic and pathologic features. As such, these cases represent a unique opportunity to learn the pathologic basis of diagnostic imaging. One radiology resident is assigned full-time to the preparation and presentation of the cases, reflecting the level of effort that goes into this 60-minute conference. With the aid of a sometimes misleading history, a participant who has not previously seen the case discusses the relevant radiologic findings and provides a differential diagnosis. The pathologist then reveals the diagnosis, and in a spirited interchange between the presenter, the pathologist, the participant, the moderator, and the audience, the salient pathologic features relevant to the radiologic features are brought to light.

For the cases in this book, we have retained the case presentation format of the original conference. Each case begins by challenging the reader with a series of images. The reader is provided with a differential diagnosis on the next page to compare with his own. These differential diagnoses are drawn from the original case discussions at the conference and should not necessarily be taken as definitive for similar cases. The pathology is shown, and the diagnosis and discussion are provided on the following pages.

REFERENCES

1. Annual report (1927) of the General Executive Committee of the Massachusetts General Hospital. Cited by McNeill JM, Robbins LL (eds). X-ray seminar cases of the Massachusetts General Hospital. Boston, Little, Brown, 1971:v.

2. Chew FS: The 50 most frequently cited papers in the past 50 years. AJR 1988; 150:227–233.

3. Chew FS. Smith PL, Barboriak DP. Candidal splenic abscesses. AJR 1991; 156:474.

4. Courey RW. Osteoblastic lesions of unusual nature. JAMA 1972; 219:377–378.

5. Hampton AO, Castleman B. Correlation of postmortem chest teleroentgenograms with autopsy findings: with special reference to pulmonary embolism and infarction. Am J Roentgenol 1940; 43:305–326.

6. Holmes GW, Ruggles HE. Roentgen interpretation: a manual for students and practitioners. Philadelphia: Lea & Febiger, 1919.

7. Lingley JR. Case report from the weekly seminar, Department of Roentgenology, Massachusetts General Hospital. Am J Roentgenol 1938; 40:126–128.

8. Lingley JR. Case report from the weekly seminar, Department of Roentgenology, Massachusetts General Hospital. Am J Roentgenol 1939; 43:438–441.

9. McNeill JM. A history of radiology at the Massachusetts General Hospital 1896–1971 [pamphlet]. Department of Radiology, MGH, 1971:37 pp.

10. McNeill JM. X-ray seminar [letter]. JAMA 1972; 219:388.

11. McNeill JM, Robbins LL (eds). X-ray seminar cases of the Massachusetts General Hospital. Boston: Little, Brown, 1971.

12. Merrill AS. A brief history of the Department of Roentgenology of the Massachusetts General Hospital. Am J Roentgenol 1936; 36:727–736.

13. Roster of Dr. George W. Holmes' associates and students. Am J Roentgenol 1936; 36:987–991.

14. Scanlan RL, Rigler LG. In memoriam. John D. Camp, M.D. 1898–1969. Radiology 1969; 93:447–448.

15. Weylman WT, Simon H. Tumor or varices. JAMA 1961; 177:202–203.

16. Wyman SM. In memoriam. J. Reginald Lingley, M.D. Radiology 1980; 135:796.

17. Wyman SM. Personal communication.

Contributors

Daniel P. Barboriak, M.D.

Stephen M. Bloch, M.D.

James H. Brown, M.D.

William B. Crenshaw, M.D.

David G. Disler, M.D.

Elizabeth L. Gerard, M.D.

David C. Harrison, M.D.

Thomas B. Kinney, M.D.

Mark H. Lerner, M.D.

Carey S. Linker, M.D., Ph.D.

William W. Mayo-Smith, M.D.

William E. Palmer, M.D.

Martin R. Prince, M.D., Ph.D.

Mitchell S. Rivitz, M.D.

Richard L. Robertson, Jr., M.D.

Pamela W. Schaefer, M.D.

Fred A. Scialabba, M.D.

Peter L. Smith, M.D.

Ralph Weissleder, M.D., Ph.D.

Wendy E. Zimmer, M.D.

Contents

Contents

Case 1

HISTORY

A 34-year-old woman presented with right wrist pain and limitation of motion.

RADIOLOGY

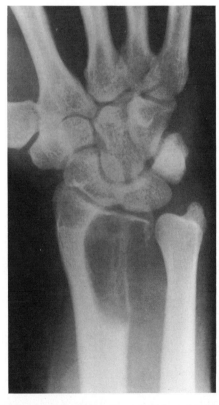

Figure 1-1. Posteroanterior (PA) radiograph of the wrist demonstrates a lytic lesion of the distal radius. The margins between the lesion and the adjacent bone are well defined and not sclerotic. A faintly and incompletely mineralized periosteal shell is seen protruding into the dorsal and medial soft tissues. The lesion extends to within 1 mm of both the radial carpal and radial ulnar articular surfaces.

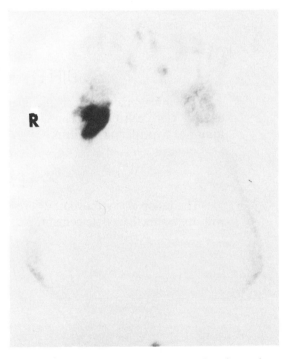

Figure 1-2. Radionuclide bone scan shows a solitary focus of markedly increased tracer accumulation.

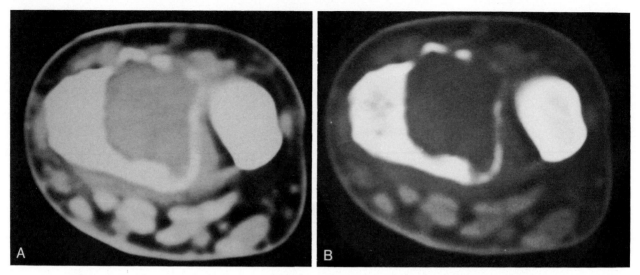

Figure 1-3*A*. CT scan at the level of the distal radial ulnar joint demonstrates a mass of soft tissue density (not cystic) occupying the distal radius. *B*. Bone windows reveal an expanded, incompletely mineralized periosteal shell.

DIFFERENTIAL DIAGNOSIS

The differential diagnosis includes aneurysmal or unicameral bone cyst, metastatic disease, giant cell tumor, chondromyxoid fibroma, desmoplastic fibroma, and brown tumor of hyperparathyroidism.

PATHOLOGY

The lesion was removed by curettage, and the resulting defect in bone was packed with methylmethacrylate cement.

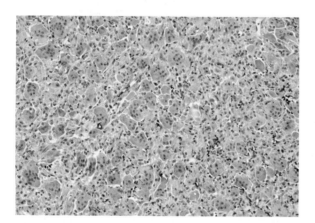

Figure 1-4. The lesion contains numerous multinucleated osteoclast-type giant cells. Between the giant cells are mononuclear stromal cells that tend to be oval or spindle shaped.

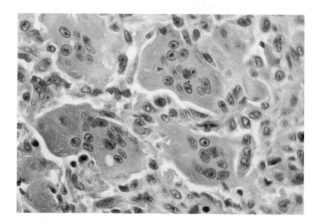

Figure 1-5. The nuclei of the stromal cells are identical in morphology to the nuclei of the giant cells.

DIAGNOSIS

The final pathologic diagnosis was giant cell tumor.

DISCUSSION

The giant cell tumor, or osteoclastoma, is an uncommon lesion. It represents only 4% of all bone tumors, yet it is still the second most common benign tumor of bone. Although it is classified as a benign tumor, metastases may occur rarely.

The giant cell tumor is distinguished on histologic examination by a vascular network of multinucleated giant cells intermixed with plump stromal cells. The giant cells are not thought to represent the neoplastic element; the background mononuclear fibrous cells determine the biologic behavior of these lesions. The exact origin of the giant cells and mononuclear cells is unclear.

The lesions are usually found in close proximity to a joint, often adjacent to an articular cortex. Although there is some disagreement about whether the lesions arise primarily in the epiphysis or the metaphysis, the tumors commonly spread through both and occasionally break through the articular surface, invading the joint. More than 50% arise in the femur, tibia, or fibula about the knee, and 15% occur at the wrist. Other less common sites include the spine, sacrum, and shoulder. The most common presentation is a tender, swollen, warm joint or a pathologic fracture.

Radiographic features are usually distinctive and diagnostic. The tumors are seen after epiphyseal closure and may extend almost to the articular surface. Very rarely, they may be located in the shaft. Growth can be rapid, resulting in expansion and osteolysis. The tumors lack osteogenic capability. Computed tomography of giant cell tumor most commonly shows an expanded or "pushed-out" cortex, which is remodeled around the lesion by means of periosteal new bone formation. Less often, there is a clear cortical defect with the tumor extending into the soft tissues. An appearance suggesting trabeculation is uncommon but is seen most often in treated tumors; this appearance does not represent true trabeculae but rather reinforced peripheral neocortex. Periosteal reaction is limited. Angiography is useful prior to surgery to assess vascularity. Most tumors are hypervascular. Increased uptake, particularly at the periphery of the lesion, is seen on radionuclide bone scans.

Prognosis does not relate to the histologic grade of the tumor. Although classified as a benign tumor, up to 10% of giant cell tumors develop metastases and are primarily malignant, and an additional 5% become malignant upon recurrence. Local recurrence is not uncommon, depending upon the choice of therapy. Treatment choices include curettage and packing with allograft, autograft, or methylmethacrylate cement, curettage with freezing with liquid nitrogen, resection with allograft replacement, and amputation.

REFERENCES

Brown KT, Kattapuram SV, Rosenthal DI. Computed tomography analysis of bone tumors: patterns of cortical destruction and soft tissue extension. Skel Radiol 1986; 15:448.

Dahlin DC. Giant cell tumor of bone: highlights of 407 cases. AJR 1985; 144:955–960.

Hudson TM. Radiologic-pathologic correlation of musculoskeletal lesions. Baltimore: Williams & Wilkins, 1987:209–237.

Kattapuram SV, et al. Giant cell tumor of bone: radiographic changes following local excision and allograft replacement. Radiology 1986; 161:493–498.

Moser RP Jr, Kransdorf MJ, Gilkey FW, et al. Giant cell tumor of the upper extremity. Radiographics 1990; 10:83–102.

Case 2

HISTORY

A 27-year-old man complained of persistent frontal headaches and rapidly progressive left visual loss.

RADIOLOGY

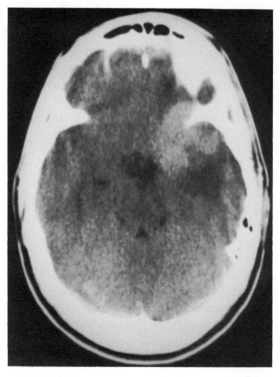

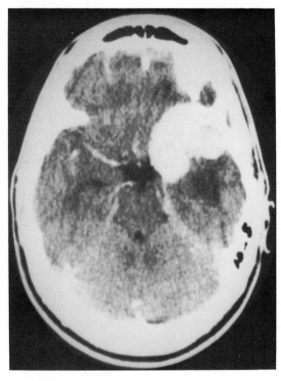

Figure 2-1. A noncontrast cranial CT scan shows a well-circumscribed mass of relatively high attenuation contiguous with the left greater sphenoid wing. No bone destruction is seen. Edema surrounds the mass.

Figure 2-2. The mass enhances homogeneously.

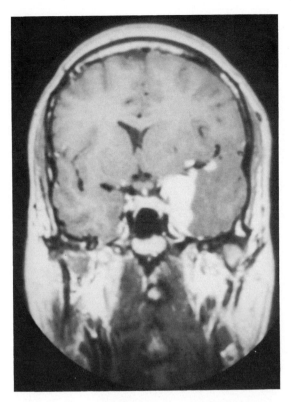

Figure 2-3. Gadolinium-enhanced coronal T1-weighted MR image demonstrates homogeneous enhancement. The mass is extra-axial. There is enhancement both of the basilar meninges along the floor of the left middle cranial fossa and of focal deposits in the left sylvian fissure.

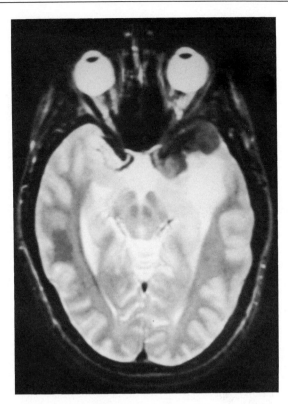

Figure 2-4. The mass loses signal intensity on T2-weighted images. Abnormal hypointense signal extends anteriorly to the left optic canal and surrounds the optic nerve.

DIFFERENTIAL DIAGNOSIS

The differential diagnosis includes meningioma with satellite foci, carcinomatous meningitis, lymphoma, leukemia, sarcoidosis, syphilis, and tuberculous and fungal meningitis.

PATHOLOGY

A biopsy of the mass was performed through a left frontal craniotomy.

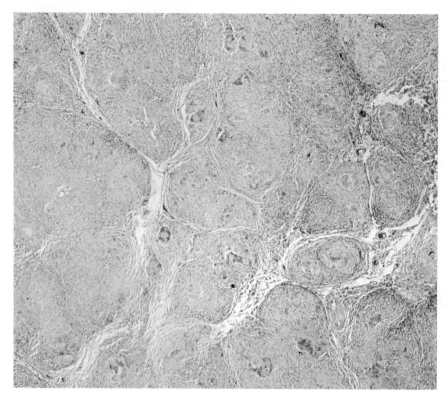

Figure 2-5. At low power there are clusters of well-formed noncaseating granulomas.

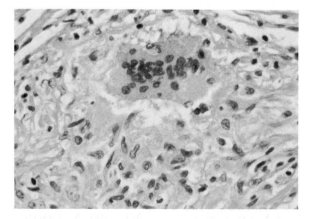

Figure 2-6. At high power a multinucleated giant cell is present within a granuloma.

DIAGNOSIS

The final pathologic diagnosis was sarcoidosis with involvement of the central nervous system.

DISCUSSION

Sarcoidosis is a multisystemic granulomatous disease of unknown etiology and pathogenesis. The characteristic microscopic lesion of sarcoid is the noncaseating granuloma, which consists of concentric arrangements of plump epithelioid cells surrounded by a rim of fibroblasts. Definitive diagnosis requires demonstration of these granulomas in the absence of another granulomatous disease (such as tuberculosis, fungal infection, or foreign body reaction). Blacks are affected 10 times more frequently than whites, females twice as often as males. Peak incidence occurs in the third to fourth decades. Although practically any organ can be involved, pulmonary disease is most common. Neurologic symptoms, which are seen in about 5% of patients, result from cranial neuropathy, aseptic meningitis, hydrocephalus, and parenchymal brain involvement.

Isolated involvement of the central nervous system by sarcoidosis is rare and is seen in only 12% of patients who have involvement of the central nervous system. In neurosarcoidosis, granulomatous inflammation involves the meninges or brain parenchyma. Meningeal disease is more common and results in a chronic nonpurulent process that may be diffuse and nodular or well circumscribed and masslike. The basal leptomeninges, in which impingement of contiguous cranial nerves, the pituitary stalk, or the periaqueductal region can occur, are most frequently involved. Communicating or obstructing hydrocephalus is a common complication. Parenchymal involvement occurs less frequently and may result from infiltration of granulomatous inflammatory tissue from the subarachnoid space along the Virchow-Robin spaces. Parenchymal deposits may be multiple and small or masslike and similar to a neoplasm.

The lesions of neurosarcoidosis on CT scans are isodense or slightly hyperdense compared with brain and may contain calcifications. Use of intravenous contrast produces homogeneous enhancement in active inflammations and spotty enhancement in end-stage fibrosis. Intraparenchymal lesions tend to be located peripherally and demonstrate minimal surrounding edema.

The MR appearance of intracranial sarcoidosis is highly variable. Lesions may be isointense or hypointense to cortex on T1-weighted images and hyperintense or (not infrequently) hypointense on T2-weighted images. The explanation for this variability is unknown and may depend on the amount of connective tissue stroma and fibrosis that is present. The use of gadolinium contrast markedly increases the sensitivity of MR to leptomeningeal involvement by sarcoid. Because CT and noncontrast MR may fail to detect leptomeningeal involvement, contrast-enhanced MR has become the imaging method of choice.

Sarcoidosis is frequently responsive to high-dose steroid therapy. In some cases the response is dramatic, and enhancing intracranial nodules may disappear.

REFERENCES

Hayes WS, Sherman JL, Stern BJ, et al. MR and CT evaluation of intracranial sarcoidosis. AJR 1987; 143:1043–1049.

McDonald WI. Magnetic resonance imaging in central nervous system sarcoidosis. Neurology 1988; 38:378–383.

Miller DH, Kendall BE, Barter S, et al. Sarcoidosis and its neurological manifestations. Arch Neurol 1985; 42:909–917.

Mirfakhraee M, Crofford MJ, Guinto FC, et al. Virchow-Robin space: a path of spread in neurosarcoidosis. Radiology 1986; 158:715–720.

Sherman JL, Stern BJ. Sarcoidosis of the CNS: comparison of unenhanced and enhanced MR images. AJR 1990; 155:1293–1301.

Wiederholt WC, Siekert RG. Neurological manifestations of sarcoidosis. Neurology 1968; 15: 1147–1154.

Case 3

HISTORY

A 53-year-old man presented with microscopic hematuria.

RADIOLOGY

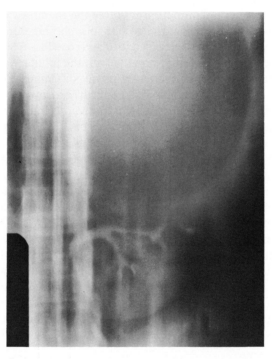

Figure 3–1. Linear tomogram from an excretory urogram shows a large lucent mass with an enhancing rim in the upper pole of the kidney.

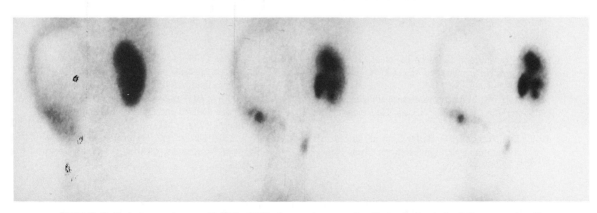

Figure 3–2. Posterior renal scan with ^{99m}Tc-DPTA shows a large nonfunctioning lesion in the left upper pole with a rim of activity and functioning kidney below.

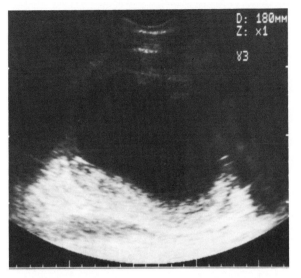

Figure 3–3. Sonogram shows a cystic mass with a thick wall. The inner margin of the wall is irregular and not well defined.

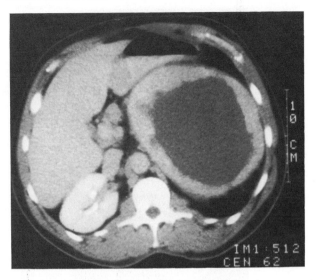

Figure 3–4. Contrast-enhanced CT scan shows the mass has a well-circumscribed margin, a nonenhancing low-attenuation center consistent with fluid, an irregular inner wall, calcification, and a smooth exterior margin.

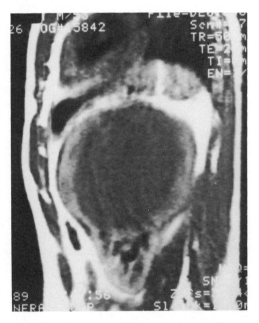

Figure 3–5. T1-weighted sagittal MR image shows a 15-cm, well-circumscribed, cystic mass with an irregular rim of variable thickness. The central portion of the mass has low signal intensity.

DIFFERENTIAL DIAGNOSIS

The differential diagnosis includes renal cell carcinoma, metastasis, abscess, complex renal cyst, obstructed upper pole, angiomyolipoma, adenoma, and oncocytoma.

PATHOLOGY

A radical left nephrectomy was performed.

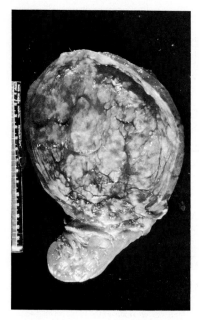

Figure 3-6. The well-circumscribed cystic mass has a gray-tan wall.

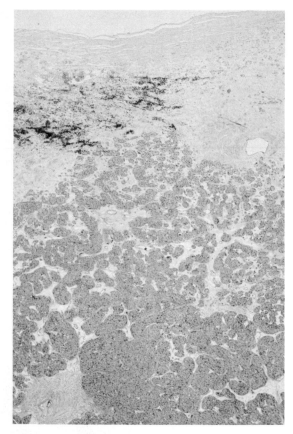

Figure 3-7. The cyst lumen (upper portion) is surrounded by nests of tumor cells.

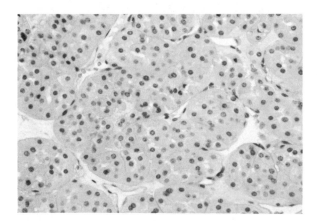

Figure 3-8. The large polyhedral eosinophilic tumor cells grow in round nests and are frequently separated from each other by capillaries.

epithelium of the proximal tubules

DIAGNOSIS

The final pathologic diagnosis was oncocytoma, cystic variant.

DISCUSSION

Renal oncocytoma is an uncommon benign tumor that originates in the epithelium of the proximal tubules. Although renal oncocytoma is often detected as an incidental renal mass in asymptomatic adults, it must be differentiated from other renal tumors, particularly renal cell carcinoma. Radiologic features typical of oncocytoma, including

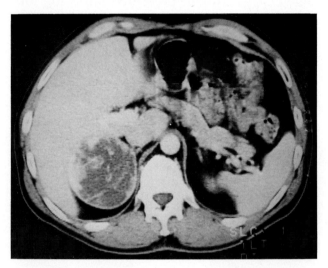

Figure 3-9. A CT scan without contrast demonstrates the central stellate scar that is typical of oncocytoma. This feature, while characteristic, is not sufficiently diagnostic to eliminate the need for biopsy.

the appearance of a solid mass with homogeneous enhancement, sharp margination, central stellate scar detectable by sonography, CT, or MR (Fig. 3-9), and an angiographic spoked-wheel pattern, may occur in patients with renal cell carcinoma. Cystic necrosis and calcification are rare in oncocytoma and more common in renal cell carcinoma. On MR, these lesions can be distinguished only if tumor thrombus is demonstrated in the renal vein or inferior vena cava.

Treatment is surgical enucleation or heminephrectomy. If preoperative differentiation from renal cell carcinoma is uncertain, radical nephrectomy may be necessary.

REFERENCES

Ball DS, Friedman AC, Hartman DS, et al. Scar sign of renal oncocytoma: magnetic resonance imaging appearance and lack of specificity. Urol Radiol 1986; 8:46–48.

Levine E, Huntrakoon M. Computed tomography of renal oncocytoma. AJR 1983; 141:741–746.

Neisius D, Braedel HU, Schindler E, et al. Computed tomographic and angiographic findings in renal oncocytoma. Br J Radiol 1988; 61:1019–1025.

Palmer WE, Chew FS. Renal oncocytoma. AJR 1991; 156:1144.

Quinn MJ, Hartman DS, Friedman AC, et al. Renal oncocytoma: new observations. Radiology 1984; 153:49–53.

Case 4

HISTORY

A 20-year-old male college student presented following four episodes of hemoptysis during the past year.

RADIOLOGY

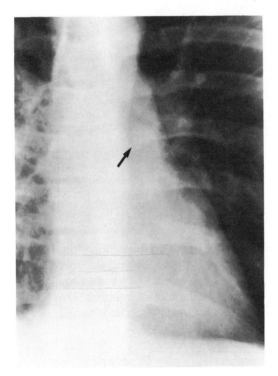

Figure 4-1. Chest radiograph shows a mass in the left main stem bronchus (arrow).

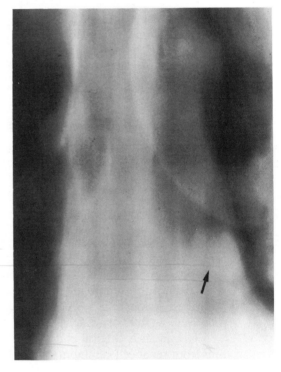

Figure 4-2. Anteroposterior linear tomogram shows the mass (arrow).

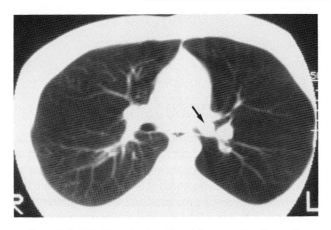

Figure 4-3. CT of the chest confirmed the presence of a single endobronchial lesion and revealed no extrabronchial extension or mediastinal lymphadenopathy. The lungs were clear.

DIFFERENTIAL DIAGNOSIS

The differential diagnosis includes bronchial carcinoid, mucoepidermoid, adenoid cystic carcinoma, hamartoma, and mesenchymal tumors.

PATHOLOGY

A sleeve resection of the left main stem bronchus was performed. Six regional lymph nodes were sampled and found to be free of tumor.

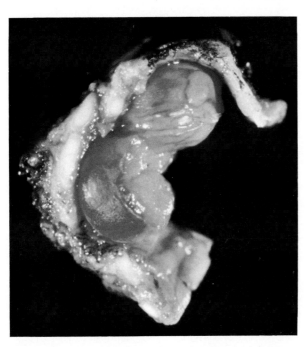

Figure 4-4. The removed segment of bronchus shows a bulging, glistening ovoid mass arising from the mucosal surface of the left main stem bronchus.

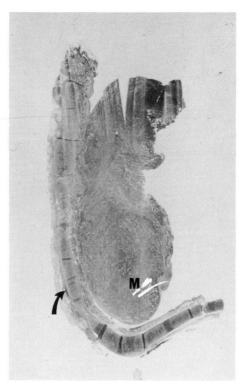

Figure 4-5. The lesion (M) Does not invade the underlying cartilaginous ring (arrow).

DIAGNOSIS

The final pathologic diagnosis was bronchial carcinoid.

DISCUSSION

The classic bronchial carcinoid tumor, formerly called bronchial adenoma, is a low-grade malignant neoplasm that shares histologic features with Kulchitsky cells, a neuroendocrine argentaffin cell of the bronchial and bronchiolar mucosa. The carcinoid tumor is further characterized by an organoid growth pattern consisting of a rich vascular stroma, minimal nuclear pleomorphism, minimal mitotic activity, and an absence of necrosis. Among the three subtypes of the pulmonary neuroendocrine tumors, also called Kulchitsky cell carcinomas (the others being atypical carcinoid tumor and neuroendocrine carcinoma), this tumor is the lowest grade (type I of the three subtypes). The lesion occurs in adults and is rare in adolescents. The prognosis is favorable following surgical resection with clear margins.

Bronchial carcinoids usually involve subsegmental or more proximal bronchi. Because the lesions grow slowly into the bronchial lumen, the typical presentation is segmental or lobar atelectasis, leading to indolent symptoms of coughing, wheezing, recurrent infections, or hemoptysis. When directly visualized, the lesions are seen to be polypoid intraluminal masses smaller than 3 cm in diameter. A more peripheral lesion presents as an asymptomatic pulmonary nodule because the region of distal atelectasis is radiologically and clinically insignificant. Even in those with metastatic disease (10% of cases), carcinoid syndrome (intermittent diarrhea, flushing, and cyanosis) is uncommon.

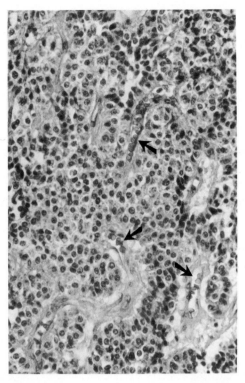

Figure 4-6. The tumor is composed of trabeculae and islands of tumor cells that have centrally placed nuclei and moderate amounts of eosinophilic cytoplasm.

REFERENCES

Forster BB, Muller NL, Miller RR, et al. Neuroendocrine carcinomas of the lung: clinical, radiologic, and pathologic correlation. Radiology 1989; 170: 441–445.

McCaughan BC, Martini N, Bains MS. Bronchial carcinoids. Review of 124 cases. J Thorac Cardiovasc Surg 1985; 89:8–17.

Warren WH, Faber LP, Gould VE. Neuroendocrine neoplasms of the lung. A clinicopathologic update. J Thorac Cardiovasc Surg 1989; 98:321–332.

Case 5

HISTORY

During oncologic staging of a 70-year-old man with prostatic carcinoma, a round, well-defined splenic mass was discovered incidentally on abdominal CT.

RADIOLOGY

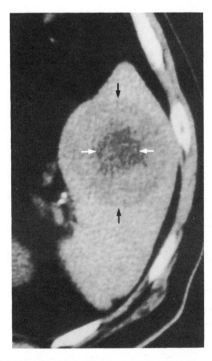

Figure 5–1. Noncontrast CT scan shows a rounded splenic lesion with lower attenuation in the center (white arrows) than in the periphery (black arrows).

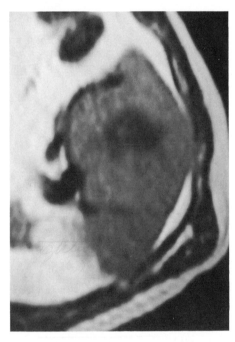

Figure 5–2. On a T1-weighted MR image, the center of the lesion has low signal intensity, but the periphery is nearly isointense with the spleen.

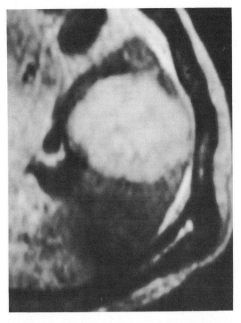

Figure 5-3. With T2 weighting the lesion shows a hyperintense signal.

DIFFERENTIAL DIAGNOSIS

The differential diagnosis includes metastasis, primary benign or malignant neoplasm, lymphoma, and abscess.

PATHOLOGY

Splenectomy was performed.

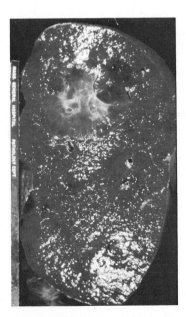

Figure 5-4. The bisected spleen demonstrates an unencapsulated hemorrhagic mass with a central tan-white, stellate scar.

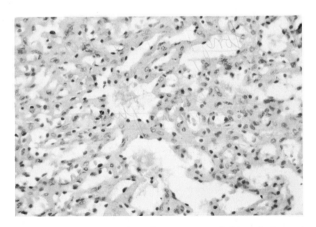

Figure 5-5. The lesion consists of numerous small, thin-walled vascular spaces that are focally filled with red blood cells. The lining endothelial cells are cytologically benign.

DIAGNOSIS

The final pathologic diagnosis was splenic hemangioma.   *most common neoplasm in the spleen.*

DISCUSSION

A cavernous hemangioma is an unencapsulated mass of dilated, endothelially lined vascular channels filled with slowly flowing blood. Typically 1 to 2 cm in size, they can be much larger. Sonograms may demonstrate an inconsistent and nonspecific appearance of echogenicity and sharp margination, sometimes with cystic regions. Plain CT shows a low attenuation mass; with intravenous contrast infusion, the vascular channels slowly fill from the periphery inward. Larger lesions fill more slowly and may do so incompletely and inhomogeneously. Similarly, because of the slow blood flow, nuclear imaging with ^{99m}Tc-labeled red blood cells shows slow accumulation of activity in the lesion followed by slow washout. A nuclear scan with ^{99m}Tc-labeled sulfur colloid shows a photopenic defect because the radiopharmaceutical is accumulated only by the functional splenic tissue. T2-weighted MR images show a bright signal similar to that produced by bile, cerebrospinal fluid (CSF), or gastric fluid because of long T2 relaxation times; this quality generally distinguishes an hemangioma from a solid neoplasm. However, regions of liquefactive necrosis in solid tumors are also bright on T2-weighted MR images.

Most splenic hemangiomas are discovered incidentally, and their clinical importance generally lies in the need to differentiate them from other conditions, particularly metastases. Occasionally they may present with splenomegaly, abdominal pain, dyspnea, diarrhea, or constipation. Spontaneous rupture with hemorrhage is a risk with larger lesions. There is no malignant potential. Hemangiomas are not treated unless they are symptomatic or very large and pose an increased risk of hemorrhage; treatment is splenectomy. Occasionally histologic examination is necessary for diagnosis. Although unusual, they are nonetheless the most common primary splenic neoplasm.

REFERENCES

Hahn PF, Weissleder R, Stark DD, et al. MR imaging of focal splenic tumors. AJR 1988; 150:823–827.

Husni EA. The clinical course of splenic hemangioma. Arch Surg 1961; 83:681–688.

Ros PR, Moser RP Jr, Dachman AH, et al. Hemangioma of the spleen: radiologic-pathologic correlation in ten cases. Radiology 1987; 162:73–77.

Long T2 relaxation time - T2 weighted
bile
CSF
gastric fluid
hemangioma

Case 6

HISTORY

A female infant presented at birth with a large soft right neck mass extending into the supraclavicular region.

RADIOLOGY

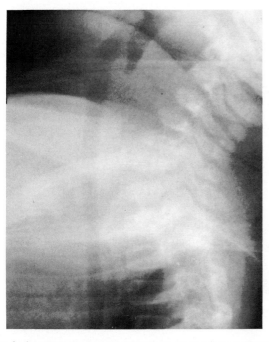

Figure 6-1. Lateral chest radiograph shows abnormal prevertebral soft tissue displacing the trachea and hypopharynx anteriorly.

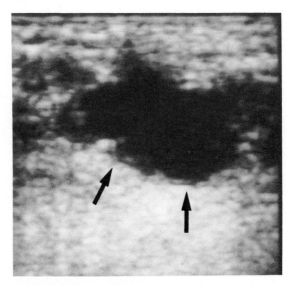

Figure 6-2. Real-time ultrasound of the right supraclavicular component demonstrates a complex cystic collection (arrows).

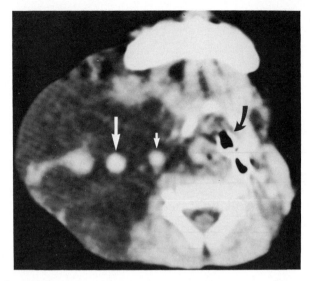

Figure 6-3. During intravenous contrast administration, cervical CT scan shows irregular enhancement of a complex cystic mass that separates the right carotid artery (small white arrow) and jugular vein (large white arrow) and displaces the esophagus and narrowed trachea (curved black arrow) to the left.

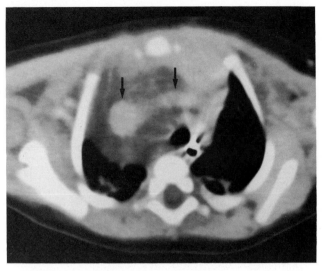

Figure 6-4. At the level of the superior mediastinum, the mass encases the right brachiocephalic vessels (arrows). There is right axillary extension.

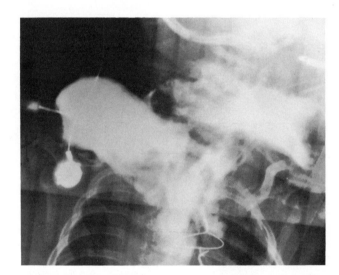

Figure 6-5. Injection of contrast into the right supraclavicular mass shows communication with both cervical and mediastinal components.

DIFFERENTIAL DIAGNOSIS

The differential diagnosis includes cystic hygroma, lymphangiosarcoma, hemangioma, lymphadenitis, pyogenic abscess, cystic teratoma, and necrotic sarcoma.

PATHOLOGY

The mass was excised.

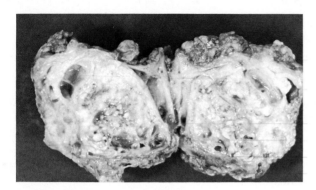

Figure 6-6. The removed mass contains numerous cystic spaces that contain watery fluid.

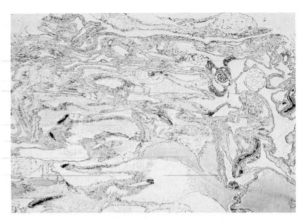

Figure 6-7. The lesion consists of an interconnecting network of dilated lymphatic spaces that have lymphocytes within their septa.

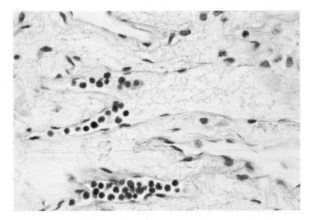

Figure 6-8. The lymphatic spaces are lined by benign endothelial cells and contain proteinaceous material and lymphocytes within the lumen.

DIAGNOSIS

The final pathologic diagnosis was cystic hygroma.

DISCUSSION

Cystic hygroma (cavernous lymphangioma) is a rare benign congenital abnormality that occurs with equal sex distribution in otherwise healthy children and results from malformation of the developing lymphatic system. Embryologic theories propose that primitive endothelial lymph buds begin to dilate abnormally between the sixth and eighth gestational weeks and gradually form cystic sacs. These dilated sacs may either be separate from the normal lymphatic system or communicate with it via partially obstructed ducts.

Cystic hygromas involve the neck or lower face in 80% of patients. Rare locations include the mediastinum, retroperitoneum, abdominal viscera, pelvis, and scrotum. Although histologically they are benign, hygromas lack encapsulation and infiltrate normal tissue planes. Mediastinal hygromas typically result from extension of cervical lesions and may be complicated by chylothorax and chylopericardium.

Approximately 50% to 65% of lesions present at birth and 90% present within 2 years. Most hygromas are clinically asymptomatic but visually obvious because of the resulting cosmetic deformity. When symptoms occur, they result from local mass effect and include respiratory distress, dysphagia, and vascular insufficiency. The neck mass enlarges in proportion to the infant's growth until infection or internal hemorrhage causes rapid, painful expansion. Spontaneous regression of hygromas is uncommon. Therapy consists of complete resection to prevent relentless growth, mass effect, and infection. Incomplete resection often results in recurrence.

Imaging methods include conventional radiography, sonography, CT, and MR. A lateral plain film of the neck may show prominent retropharyngeal tissue suggestive of hematoma or abscess formation, both of which are more common than cystic hygroma. Sonography, CT, and MR distinguish between cystic and solid neck masses. If unilocular, hygromas are similar in appearance to other congenital masses such as branchial cleft and thyroglossal duct cysts. Hygromas are more commonly multilocular and may be indistinguishable from tuberculous adenitis, teratoma, and vascular lesions such as arteriovenous malformation and hemangioma.

The sonographic appearance depends on the degree of dilatation of the lymphatic spaces. The endothelial-lined cystic spaces, which may decompress after surgical incision, range in size from macroscopic cavernous chambers to microscopic tubular channels. Sonography typically shows a lobulated, multilocular cystic mass with septa of variable thickness. Solid echogenic components and focal nodular wall thickening represent disorganized lymphatic tissue. Prenatal sonography may detect fetal cystic hygroma during the second or third trimester.

CT is used to evaluate the mediastinal extension of large hygromas and defines the relationship of the tumor to the trachea, esophagus, and neurovascular bundles. The cystic loculations usually are of water density. The cyst walls and septa may enhance slightly. When infiltrative, these lesions are poorly circumscribed and obliterate the surrounding fascial planes. MR spin-echo pulse sequences characterize the cystic components of hygromas. Although the majority of cysts exhibit signal intensities typical of simple fluid, variable T1-weighted signal intensities indicate the presence of blood, chyle, or protein in the lymphatic fluid. Multiplanar imaging precisely evaluates mediastinal, supraclavicular, and axillary extension as well as the relationship of the tumor to the thoracic inlet, chest wall, and brachial plexus.

REFERENCES

Glazer HS, Siegel MJ, Sagel SS. Low-attenuation mediastinal masses on CT. AJR 1989; 152: 1173–1177.

Pijpers L, Reuss A, Stewart PA, et al. Fetal cystic hygroma: prenatal diagnosis and management. Obstet Gynecol 1988; 72:223–224.

Sheth S, Nussbaum AR, Hutchins GH, et al. Cystic hygromas in children: sonographic-pathologic correlation. Radiology 1987; 162:821–824.

Siegel MJ, Glazer HS, Amour TES, et al. Lymphangiomas in children: MR imaging. Radiology 1989; 170:467–470.

Silverman PM, Korobkin M, Moore AV. Computed tomography of cystic neck masses. J Comput Assist Tomogr 1983; 7:498–502.

Case 7

HISTORY

A 29-year-old male who was known to have multiple hereditary exostoses (osteochondromatosis) complained of pain in the right hip and an enlarging mass.

RADIOLOGY

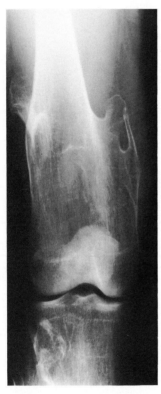

Figure 7-1. There are multiple osteocartilaginous exostoses involving the distal femur, the proximal tibia, and the fibula.

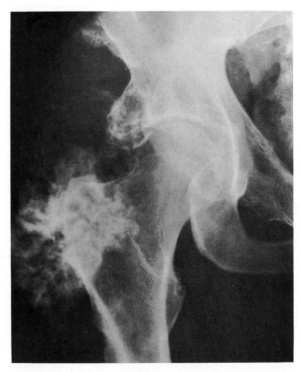

Figure 7-2. Anteroposterior (AP) view of the right hip demonstrates a large osteochondroma arising from the proximal femur. The more distal part of the lesion appears densely mineralized centrally. The proximal part of the lesion contains a lucent center that is partially surrounded by a mineralized shell.

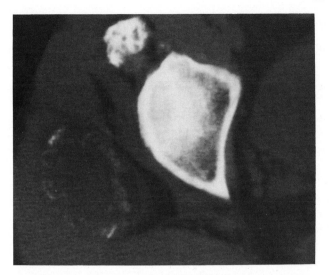

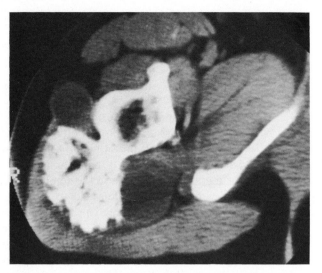

Figure 7-3. CT scan through the proximal portion of the lesion demonstrates the faintly mineralized peripheral shell, which has an undulating, polycyclic contour suggesting nodular growth. The lesion has lower attenuation than the surrounding muscle.

Figure 7-4. CT scan through the midportion of the lesion demonstrates cortical continuity between the mineralized part of the tumor and the femoral cortex. Incidental note is made of a second small anterior osteochondroma. Two small rounded areas of low attenuation with no internal or peripheral mineralization are also present. The anterior and posterior portions of these low attenuation areas were shown to communicate with each other more caudally.

DIFFERENTIAL DIAGNOSIS

The differential diagnosis includes benign exostosis, possibly with malignant degeneration.

PATHOLOGY

The lesion was resected.

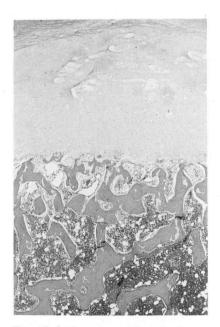

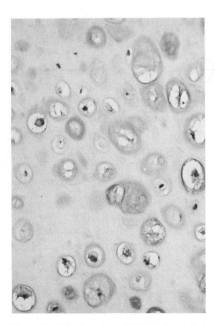

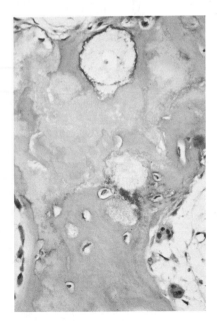

Figure 7-5. The surface of the lesion is composed of hyaline cartilage that is undergoing endochondral ossification at its base. The cartilage is attached to a bony stalk.

Figure 7-6. Further magnification shows that the hyaline cartilage of the cap is hypocellular and contains uniform round, small, bland chondrocytes.

Figure 7-7. The base of the cartilage cap serves as "scaffolding" for the deposition of newly formed bone.

DIAGNOSIS

The final diagnosis was multiple hereditary exostoses with bursa formation.

DISCUSSION

[handwritten margin note: tubular bones, metaphysis, never epiphysis]

Osteochondroma (osteocartilaginous exostosis) is the most common benign skeletal lesion. It consists of a projection of bone with a cartilage cap. Often solitary, it can occur in any bone that is preformed in cartilage and is most common in the long tubular bones, particularly those about the knee. It is almost always found in the metaphysis, rarely in the diaphysis, and never in the epiphysis. Osteochondromas most often present in the first or second decade of life as slowly growing painless masses.

An osteochondroma can almost always be easily diagnosed by x-ray examination. Because the lesion arises as an abnormal orientation of a portion of the growth plate, the cortex of the parent bone is incomplete where it merges with the base of the lesion. The cap consists of hyaline cartilage and exhibits endochondral ossification at its junction with cancellous bone. The cap varies in size with age; it can be up to 3 cm thick during the growth period and is often absent in adults. Islands of calcified cartilage are also found deeper within cancellous bone. Growth of the lesion ceases after puberty.

The lesions may be pedunculated or sessile (broad flat base). Local widening of the metaphysis is a frequent finding even with solitary osteochondromas. Because they commonly occur at or near sites of tendon or ligament attachment, their orientation is determined by the direction of muscle pull, and thus most point away from the adjacent joint.

Hereditary multiple exostoses is one of the most common abnormalities of skeletal development. Multiple (sometimes more than 100) osteochondromas are discovered in these patients, usually between the ages of 2 and 10 years. The lesions are often bilaterally symmetric and occur in any bone formed by endochondral ossification. The bones about the knee are most often involved. The condition is inherited as an autosomal dominant trait with a male to female predominance of 2 : 1. Bone modeling is abnormal, and failure of tubulation of the metaphysis is characteristic. Other common findings include shortening of the ulna (with bayonet deformity) and fibula, bilateral coxa valga, and widening of the proximal femoral metaphyses.

Complications of osteochondromas include neural compression, particularly spinal stenosis; fracture; formation of a bursa around the lesion, which can become inflamed, painful, or distended with fluid; vascular injury leading to pseudoaneurysm formation, joint dysfunction, or pressure erosion of adjacent bones; and malignant degeneration, said to occur in fewer than 1% of solitary osteochondromas and in 2% to 27% of patients with multiple hereditary osteochondromas.

Malignant degeneration to peripheral chondrosarcoma occurs most often in the age range of 20 to 40 years and may be recognized by growth of the lesion, pain, swelling, and the presence of a soft tissue mass. Chondrosarcoma arising in this setting is almost always of low grade and slow growing and is associated with recurrence rather than metastasis. Histologic evidence of malignancy can be quite subtle. Rosenthal et al (1984) state that, with regard to evaluation of cartilage lesions, the most aggressive feature, be it pathologic, clinical, or radiologic, is the most important factor.

Radiologic signs suggestive of malignant transformation include growth of a previously stable lesion; formation of a soft tissue mass, which may exhibit calcification in rings and spicules (suggesting a low-grade lesion) or amorphous and irregular calcification or no calcification (suggesting a higher grade or myxoid tumor); thickening and irregularity of the cartilage cap to at least 1 to 3 cm (controversial); irregular, dispersed cap calcification that is separate from the densely calcified area deep to the cap; and destruction and erosion of adjacent bone. Benign lesions may have homogeneous, stippled calcification.

CT is valuable in evaluating calcification, the soft tissue mass, and the relation of the lesion to the parent bone. The cartilage cap frequently cannot be distinguished from muscle, particularly when it is thin. MR can detect caps (high signal on T2-weighted images) as thin as 3 mm and can accurately assess their thickness. Both CT and MR are important for selection of a biopsy site and staging.

Benign osteochondromas are treated by marginal resection. Low-grade peripheral chondrosarcomas require wider margins.

REFERENCES

Hudson TM. Radiologic-Pathologic Correlation of Musculoskeletal Lesions. Baltimore: Williams & Wilkins, 1987:109–121.

Lee JK, et al. MR imaging of solitary osteochondromas: report of eight cases. AJR 1987; 149: 557–560.

Norman A, Sissons HA. Radiographic hallmarks of peripheral chondrosarcoma. Radiology 1984; 151:589–596.

Rosenthal DI, et al. Chondrosarcoma: correlation of radiological and histological grade. Radiology 1984; 150:21–26.

Case 8

HISTORY

A 16-year-old Indian male complained of having headaches for several months.

RADIOLOGY

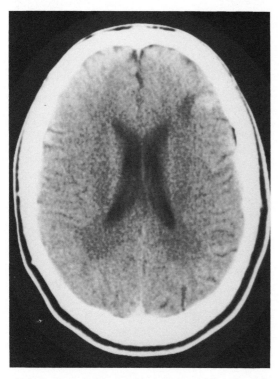

Figure 8-1. Noncontrast CT scan demonstrates a 1.5-cm hyperdense focus in the peripheral left frontal lobe. There is a small amount of adjacent edema.

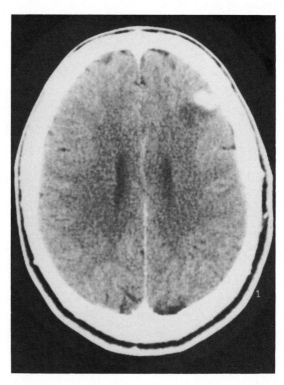

Figure 8-2. CT scan after contrast administration shows homogeneous enhancement.

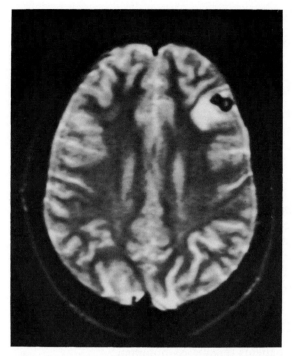

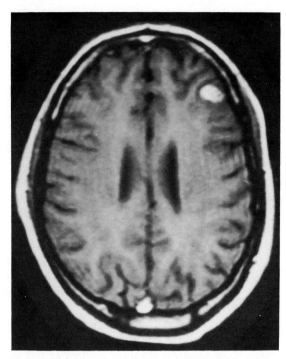

Figure 8-3. Axial late echo T2-weighted MR image shows a dumbbell-shaped region of low signal intensity with a central focus of high signal. There is surrounding edema.

Figure 8-4. Postgadolinium T1-weighted axial image shows dense enhancement of the lesion.

DIFFERENTIAL DIAGNOSIS

The differential diagnosis includes oligodendroglioma, low-grade astrocytoma, cysticercosis, sarcoidosis, and tuberculoma or other granulomatous disease.

PATHOLOGY

A left frontal biopsy was performed.

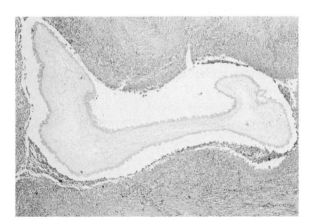

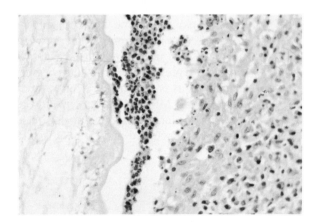

Figure 8-5. The lesion is composed of a marked inflammatory infiltrate that surrounds an organism.

Figure 8-6. The inflammatory infiltrate is rich in eosinophils that in turn are surrounded by a layer of macrophages, chronic inflammatory cells, and reactive fibrosis.

DIAGNOSIS

The final pathologic diagnosis was cysticercosis.

DISCUSSION

Neurocysticercosis is a manifestation of infestation with the pork tapeworm (Cestoda) *Taenia solium*. The disease is common in parts of Central and South America, Asia, Africa, and Mexico. In endemic areas it is the most common cause of seizures in young adults. Between 13 and 34% of cerebral lesions in Mexico and Central America are due to cysticercosis. The incidence of the disease in the United States is rising, particularly in the Southwest.

Ingestion of *T. solium* eggs, usually by the fecal-oral route or through regurgitation from the intestine, can result in cysticercosis. The embryos that hatch from the ingested eggs pass through the stomach wall into the bloodstream. These embryos may then spread hematogenously into the eyes, skin, muscles, or brain and develop into cystic larvae (cysticerci). The cysticercus consists of a cystic structure containing an invaginated mural nodule called a scolex. The central nervous system is involved in 60 to 90% of patients with cysticercosis.

Viable cysts within the central nervous system produce little host reaction. Dying cysts, however, elicit intense inflammation, and symptoms (most commonly headaches or seizures) are most evident at this stage. Many patients remain asymptomatic.

Cysticerci seen on CT or MR examinations have a propensity to involve the gray matter and overlying leptomeninges. As a result, many lesions occur near the inner table of the skull. The cysts are typically about 1 cm in diameter and have attenuation and signal properties similar to those of cerebrospinal fluid (CSF) on CT and MR studies, respectively. Intraventricular and spinal involvement is less common. Involvement of the meningobasal subarachnoid space can produce a large, multilobular, nonviable, degenerated cyst lacking a mural nodule called a racemose cyst. These are most frequently found in the cerebellopontine angle and suprasellar regions.

Cysticercosis has a distinctive natural history that can be followed by CT and MR imaging. Initially, an acute encephalitic phase can be seen, characterized by multiple enhancing nodules surrounded by severe cerebral edema. In the chronic stage of infestation, if the organisms remain viable, nonenhancing cystic lesions without surrounding edema are seen. On MR the cyst fluid follows CSF signal intensities. A mural nodule may be seen on either CT or MR. As the larvae die, the cyst fluid becomes more jellylike, and the capsular membrane thickens. This membrane ring enhances on CT, and surrounding cerebral edema is commonly present. On MR the thickened capsular membrane appears as a dark rim on T2-weighted images. Following this stage, the cystic component continues to regress, and calcification begins to appear within the scolex. Eventually, a dense calcific focus is seen on CT, corresponding to larval involution.

CT and MR each have a role in the evaluation of neurocysticercosis. CT is clearly superior in demonstrating end-stage calcification, whereas MR is more sensitive in detecting subarachnoid and intraventricular cysts.

REFERENCES

Kramer LD, Locke GE, Byrd SE, et al. Cerebral cysticercosis: documentation of natural history with CT. Radiology 1989; 171:459–462.

Lotz, J, Hewlett R, Alheit B, et al. Neurocysticercosis: correlative pathomorphology and MR imaging. Neuroradiology 1988; 30:35–41.

Mazer S, Antoniuk A, Ditzel LFS, et al. The computed tomographic spectrum of cerebral cysticercosis. Comput Radiol 1983; 7:373–378.

Rodriquez-Carbajal J, Salgado P, Gutierrez-Alvarado R, et al. The acute encephalitic phase of neurocysticercosis: computed tomographic manifestations. AJNR 1983; 4:51–55.

Suh DC, Chang KH, Han MH, et al. Unusual MR manifestations of neurocysticercosis. Neuroradiology 1989; 31:396–402.

Suss RA, Maravilla KR, Thompson J. MR imaging of intracranial cysticercosis: comparison with CT and anatomopathologic features. AJNR 1986; 7:235–242.

Zee C, Segall HD, Boswell W, et al. MR imaging of neurocysticercosis. J Comput Assist Tomogr 1988; 12:927–934.

Case 9

HISTORY

A 36-year-old man presented with sudden onset of right flank pain but no hematuria.

RADIOLOGY

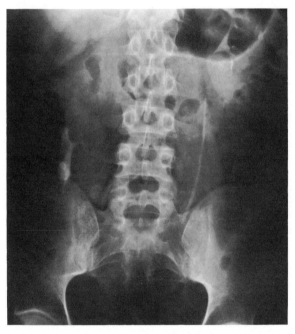

Figure 9-1. An intravenous urogram shows inferior displacement of the right kidney by a mass of low attenuation in the suprarenal region.

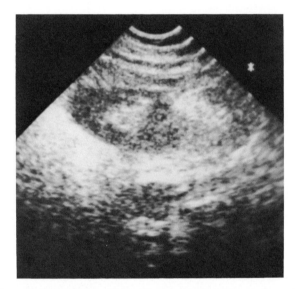

Figure 9-2. Sonography shows a 5-cm hyperechoic mass in the region of the right adrenal gland. The echogenicity of the lesion is similar to that of the adjacent retroperitoneal fat.

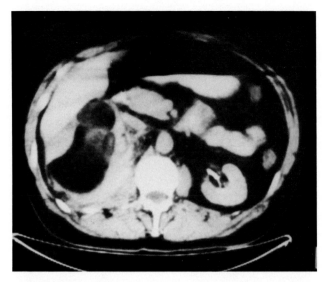

Figure 9-3. CT shows a heterogeneous lesion with fat and curvilinear soft tissue attenuation that is sharply marginated anteriorly. The lesion indents the underside of the liver.

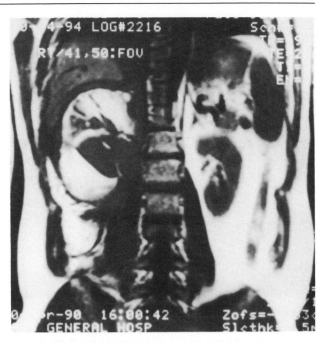

Figure 9-4. T1-weighted coronal MR image shows a fatty mass displacing the liver and right kidney. Regions of lower signal extend into and around the lesion.

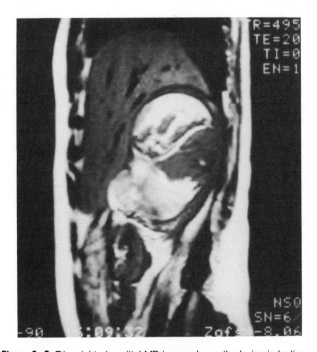

Figure 9-5. T1-weighted sagittal MR image shows the lesion indenting the liver from below and displacing the right kidney inferiorly.

DIFFERENTIAL DIAGNOSIS

The differential diagnosis includes retroperitoneal lipoma and liposarcoma, adrenal myelolipoma, pedunculated renal angiomyelolipoma, metastasis, adrenocortical carcinoma, and teratoma.

PATHOLOGY

An 18.5- × 15- × 9-cm mass consisting of adipose and myeloid tissue was resected.

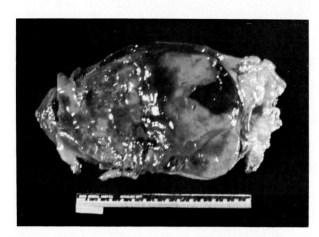

Figure 9-6. Extensive infarction and acute and organizing hematoma were present. A large oval hemorrhagic tan mass expands and replaces much of the adrenal. These hematomas correlate with the soft tissue portions of the lesion identified on CT and MR image.

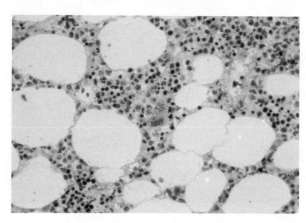

Figure 9-7. Microscopy of a viable portion of the lesion shows that the tumor consists of scattered large mature adipocytes surrounded by hematopoietic elements.

DIAGNOSIS

The final pathologic diagnosis was adrenal myelolipoma.

DISCUSSION

Adrenal myelolipoma is an uncommon benign, endocrinologically inactive tumor of unknown pathogenesis composed of adipose and myeloid tissue. In most lesions the fatty component is predominant and is recognizable on imaging. Such lesions are lucent on radiography and hyperechoic on sonography and show low attenuation on CT. On MR imaging they are bright on T1-weighted images and intermediate on T2-weighted images. Tumors composed primarily of myeloid tissue may be hypoechoic on sonography and have the imaging characteristics of red marrow on other imaging techniques.

In complicated cases in which infarction or hematoma is present the margins of the lesions may be irregular and infiltrative, with blood dissecting through the retroperitoneum. The imaging findings of acute, subacute, or chronic hematoma are then superimposed on the lesion. When lesions are fatty, well marginated, uncomplicated, and in the position of the adrenal gland, a specific radiologic diagnosis is possible. However, the mere presence of fat in an adrenal mass is insufficient for diagnosis because a metastasis or other aggressive lesion may engulf fat as it spreads.

Adrenal myelolipoma is usually an incidental diagnosis in adults undergoing imaging for unrelated clinical indications. Virtually all lesions originate in the adrenal cortex. In autopsy series its prevalence is between 0.08 and 0.2% with an equal sex distribution. Nearly half of resected lesions in one literature survey were 10 cm or larger. Symptoms, when present, typically relate to a simple mass effect, but spontaneous bleeding can cause acute flank pain or even hemodynamic shock. Bleeding is more likely in lesions composed primarily of myeloid tissue.

Surveillance has been suggested for incidentally discovered adrenal myelolipomas. However, if metastases are suspected, if endocrinologic assays are abnormal, or if radiologic findings are inconsistent with uncomplicated myelolipoma, a histologic diagnosis is necessary. CT- or ultrasound-guided percutaneous needle biopsy can provide tissue. Surgical excision is reserved for myelolipomas causing a mass effect or bleeding.

REFERENCES

Asch MR, Poon PY, McCallum RW, et al. Myelolipoma: radiographic findings in seven patients. J Can Assoc Radiol 1989; 40:247–250.

Dieckmann KP, Hamm B, Pickartz H, et al. Adrenal myelolipoma: clinical, radiologic, and histologic features. Urology 1987; 29:1–8.

Greene KM, Brantly PN, Thompson WR. Adenocarcinoma metastatic to the adrenal gland simulating myelolipoma: CT evaluation. J Comput Assist Tomogr 1985; 9:820–821.

Musante F, Derchi LE, Zappasodi F, et al. Myelolipoma of the adrenal gland: sonographic and CT features. AJR 1988; 151:961–964.

Palmer WE, Gerard-McFarland EL, Chew FS. Adrenal myelolipoma. AJR 1991; 156:724.

Case 10

A 35-year-old woman presented with a cough.

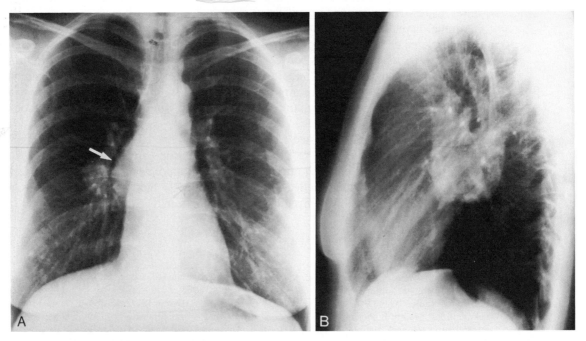

Figure 10–1. *A, B.* Chest radiographs reveal a 6.5-cm subcarinal mass and right hilar lymphadenopathy. The bronchus intermedius is narrowed (arrow).

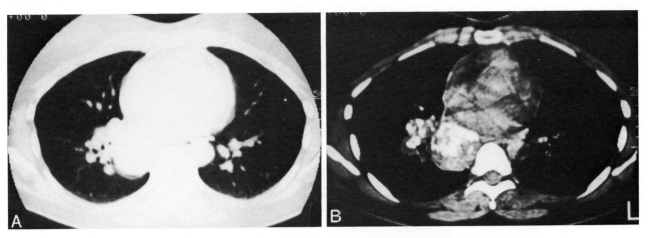

Figure 10-2. Noncontrast chest CT scan confirms the large posterior mediastinal, right hilar, and subcarinal lymph node mass with extensive calcification that encases the bronchus intermedius. No paratracheal adenopathy is seen. The left hilum is normal.

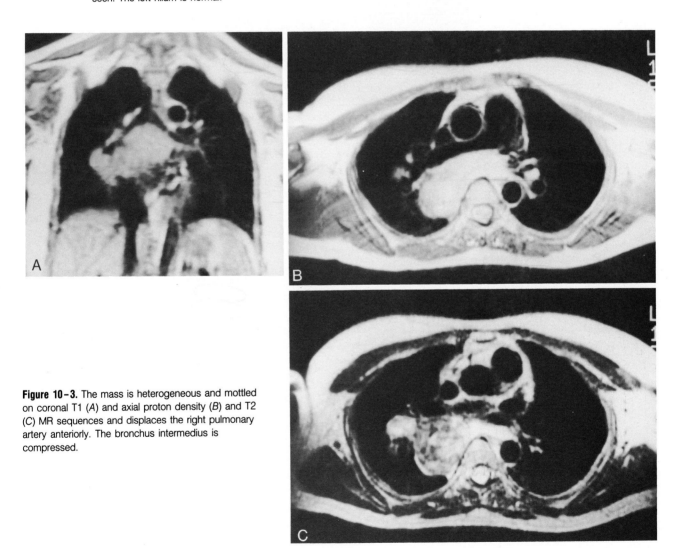

Figure 10-3. The mass is heterogeneous and mottled on coronal T1 (*A*) and axial proton density (*B*) and T2 (*C*) MR sequences and displaces the right pulmonary artery anteriorly. The bronchus intermedius is compressed.

DIFFERENTIAL DIAGNOSIS

The differential diagnosis includes tuberculosis, histoplasmosis, metastatic disease, lymphoma (treated), and complicated bronchogenic cyst or teratoma.

PATHOLOGY

The right middle and lower lobes were resected.

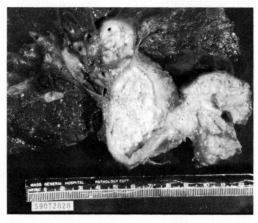

Figure 10-4. The beefy red pulmonary parenchyma surrounds the hilar region, which contains soft tan-pale yellow lymph nodes.

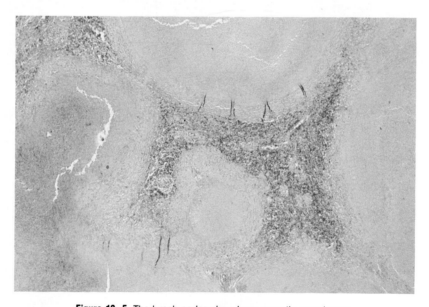

Figure 10-5. The lymph nodes show large necrotic granulomas.

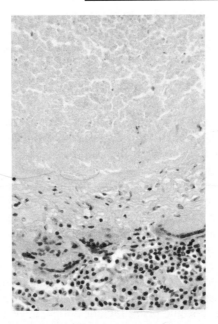

Figure 10-6. The granulomas are surrounded by epithelioid histiocytes and scattered multinucleated giant cells.

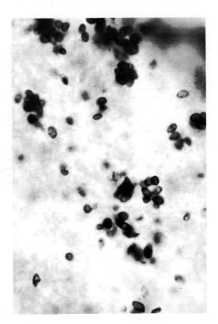

Figure 10-7. A special silver stain for fungi shows small budding yeast.

DIAGNOSIS

The final pathologic diagnosis was mediastinal histoplasmosis.

DISCUSSION

Histoplasma capsulatum is a fungus that exists in its mycelial form as a saprophyte in soil that has a high nitrogen content and as an oval, 2- to 5-μm yeast form in infected animals and humans. The organism is distributed throughout the world but is seen most commonly in North America, especially in the Ohio, Mississippi, and St. Lawrence River valleys. Infection can be acquired during a brief visit to an endemic area. The infection occurs equally in males and females of all ages but is particularly virulent in the very young and very old and in immunocompromised people. The clinical manifestations of infection include asymptomatic disease, acute histoplasmosis, flulike disease, or diffuse nodular disease, and chronic syndromes of pulmonary or mediastinal involvement leading to pericarditis, esophageal or tracheal encroachment, or pulmonary vessel or superior vena cava obstruction. Nodal disease can involve the mediastinum, the hila, or intrapulmonary nodes. Nodal disease can be asymptomatic during the acute phase; manifestations during the healing or chronic phase include cough, atelectasis, hemoptysis (secondary to broncholithiasis), postobstructive pneumonitis, and right middle lobe syndrome.

The initial response to the inhaled *Histoplasma* organism is acute inflammation, with rapid aggregation of lymphocytes and macrophages. Hypersensitivity and granulomatous inflammation develop over a period of 1 or 2 weeks, followed by necrosis and fibrosis. Healing can be rapid, but some foci of disease may enlarge and coalesce with other foci. A severe immune response may result in mediastinal granuloma formation: an encapsulated fibrous mass of adenitis surrounding a core of caseating lymph nodes. Calcification is usually profuse and exuberant. Organisms are rarely identified. The nodal involvement may be identical to that seen in tuberculosis, coccidioidomycosis, cryptococcosis, or other fungal diseases. Although the masses can be identified on plain radiographs, CT can demonstrate the nature and extent of the calcification and the involvement of contiguous structures. Identification of nodal calcification is important because it usually indicates a benign process. MR and contrast CT can identify the patency of blood vessels.

Antibiotics are usually not useful in mediastinal granuloma because the predominant inflammatory response is one of fibrotic encapsulation. Steroids are generally contraindicated because of the risk of dissemination of disease. Surgical exploration and debridement are the best means of identifying the etiologic agent, but the organism can be identified in only 30% of cases. Surgery may also be indicated for complications such as compression of the airway, esophagus, or vessels.

REFERENCES

Fishman AP (ed). Pulmonary Diseases and Disorders (2nd ed). New York: McGraw-Hill, 1988.

Heitzman ER. The Mediastinum: Radiologic Correlations with Anatomy and Pathology (2nd ed). St. Louis: Mosby, 1988.

Nardell EA, Mark EJ. A 57-year-old man with increasing dyspnea and a mediastinal mass. N Engl J Med 1989; 320:380–389.

Case 11

HISTORY

A 46-year-old female complained of low back pain and progressive constipation.

RADIOLOGY

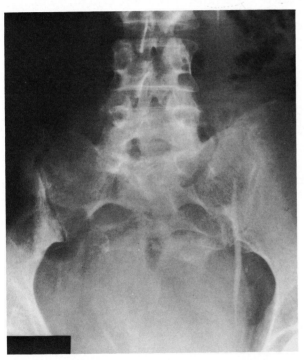

Figure 11-1. Anteroposterior radiograph of the pelvis obtained during an intravenous pyelogram demonstrates destruction of the distal sacrum and proximal coccyx.

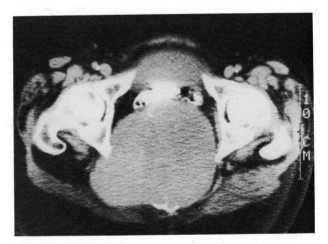

Figure 11-2. CT scan demonstrates the large pelvic soft tissue mass that has protruded through the greater sciatic notch on the right, displacing the sciatic nerve.

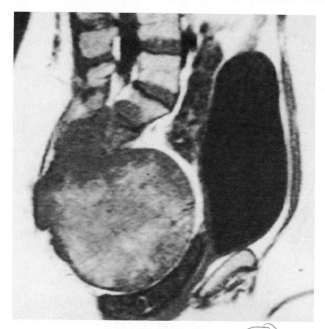

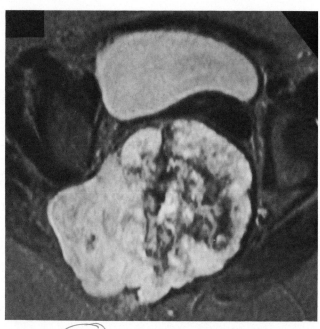

Figure 11-3. Sagittal view of the sacrum and coccyx with T1 weighting demonstrates a huge soft tissue mass eroding anteriorly from the sacrum. The upper end of the lesion is in the mid-S1 segment. One component of the soft tissue mass protrudes posteriorly into the sacral spinal canal.

Figure 11-4. Axial T2-weighted spin-echo images (TR = 2130, TE = 120) show the large anterior soft tissue mass arising from the distal sacrum. There is involvement of the right wing of the S1 and S2 segments.

DIFFERENTIAL DIAGNOSIS

The differential diagnosis includes giant cell tumor, aneurysmal bone cyst, chordoma, chondrosarcoma, osteosarcoma, multiple myeloma (plasmacytoma), sacrococcygeal teratoma, metastasis, and ependymoma.

PATHOLOGY

The lesion was resected.

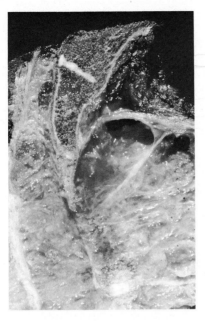

Figure 11-5. Cross section of resection specimen shows the relationship between the glistening focally cystic gray-tan tumor that has destroyed the sacrum and abuts the adjacent vertebral body.

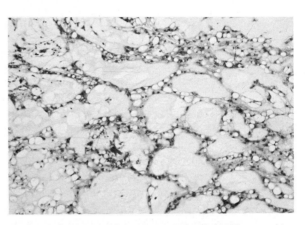

Figure 11-6. The tumor has a very prominent pale blue myxoid background within which are interconnecting cords of tumor cells.

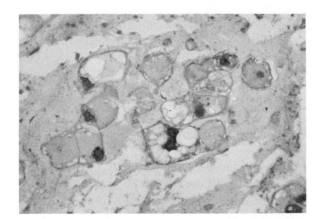

Figure 11-7. The tumor cells have abundant eosinophilic cytoplasm and eccentric nuclei. The cytoplasm of some of the tumor cells have numerous vacuoles typical of the physaliferous cell.

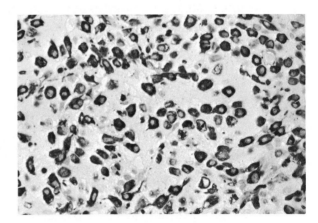

Figure 11-8. Immunohistochemistry shows that the tumor cells stain strongly with the antibody to the cytoskeletal intermediate filament keratin.

DIAGNOSIS

The final pathologic diagnosis was chordoma.

DISCUSSION

Chordoma is an uncommon, slowly growing, locally invasive neoplasm that is believed to arise from remnants of the primitive notochord. In the embryo the notochord is a tubular structure anterior to the neural tube. The skull and developing vertebrae envelope the notochord and extrude it into the intervertebral spaces, where it becomes the nucleus pulposus. Although the majority of notochordal tissue is therefore found in the interspaces, chordoma usually originates from intraosseous rests. Chordoma generally occurs at one of the ends of the spine: sacral-coccygeal (50%), spheno-occipital (35%), or cervical (especially C2)/thoracic/lumbar (15%), where it presumably arises from entrapped disc remnants within the compound segments. (The sacrum, clivus, and C2 are all composed of more than one segment.)

This tumor comprises 2 to 4% of all bone tumors and 20% of spinal tumors. The peak incidence of sacrococcygeal chordoma occurs in the sixth to seventh decades. Males are affected twice as frequently as females. Because of its effect upon the neighboring vital structures, spheno-occipital chordoma is recognized clinically approximately one decade earlier. Chordoma is uncommon in patients less than 35 years old, although tumors have been encountered during childhood. These are usually limited to the spheno-occipital region or cervical spine. Hematogenous metastases (usually to lung and liver) are more common than spread to local lymph nodes. Metastases occur in the later stages of disease and are more often associated with cervical, thoracic, or lumbar tumors than with a sacrococcygeal primary.

The symptoms of sacrococcygeal chordoma develop insidiously over months to years. Patients usually complain of low back pain. As the tumor enlarges anteriorly it may compress the rectum and bladder, leading to constipation and urinary urgency or incontinence. Although physical examination practically always demonstrates a fixed presacral mass, sacrococcygeal tumors rarely produce a palpable postsacral mass. Impingement upon nerves results in radicular pain and paresthesias. The most significant neurologic symptoms, however, develop in patients with tumors originating in the higher segments and result from cranial nerve and spinal cord compression.

Plain films usually demonstrate sacral destruction and a pelvic soft tissue mass. The bony margins of the lesion are relatively well defined, often sclerotic, and sometimes expanded. A midline location is frequent but not invariable. Progressive erosion of the sacral "pillars" may result in pelvic instability. Sacrococcygeal tumors may attain a huge size within the capacious pelvic cavity. The average size at presentation is 10 cm. The soft tissue matrix may contain sequestra of necrotic bone, dystrophic calcification, or reactive bone formation. Although CT scanning is better for evaluation of bone destruction and calcification, the multiplanar imaging of MR permits assessment of tumor invasion into adjacent structures and cranial extension into the spinal canal.

Chordomas are usually soft in consistency, lobulated in contour, cystic in cross section, and grayish in color. They are surrounded by a pseudocapsule. The characteristic cell (physaliferous cell) is vacuolated and distended by intracytoplasmic mucin (similar to a mucin-producing adenocarcinoma). Another characteristic finding is syncytial stranding of cells within a mucoid matrix. Of note, chordoma may closely resemble chondrosarcoma radiographically, histologically, and by chemical staining.

Treatment of sacrococcygeal chordomas ideally consists of complete surgical excision. Preoperative radiation may also be used. Unfortunately, the large size of these tumors, their soft, gelatinous consistency, and their proximity to vital organs often contribute to subtotal resection. High sacral amputation may result in pelvic instability, denervation of the bladder and rectum with urinary and fecal incontinence, and genital dysfunction. Even when surgical excision is considered complete, chordomas frequently recur, sometimes as late as 20 years after initial excision. The 5-year survival rate is 50 to

60%. Because the tumor is relatively radioresistant, radiation therapy plays its most important role in palliation of primary or recurrent disease. As elsewhere, radiation-induced sarcoma is a hazard among long-term survivors.

REFERENCES

Dahlin DC, Unni KK. Bone Tumors: General Aspects and Data on 8542 Cases (4th ed). Springfield, IL: Charles C Thomas, 1986:379–393.

Hudson TM. Radiologic-Pathologic Correlation of Musculoskeletal Lesions. Baltimore: Williams & Wilkins, 1987:287–303.

Meyer JE, et al. Chordomas: their CT appearance in the cervical, thoracic and lumbar spine. Radiology 1984; 153:693–699.

chordoma – 2%
4% of all bone tumors

Case 12

HISTORY

A 69-year-old female presented with recurrent fainting spells. These were associated with diaphoresis and personality change and occurred in the late mornings and afternoons.

RADIOLOGY

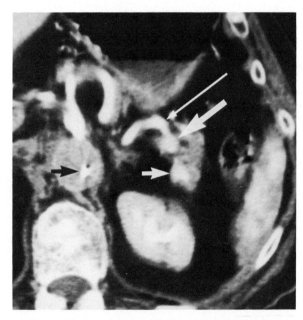

Figure 12-1. Dynamic CT scan performed during selective celiac arteriography demonstrates the catheter (black arrow) in the aorta. The normal splenic artery (thin white arrow) and vein (large white arrow) are adjacent to a 1.1-cm hypervascular mass (small white arrow) located in the tail of the pancreas.

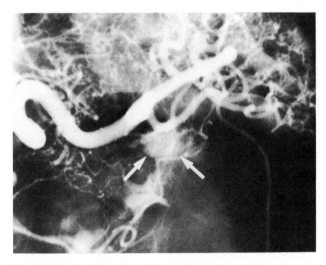

Figure 12-2. Selective celiac arteriography confirms, in the venous phase, an elliptical hypervascular lesion (arrows) located in the region of the pancreatic tail.

DIFFERENTIAL DIAGNOSIS

The differential diagnosis includes islet cell tumor (neoplasm secreting insulin, glucagon, somatostatin, or pancreatic polypeptide), ectopic endocrine tumor (neoplasm secreting gastrin, vasoactive intestinal polypeptide (VIP), adrenocorticotropic hormone (ACTH), antidiuretic hormone (ADH), or parathyroid hormone), pancreatic adenocarcinoma, and metastasis.

PATHOLOGY

Laboratory tests indicated fasting hypoglycemia and hyperinsulinemia. The lesion was excised.

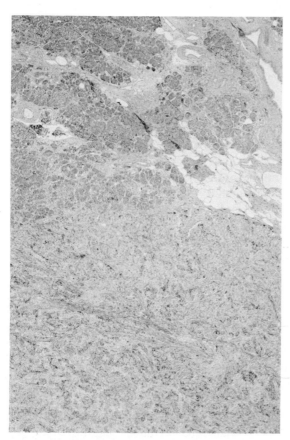

Figure 12-3. The specimen shows an ill-defined tumor adjacent to residual pancreatic parenchyma.

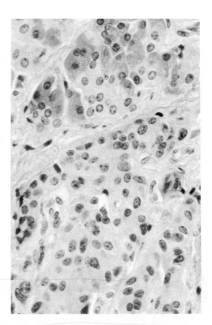

Figure 12-4. The tumor is composed of intermediate-size round cells that have a moderate amount of eosinophilic cytoplasm and centrally located nuclei. The tumor cells are morphologically similar to those composing the islets of Langerhans.

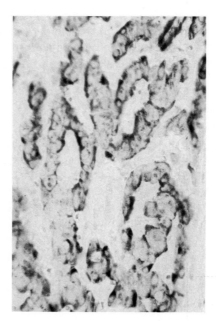

Figure 12-5. Immunohistochemistry shows that the tumor cells stain with antibodies to insulin.

DIAGNOSIS

The final pathologic diagnosis was pancreatic insulinoma.

most common islet cell tumor

DISCUSSION

The pancreas is composed of acinar (exocrine) and islet (endocrine) cells. Islet cells arise from the amine precursor uptake and decarboxylation (APUD) system of cells, which synthesize and store polypeptide hormones. Islet cells are grouped into clusters, the islets of Langerhans, which comprise approximately 2% of total pancreatic weight and are distributed unevenly throughout the pancreas. The pancreatic tail contains the greatest proportion.

The majority of islet cell neoplasms, adenomas as well as carcinomas, release at least a small amount of the hormonal polypeptide. Islet cell tumors are designated as nonfunctioning if humoral activity remains below the threshold of clinical symptoms and laboratory detection. Because excessive autonomous hormone production results in clinical endocrinopathy, functioning tumors typically present as small masses. Ninety percent of functioning tumors measure less than 5.0 cm in diameter at diagnosis, and 50% measure less than 1.0 cm. Nonfunctioning tumors continue to grow until signs and symptoms develop owing to the mass effect. With the exception of insulinomas, islet cell neoplasms possess significant malignant potential and often have metastasized by the time they are diagnosed. Malignant islet cell disease is defined radiographically by the presence of local tumor invasion or distant metastases. Metastases of a functioning islet cell carcinoma usually release the same polypeptide.

β cells

Although insulinoma is the most common islet cell tumor, it arises from beta cells, which comprise only 20% of the islet cell population. The tumor occurs with equal sex distribution during the fourth and fifth decades but develops earlier in patients who have the syndrome of multiple endocrine adenoma type I (MEA I). Insulinomas are 90% sporadic (10% associated with MEA I), 90% benign, and 90% solitary. Clinical symptoms result from hyperinsulinemia and fasting hypoglycemia. Functioning islet cell tumors are treated by surgical enucleation or subtotal pancreatic resection. Metastatic disease may require a combination of surgical debulking of both primary and secondary lesions, cytotoxic chemotherapy, and selective arterial embolization.

The goals of radiologic imaging include preoperative localization of an adenoma that may not be palpable by the surgeon, detection of synchronous tumors, and evaluation of metastatic disease. Functioning tumors remain radiographically occult in up to 25% of patients with clinical and biochemical evidence of hyperinsulinoma. Without precise intraoperative localization of occult insulinomas, patients may undergo blind distal pancreatectomy and remain at risk for persistent hyperinsulinism, thus requiring additional surgery.

Imaging methods include sonography, CT, angiography, and transhepatic portal vein catheterization with pancreatic venous sampling. The success of preoperative sonography depends on body habitus, overlying bowel gas, tumor size, and intrapancreatic location. The tumor is usually round or oval, sharply defined, and hypoechoic relative to normal pancreas. When intraoperative sonography is performed, tumor detection improves significantly, in part because the pancreatic tail can be examined.

Insulinomas are isodense with normal pancreatic tissue and are undetectable on noncontrast CT unless the pancreatic contour is deformed. Dynamic rapid-sequence scanning during intravenous bolus infusion increases soft tissue contrast resolution and localizes tumors that measure more than 2 cm in diameter. CT also provides information about tumor stage and resectability. The most common metastatic sites include the liver, retroperitoneum, and regional lymph node groups.

*liver
retroperitoneum
LN groups*

On angiography, insulinomas exhibit a well-circumscribed, hypervascular, and uniformly dense stain in the capillary phase. The complete pancreatic arteriogram includes selective injections of the celiac, superior mesenteric, splenic, gastroduodenal, dorsal pancreatic, and pancreaticoduodenal arteries. Well-defined lesions as small as 0.5 cm may be detectable by using selective angiography with digital subtraction technique. The most powerful diagnostic technique combines CT and angiography. CT angiography (CTA) is used when an insulinoma is strongly suspected but cannot be detected by angiography alone. The patient is transported to the CT suite with a catheter in the celiac axis and scanned during intra-arterial contrast administration.

REFERENCES

Ahlstrom H, Magnusson A, Grama D, et al. Preoperative localization of endocrine pancreatic tumours by intra-arterial dynamic computed tomography. Acta Radiol 1990; 31:171–175.

Freison B. Tumors of the endocrine pancreas. N Engl J Med 1982; 306:580–590.

Galiber KG, Reading CC, Charboneau JW, et al. Localization of pancreatic insulinoma: comparison of pre- and intraoperative ultrasound with CT and angiography. Radiology 1988; 166:405–408.

Merine DS, Fishman EK, Siegelman SS. Combined computerized tomography and angiography in the diagnosis of insulinoma. South Med J. 1990; 83:595–596.

Rossi P, Allison DJ, Bezzi M. Endocrine tumors of the pancreas. Radiol Clin North Am 1989; 27:129–161.

Stark DD, Moss AA, Goldberg HL, et al. CT of pancreatic islet cell tumors. Radiology 1984; 150:491–494.

van Heerden JA, Service FJ. The surgical aspects of insulinomas. Ann Surg 1979; 189:677–682.

Case 13

HISTORY

A 4-week-old male infant presented because of transient tachypnea at birth.

RADIOLOGY

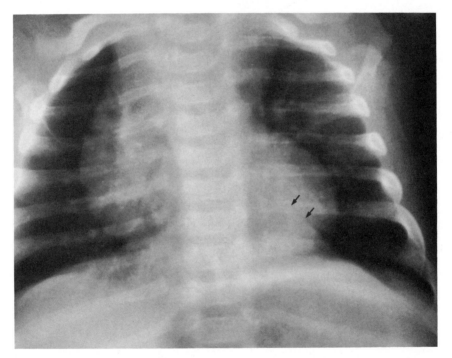

Figure 13-1. Posteroanterior (PA) chest radiograph demonstrates a sharply defined, pyramidal, left retrocardiac opacity (arrows). The lungs and mediastinum are otherwise normal.

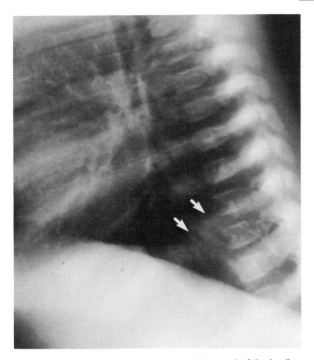

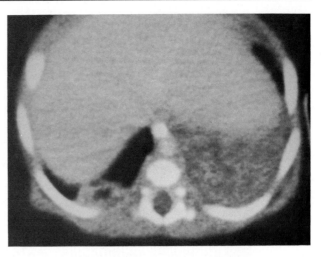

Figure 13-3. Following intravenous contrast administration, thoracic CT scan shows a left paravertebral mass. Heterogeneous enhancement suggests cystic change. There is right basilar atelectasis.

Figure 13-2. Lateral view shows the margin (arrows) of the basilar opacity.

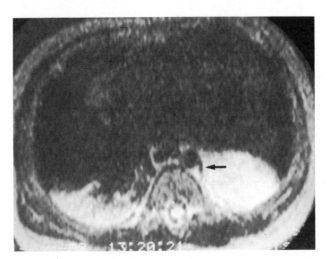

Figure 13-4. Axial T2-weighted MR image (TR = 2350, TE = 120) shows nonspecific, increased signal intensity similar to that of the atelectatic lung at the right base. A linear signal void (arrow) extends posteriorly from the left lateral aspect of the aorta and suggests a feeding vessel.

DIFFERENTIAL DIAGNOSIS

The differential diagnosis includes bronchopulmonary sequestration, bronchogenic or gastrointestinal duplication cyst, cystic adenomatoid malformation, neuroblastoma, diaphragmatic herniation (Bochdalek), and pulmonary atelectasis or consolidation.

PATHOLOGY

Thoracotomy was performed, and the lesion was resected.

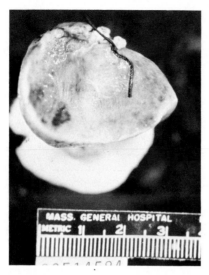

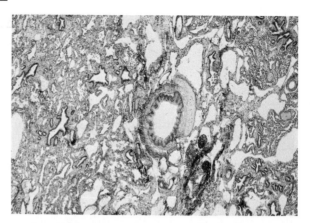

Figure 13-6. The pulmonary tissue contains bronchioles with cartilage rings and numerous alveolar spaces.

Figure 13-5. The gross tissue specimen shows compressed pulmonary parenchyma with an attached black suture.

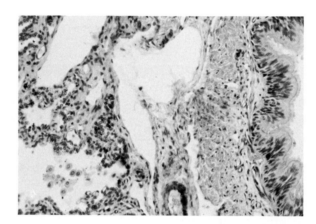

Figure 13-7. Surrounding the bronchi and extending into the interstitium are dilated lymphatics. Within the alveoli are alveolar macrophages.

DIAGNOSIS

The final pathologic diagnosis was extralobar bronchopulmonary sequestration.

systemic circulation

DISCUSSION

Bronchopulmonary foregut malformations, including pulmonary sequestration, comprise a continuum of congenital abnormalities united by a common embryogenesis. Bronchopulmonary sequestration represents dysplastic lung that is disconnected from the tracheobronchial tree and is vascularized by systemic instead of pulmonic arteries. The embryonic lung bud receives its blood supply from both the pulmonic arterial tree and the aorta. The normal pulmonic artery plexus grows with the lung bud as the aortic vessels regress. If the pulmonic connections become atretic and the aortic connections persist, however, the pulmonary tissue survives and becomes "sequestered" from normal lung.

Bronchopulmonary sequestration is classified as intralobar or extralobar. Intralobar sequestration represents 75% of all sequestrations. The dysplastic tissue of intralobar sequestration is contained within the visceral pleura of normal lung and usually is located within the left lower lobe. Systemic feeding vessels originate from the descending thoracic aorta. Vascular drainage into the left atrium occurs through the normal pulmonary veins and results in a left-to-left shunt. Owing to proximity to the tracheobronchial tree, infection and hemoptysis are frequent complications. Associated congenital abnormalities are rare.

The dysplastic tissue of extralobar sequestration is separated from normal lung by its own pleural sheath. Although pericardial, mediastinal, and abdominal locations are possible, 90% of extralobar sequestrations are contiguous with the left hemidiaphragm in the thorax. Systemic feeding vessels commonly originate from the thoracic or abdominal aorta (80%) or from the splenic, gastric, subclavian, or intercostal arteries. Vessels drain into the systemic circulation through the inferior vena cava, azygos, or hemiazygos veins. Associated congenital anomalies are frequent, especially left hemidiaphragmatic herniation. When the radiographic diagnosis is confident, surgery can be delayed or avoided in an asymptomatic patient. Complete surgical resection obviates infection and hemorrhage.

Radiographic imaging identifies the dysplastic lung mass, aberrant arterial supply, and anomalous venous drainage. Prenatal sonography may detect pulmonary sequestration in the fetus. The appearance is homogeneously echogenic or cystic and complex. Although these findings are nonspecific, color Doppler sonography can demonstrate the aberrant arterial supply.

A plain chest radiograph often shows a sharply circumscribed, oval or triangular opacity at the left lung base. This finding may be incidental. CT demonstrates a low attenuation soft tissue mass. Cystic spaces, if present, represent dilated bronchioles filled with gelatinous mucus or pus. Although no direct bronchial communication exists, these cysts may contain gas because of collateral ventilation and air trapping. Heterogeneous enhancement follows contrast administration. Although CT can detect the feeding artery in many cases, small anomalous vessels oriented out of the axial plane may not be visualized.

MR imaging increases soft tissue contrast resolution, characterizes the dysplastic pulmonary parenchyma, and identifies the presence of dilated mucoid-filled bronchioles. Coronal views are used to visualize the origin, size, and course of anomalous vessels from the descending thoracic and upper abdominal aorta. Gradient echo-pulse sequences sensitive to blood flow permit construction of MR angiograms. Angiography, once required for diagnosis of sequestration, evaluates anomalous arterial supply and venous drainage. Although CT or MR may demonstrate anomalous vessels, angiography remains the only imaging modality capable of showing small and multiple arteries, especially if they originate from unusual sources such as the splenic, gastric, subclavian, or intercostal arteries.

Marginalia (handwritten):
Intralobar
75%
w/in visceral pleura
LLL
descending Th. aorta
L-L shunt
infection & hemoptysis

Extralobar
own sheath
pericardial
mediastinal
abdominal
90% contiguous with L hemid.
80% splenic
gastric
subclavian
intercostal
IVC
azygos
hemiazygos

REFERENCES

Felker RE, Tonkin ILD. Imaging of pulmonary sequestration. AJR 1990; 154:241–249.

Ikezoe J, Murayama S, Godwin JD, et al. Bronchopulmonary sequestration: CT assessment. Radiology 1990; 176:375–379.

Oliphant L, McFadden RG, Carr TJ, et al. Magnetic resonance imaging to diagnose intralobar pulmonary sequestration. Chest 1987; 91:500–502.

Pessar ML, Soulen RL, Kan JS, et al. MRI demonstration of pulmonary sequestration. Pediatr Radiol 1988; 18:229–231.

West MS, Donaldson JS, Shkolnik A. Pulmonary sequestration: the value of ultrasound. J Ultras Med 1989; 8:125–129.

Case 14

HISTORY

A 14-year-old boy fell onto the right side of his back 2 months ago while skiing. He presented with persistent left anterior chest wall pain, occasional difficulty in breathing, and an enlarging mass.

RADIOLOGY

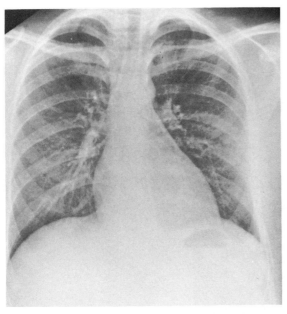

Figure 14-1. One month after sustaining a minor amount of trauma, there is an ill-defined, hazy density overlying the left lateral chest wall.

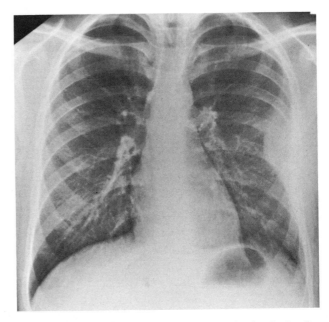

Figure 14-2. After an additional month of observation the chest wall mass has clearly increased in size, and there is a pathologic fracture of the 7th rib.

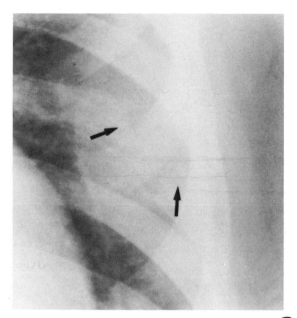

Figure 14-3. Close-up views of the left 7th rib demonstrate a lytic lesion, pathologic fracture, and periosteal response (arrows).

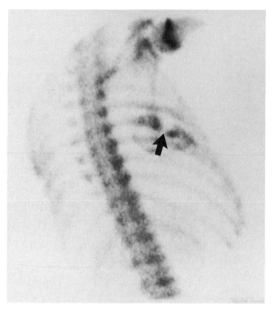

Figure 14-4. There is a focal cold area in the left 7th rib (arrow), surrounded by increased uptake both proximally and distally.

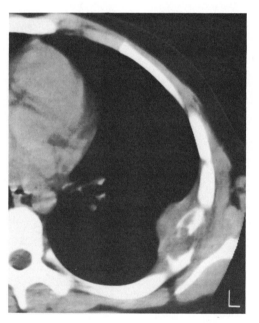

Figure 14-5. A CT scan confirms the lytic lesion of the rib and demonstrates a low attenuation soft tissue mass surrounding the bone lesion.

DIFFERENTIAL DIAGNOSIS

The differential diagnosis includes immature callus formation at the rib fracture site and pathologic fracture through a variety of tumors, including enchondroma, fibrous tumor, Ewing's sarcoma, cartilage tumor, and lymphoma.

PATHOLOGY

A biopsy of the lesion was performed.

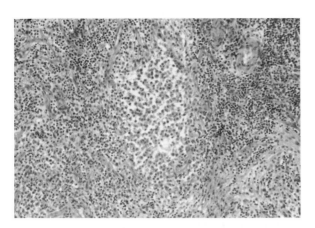

Figure 14-6. Microscopically the lesion is very cellular and consists of ovoid aggregates of medium-size cells surrounded by smaller cells.

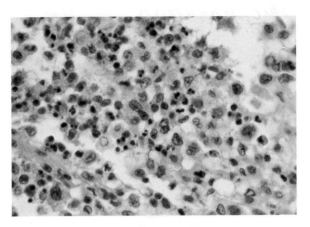

Figure 14-7. The larger ovoid cells have kidney bean-shaped, irregular hyperlobulated nuclei and a moderate amount of eosinophilic cytoplasm; they intermingle with eosinophils.

Histiocytosis (handwritten)

Letterer Siwe - acute (handwritten)
Hand-Shuller - Chronic. (handwritten)
Eosinophic granuloma - solitary bone lesion (handwritten)

DIAGNOSIS

The final pathologic diagnosis was eosinophilic granuloma.

DISCUSSION

Eosinophilic granuloma represents one end of a wide spectrum of diseases designated idiopathic inflammatory histiocytosis, or histiocytosis X. It comprises three distinct syndromes: Letterer-Siwe disease, the acute and rapidly progressive form of the disease; Hand-Schüller-Christian disease, a chronic and disseminated form involving the bones and soft tissues; and eosinophilic granuloma, usually a solitary bony lesion. Although these clinical entities differ from each other with respect to organ involvement and prognosis, they are similar in that large histiocytic cells are present within the lesions. No specific etiology for the syndrome has been determined, and it may represent a reaction to many different factors, including genetic, prenatal, immunologic, and infectious factors.

reticulum cell (handwritten)

Lesions typically consist of a proliferation of reticulum cells containing variable amounts of lipids. In eosinophilic granuloma, focal granulomas containing lipidized and nonlipidized histiocytes are seen as well as eosinophils in sheets or masses. Other types of white blood cells, fibroblasts, and foreign body or Langhans' giant cells are also seen, though this appearance can be quite variable. Necrosis can be present. Monostotic eosinophilic granuloma is more common than disseminated disease. If dissemination is to occur, it usually does so within the first 6 months of detection of disease and is more common in patients under 5 years of age; lesions that remain solitary for 12 months are not expected to disseminate.

Signs and symptoms depend on the location and extent of involvement. Pain, swelling, tenderness, and limitation of motion occur as the bone is eroded. Pathologic fractures may occur. Focal disease usually does not produce constitutional symptoms; however, fever, weight loss, malaise, and weakness are seen in diffuse disease. Other symptoms include soft tissue mass, exophthalmus, seborrhealike rash, and otitis. Laboratory findings are usually normal with solitary lesions.

Radiographically, the basic lesion is an oval or round region of osteolysis involving any part of a bone, though the epiphysis is usually spared. The radiolucency may be sharply marginated or poorly defined, and the lesion can enlarge and cause bony expansion. Lesions extend into and destroy the cortex, leading to fractures, and simulate sclerotic or "onion-skin" periosteal new bone formation. An exuberant periostitis can be seen surrounding the lesion; this has been termed the "cloak" of eosinophilic granuloma. Some lesions demonstrate a peculiar beveling of the cortex with undulating contours, giving a "hole" within a "hole" appearance. Coarsened trabeculae may be seen, and following treatment the lesions can become sclerotic. Radiographically apparent lesions do not always demonstrate increased tracer activity on radioisotope bone scans for reasons that are unclear.

Monostotic eosinophilic granuloma is treated by local excision, curettage (often with grafting), resection, and intralesional steroids. Prognosis is excellent for local disease but worse for disseminated histiocytosis. Some series report a 50 to 75% success rate, but up to 50% of patients may develop long-term disability related to skeletal abnormalities, growth failure, or other problems related to the original involvement of bones or soft tissues.

REFERENCES

Hudson TM. Radiologic-Pathologic Correlation of Musculoskeletal Lesions. Baltimore: Williams & Wilkins, 1987: 239–248.

Dahlin DC, Unni KK. Bone Tumors: General Aspects and Data on 8,542 Cases. Springfield, IL: Charles C Thomas, 1986: 452–457.

Nauert DD et al. Eosinophilic granuloma of bone: diagnosis and management. Skel Radiol 1983; 10:227–235.

Case 15

A 68-year-old male presented with progressive neurologic deterioration.

RADIOLOGY

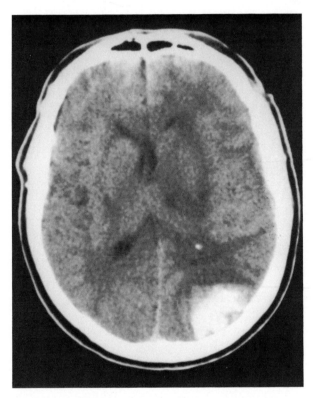 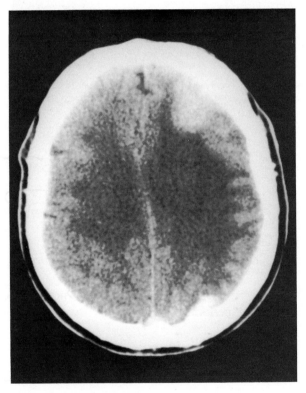

Figure 15-1. Noncontrast cranial CT scan obtained on April 13 shows high attenuation in the left parieto-occipital lobe suggestive of hemorrhage with surrounding low attenuation white matter edema. There is a mild rightward midline shift.

Figure 15-2. Another image from the same scan shows superior extension of the parieto-occipital hemorrhage as well as a second hemorrhagic focus in the left frontal lobe.

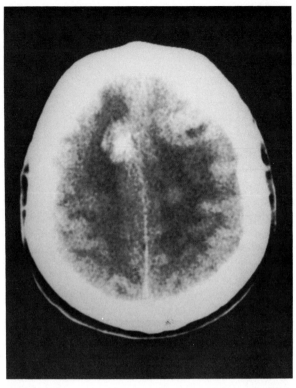

Figure 15-3. Noncontrast CT scan obtained on April 18 demonstrates both the previously visualized left frontal lobe hemorrhage and a new high attenuation hemorrhagic focus in the medial portion of the right frontal lobe. Low attenuation edema surrounds both areas of hemorrhage.

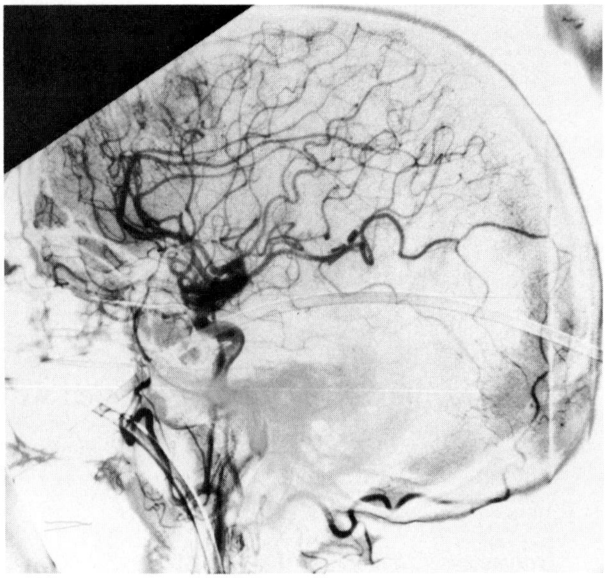

Figure 15-4. Subtraction lateral view from a left common carotid arteriogram demonstrates neovascularity and a hypervascular blush in the left frontal lobe. These findings are consistent with neoplasm.

DIFFERENTIAL DIAGNOSIS

The differential diagnosis includes metastases, multifocal neoplasm including glioblastoma or lymphoma, vascular malformations, amyloid angiopathy, and embolic disease.

PATHOLOGY

The patient died following a rapidly declining clinical course. An autopsy was performed.

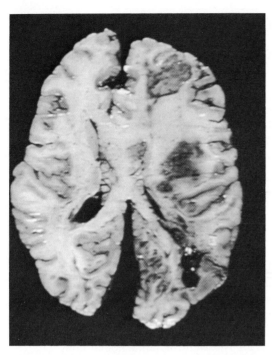

Figure 15-5. Brain section shows multiple irregular ovoid nodules of tumor present throughout the hemispheres. The tumor nodules are hemorrhagic.

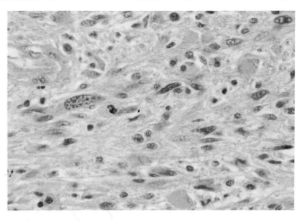

Figure 15-6. The tumor cells are pleomorphic and composed of spindle and ovoid cells that have abundant eosinophilic cytoplasm. Mitoses are conspicuous.

DIAGNOSIS

The final pathologic diagnosis was multicentric glioblastoma.

DISCUSSION

Glioblastomas are the most aggressive of the malignant gliomas. Survival is only 15 to 25% at 18 months despite therapy. Pathologically, the tumors are hypercellular, anaplastic, and highly pleomorphic. Some areas with recognizable astrocytes are often found. Focal areas of cyst formation, necrosis, and hemorrhage are not unusual. Glioblastomas are located predominantly in the supratentorial white matter but can occur anywhere in the central nervous system. Peak incidence occurs in the fifth through seventh decades, with males outnumbering females by a 3:2 margin. Presenting signs and symptoms include diffuse cerebral dysfunction, focal deficits, seizures, and elevated intracranial pressure.

The great majority of glioblastomas are solitary. They can be multifocal, with bridging tumor cells found microscopically between macroscopic foci of tumor, or multicentric, with no microscopic communication between foci. Multicentric glioblastomas constitute approximately 5% of glioblastomas. Foci of tumor can arise either synchronously or metachronously.

Hemorrhage into malignant neoplasms accounts for 10% of intracranial hematomas. Hemorrhage occurs in about 7% of glioblastomas and less frequently in ependymomas, oligodendrogliomas, and meningiomas. Three to fourteen percent of intracerebral metastases are hemorrhagic, with choriocarcinoma, melanoma, and bronchogenic, thyroid, and renal cell carcinoma the most likely primary tumors.

The CT appearance of intratumoral hemorrhage is nonspecific. Atypical location of the hemorrhage, multiplicity of hemorrhagic foci, and early enhancement suggest intratumoral hemorrhage. Features on MR imaging that favor the presence of intratumoral hemorrhage include heterogeneous signal within the hematoma due to the simultaneous presence of multiple stages of hematoma evolution; delayed hematoma evolution; an absent or incomplete hemosiderin ring; persistent mass effect in the late stages; and the presence of an enhancing nonhemorrhagic tumor component.

Differentiation of multicentric glioblastoma from multiple metastases is nearly impossible by imaging methods and generally requires a biopsy. Intracerebral lymphoma can be multifocal, but hemorrhage is distinctly uncommon.

The prognosis of multicentric glioblastoma is poor, and many patients die soon after the onset of symptoms. Surgical debulking, high-dose radiation therapy, and chemotherapy remain the major treatment options.

REFERENCES

Atlas SW, Grossman RI, Gomori JM, et al. Hemorrhagic intracranial malignant neoplasms: spin-echo MR imaging. Radiology 1987; 164:71–77.

Kieffer SA, Salibi NA, Kim RC, et al. Multifocal glioblastoma: diagnostic implications. Radiology 1982; 143:709–710.

Russel DS, Rubinstein LJ. Pathology of Tumors of the Nervous System (5th ed). Baltimore: Williams & Wilkins, 1989.

Van Tassel P, Lee Y, Bruner JM. Synchronous and metachronous malignant gliomas: CT Findings. AJNR 1988; 9:725–732.

Case 16

HISTORY

An 80-year-old woman presented with a 2-month history of low back pain. She had a history of aortic valve replacement for which she had been taking warfarin.

RADIOLOGY

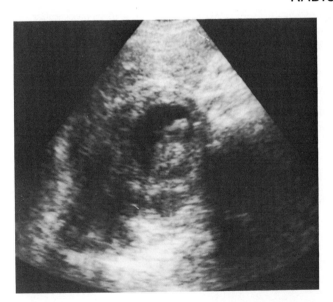

Figure 16-1. Abdominal ultrasound shows a complex right suprarenal mass measuring approximately 8- × 11-cm, which appears to be of adrenal origin. A 2.5-cm abdominal aneurysm is also noted.

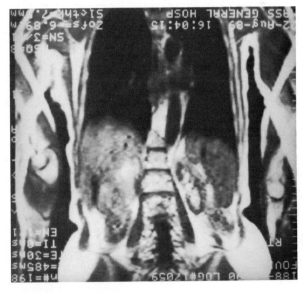

Figure 16-2. A T1-weighted coronal MR scan of the abdomen shows a mass with mixed signal intensity consistent with adrenal origin.

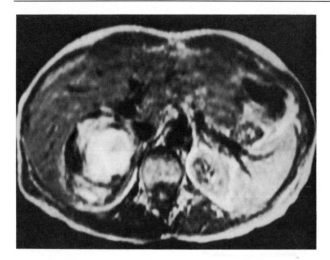

Figure 16-3. Bright uniform signal on the T2-weighted images suggests a fluid-filled structure.

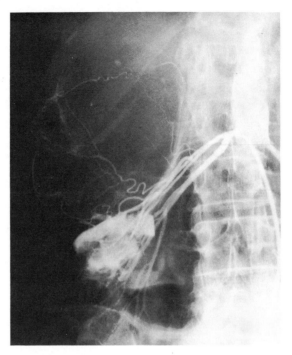

Figure 16-4. A renal angiogram shows a 9- × 10-cm hypovascular mass that pushes the right kidney inferiorly and receives some blood supply from the upper branch of the right renal artery.

DIFFERENTIAL DIAGNOSIS

The differential diagnosis includes adrenal cortical carcinoma, adrenal adenoma, exophytic renal cell carcinoma, and adrenal hemorrhage.

PATHOLOGY

A 6.5- × 6.5- × 10-cm lobulated mass was removed at surgery.

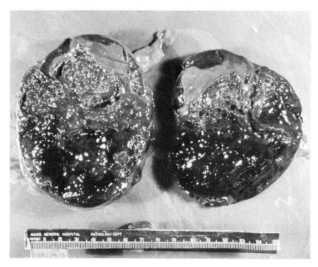

Figure 16-5. The surface of the lesion is tan-yellow with focal hemorrhage. Multiloculated cystic areas contain both recent and old hemorrhages. No neoplastic cells are seen.

DIAGNOSIS

The final diagnosis was adrenal hemorrhage.

DISCUSSION

In adult autopsy series adrenal hemorrhage has been described as having an incidence of 0.14 to 1.1%. It is often bilateral and tends to appear after a stressful event, which presumably results in intense stimulation of the gland by adrenocorticotropic hormone (ACTH). This hemorrhage may occur in the acute phase of serious systemic illness, following trauma, burns, surgery, overwhelming sepsis, or disseminated intravascular coagulation (DIC) (Fredericksen syndrome). Systemic anticoagulation increases the risk of hemorrhage, which is characteristically seen during the second or third week of anticoagulation. Adrenal hemorrhage is seen in newborns following a difficult delivery, and in children it has been documented following meningococcemia. It has been reported as a complication in 10% of patients undergoing adrenal venography. Very rarely, hemorrhage may occur in healthy patients without other risk factors.

Signs and symptoms are nonspecific and include hypotension and shock, fever, abdominal pain, nausea and vomiting, flank pain, back pain, and psychiatric symptoms. Less than 10% of patients develop adrenal insufficiency as manifested by hyponatremia, hyperkalemia, hypotension and shock. The mortality rate is usually that of the underlying disorder. Sequential imaging studies reveal a mass that may vary from 1 mm to over 15 cm in diameter and gradually decreases in size as the patient recovers.

REFERENCES

Ling D, et al. CT demonstration of bilateral adrenal hemorrhage. AJR 1983; 141:307–308.

Melby JC. Adrenal hemorrhage. N Engl J Med 1984; 311:783–790.

O'Connel TX, Aston SJ. Acute adrenal hemorrhage complicating anticoagulation therapy. Surg Gynecol Obstet 1974; 139:355–357.

Xarci VP, et al. Adrenal hemorrhage in the adult. Medicine 1978; 57:211–219.

intense stimulation of the gland by ACTH

Case 17

HISTORY

A 35-year-old human immunodeficiency virus (HIV)-positive male presented with fever, night sweats, and malaise.

RADIOLOGY

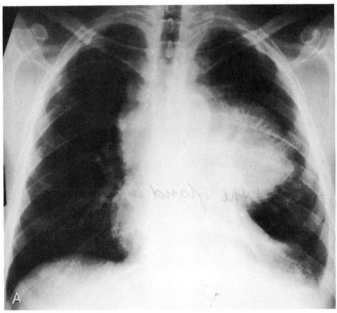

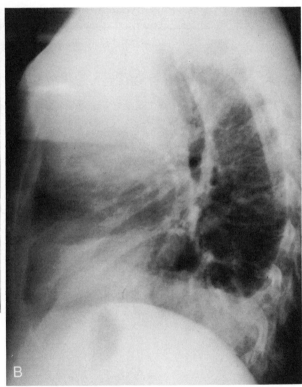

Figure 17-1. Posteroanterior (PA) and lateral views of the chest demonstrate a large anterior mediastinal mass extending asymmetrically into the left chest.

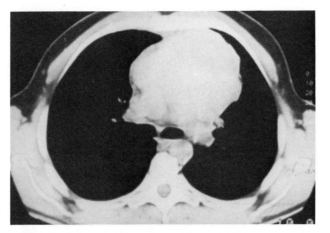

anterior mediastinal
thymoma
teratoma
choriocarcinoma
embryonal carcinoma
lymphoma

Figure 17-2. An nonenhanced CT scan of the chest confirms the presence of a large anterior mediastinal mass containing several punctate calcifications. The mass surrounds the great vessels and abuts the chest wall.

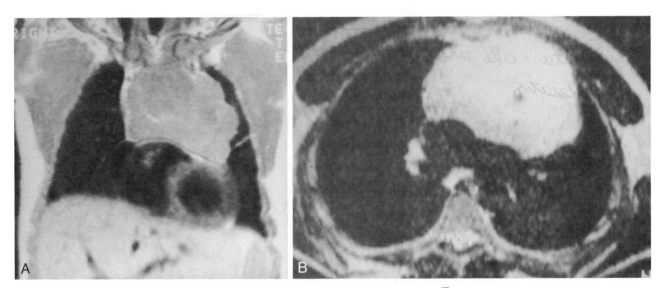

Figure 17-3. An MR image shows the mass to be of intermediate signal on the T1-weighted coronal image (*A*) and of increased signal on the T2-weighted axial image (*B*). The fat plane between the mass and the pulmonary artery has been obliterated. The mass infiltrates the anterior chest wall.

DIFFERENTIAL DIAGNOSIS

The differential diagnosis includes thymoma, teratoma, choriocarcinoma, embryonal carcinoma, and lymphoma.

PATHOLOGY

Biopsy was performed.

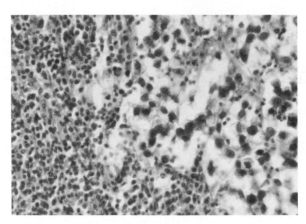

Figure 17-4. There are sheets of large tumor cells with abundant eosinophilic cytoplasm. The tumor nuclei have prominent nucleoli, and nests of tumor cells are surrounded by a prominent lymphoid infiltrate. Immunochemistry stains (not shown) were positive for placenta-like alkaline phosphatase and cytokeratin.

placenta - like alk. phosphatase
cytokeratin

DIAGNOSIS

The final pathologic diagnosis was seminoma.

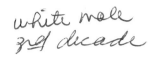

white male 3rd decade

DISCUSSION

Seminoma is the most common of the extragonadal germ cell tumors that occur in the anterior mediastinum. Other frequent sites are the sacrococcygeal region and the retroperitoneum. Anterior mediastinal seminoma is primarily a disease of white males in their third decade of life; only six cases have been reported in females. Chest pain is the most common presenting symptom, followed by acute superior vena cava syndrome and dyspnea. Twenty percent of patients are asymptomatic; in these, the tumor is discovered incidentally in a chest radiograph performed for unrelated reasons.

The pathogenesis of extragonadal germ cell tumors is disputed. One current explanation is that extragonadal germ cell tumors arise from primordial germ cells that have been misplaced during fetal development. A competing theory is that these tumors represent metastases from microscopic or involuted primary testicular tumors. The incidence of pathologically proved microscopic testicular disease in patients with anterior mediastinal tumors varies considerably, but most studies do not confirm the theory of metastases.

An association between mediastinal seminoma and acquired immune deficiency syndrome (AIDS) has not been reported; however, some reports have suggested a possible association between HIV infection and germ cell tumors of the testes.

Anterior mediastinal seminomas are usually quite large when first diagnosed. These tumors are locally aggressive and are frequently adherent to the great vessels and chest wall at surgery. Distant metastases are common in bone, lung, and liver. Anterior mediastinal seminomas have a poorer prognosis than their testicular counterparts; the 5-year survival rate is approximately 50 to 75%. Like seminomas of the testes, these tumors are radiosensitive.

bone lung liver

Anterior mediastinal seminomas are usually treated with radiotherapy. Some authors suggest surgical removal or debulking of the tumor prior to radiotherapy. The role of chemotherapy in the presence of distant metastases is unresolved.

REFERENCES

Aygun C, Slawson RG, Bajaj K, et al. Primary mediastinal seminoma. Urology 1984; 23:109–117.

Bohle A, Studer UE, Sonntag RW, et al. Primary or secondary extragonadal germ cell tumors? J Urol 1986; 135:939–943.

Lee J, Sagel S, Stanley R: Computed body tomography with MRI correlation. New York: Raven Press, 1989.

Palmer MC, Mador DR, Venner PM. Testicular seminoma associated with the acquired immunodeficiency syndrome and acquired immunodeficiency syndrome–related complex: two case reports. J Urol 1989; 142:128–130.

Raghavan D, Barrett A. Mediastinal seminomas. Cancer 1980; 46:1187–1191.

Tessler A, Catanese A. AIDS and germ cell tumors of testis. Urology 1987; 30:203–204.

Case 18

HISTORY

A 65-year-old man presented with a 3-day history of melena.

RADIOLOGY

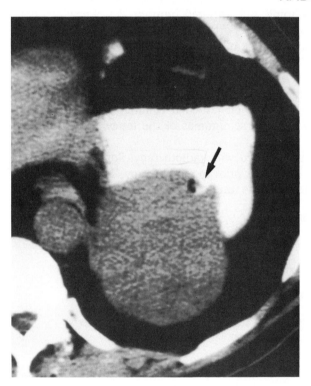

Figure 18-1. Noncontrast CT scan shows an exophytic spherical mass centered on the posterior gastric wall. Contrast and gas fill a small ulceration (arrow). The lesion is mildly heterogeneous in attenuation.

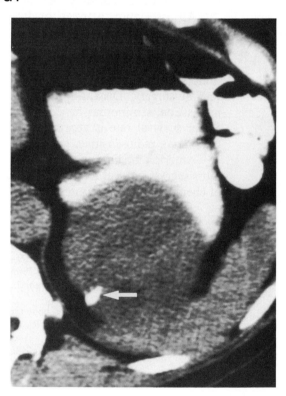

Figure 18-2. At a lower level the mass contains a focal calcification (arrow).

DIFFERENTIAL DIAGNOSIS

The differential diagnosis includes adenocarcinoma, leiomyoma, and leiomyosarcoma.

PATHOLOGY

Gastrectomy was performed.

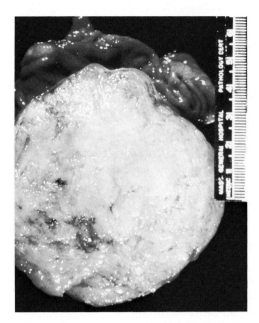

Figure 18-3. The resected mass is well circumscribed and tan-white with regions of hemorrhage and necrosis.

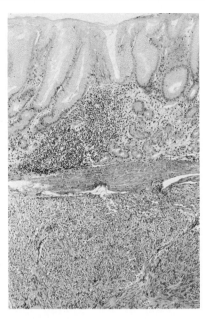

Figure 18-4. The cellular lesion does not infiltrate the overlying mucosa or muscularis mucosae.

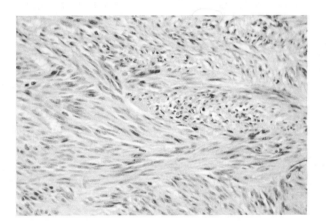

Figure 18-5. The tumor is cellular and composed of uniform elongated whorled bundles of spindle cells arranged in interesting fascicles. There is mild cytologic atypia and infrequent mitoses.

adeno ca
leiomyoma
leiomyosarcoma

DIAGNOSIS

The final pathologic diagnosis was low-grade leiomyosarcoma of the stomach.

DISCUSSION

Half of all gastrointestinal stromal tumors are gastric; approximately 80% of these are leiomyomas or leiomyosarcomas. Benign leiomyomas are common and, if small, are generally asymptomatic. Their malignant counterpart, leiomyosarcoma, is less common and accounts for only 1% of all malignant gastric neoplasms. The two tumors may be difficult to distinguish from each other clinically and radiologically. Although both leiomyomas and leiomyosarcomas may present with ulcer, bleeding, pain, nausea and vomiting, weight loss, and palpable mass, symptoms are more common in patients with leiomyosarcomas, and leiomyosarcomas tend to be larger. They grow submucosally in the gastric wall, leaving the luminal surface smooth. However, ulceration may be seen in up to 50% of cases; the ulcers tend to be small, even if the tumor itself is large.

Foci of calcification are a characteristic of both leiomyomas and leiomyosarcomas. Necrosis and hemorrhage are evident radiologically as a nonhomogeneous appearance before and after contrast enhancement; these signs occur more commonly with malignant tumors. Extragastric spread occurs with local extension and infiltration of contiguous structures, particularly the liver, omentum, and retroperitoneum, and with involvement of regional or distant lymph nodes. At presentation, extragastric spread is found in 50 to 67% of cases of leiomyosarcoma; CT is not reliable in detecting it.

Leiomyosarcomas that are 8 cm or larger in size are more likely to be associated with disseminated disease and a shorter mean survival time (15.5 months) than tumors that are smaller than 8 cm (83 months survival). The treatment is surgical, but because these lesions are asymptomatic until late in the clinical course, fewer than half are resectable.

This comparison case underscores the importance of adequate gastric distension. Abdominal CT scan can lead to a false-positive diagnosis of a gastric mass. Figures 18–6 and 18–7 show images from the barium and CT examinations of a patient with gastric pseudotumor. A second CT scan was performed to reevaluate the stomach following endoscopy, which detected no mass lesion. Gastric pseudotumor represents focal thickening of the normal gastric wall. The masslike appearance results from incomplete gastric distension or asymmetric peristalsis. Gastric pseudotumor, if not differentiated from a true mass lesion, leads to additional imaging, endoscopy, or biopsy.

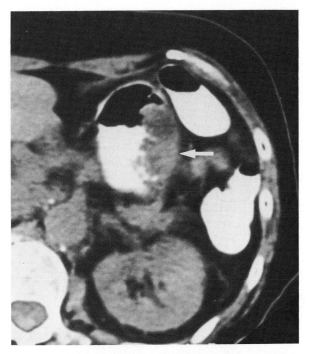

Figure 18-6. CT scan shows irregular thickening of the lateral gastric wall (arrow). There is incomplete distension of the stomach.

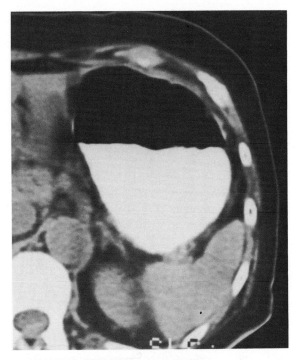

Figure 18-7. Repeat CT scan with adequate distension by oral contrast shows that the polypoid filling defect is no longer present.

REFERENCES

Andaker L, Morales O, Hojer H, et al. Evaluation of preoperative computed tomography in gastric malignancy. Surgery 1991; 109:132–135.

Berk JE, Haubrich WS, Kalser MH, et al. (eds). Bockus Gastroenterology (4th ed). Philadelphia: Saunders, 1985: 1273–1274.

Disler DG, Chew FS. Gastric leiomyosarcoma. AJR 1992; 159:58.

Megibow AJ, Balthazar EJ, Hulnick DH, et al. CT evaluation of gastrointestinal leiomyomas and leiomyosarcomas. AJR 1985; 144:727–731.

Mitros FA. Atlas of Gastrointestinal Pathology. New York: Gower Medical, 1988: 4.19–4.20.

Case 19

HISTORY

A 4-year-old child presented with recurrent pain in the right thigh.

RADIOLOGY

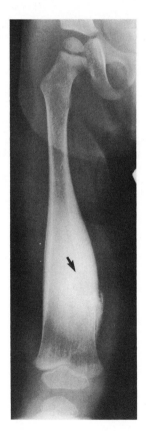

Figure 19-1. Anteroposterior (AP) radiograph shows a 1.5-cm oval lucency (arrow) involving the medial cortex of the distal right femoral diaphysis. Marked periosteal new bone surrounds the lesion. The periosteal response has widened the contour of the bone.

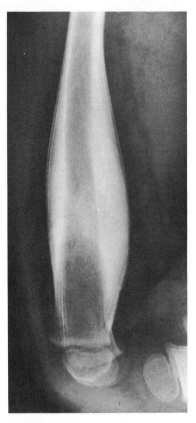

Figure 19-2. Frog lateral radiograph confirms cortical thickening and expansion with relative sparing of the medullary canal.

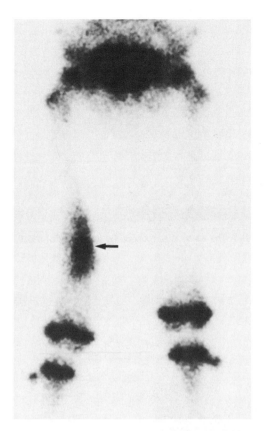

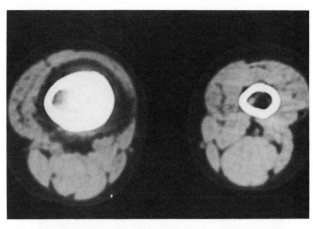

Figure 19-4. CT scan through the level of the maximum sclerosis demonstrates a "halo" of low attenuation surrounding the femur. This region presumably corresponds to fatty change and edema.

Figure 19-3. A radioisotope scan demonstrates the lucent area on the plain film as a rounded region of intensely increased uptake (arrow). The sclerotic response corresponds to a more diffuse zone of increased uptake both proximal and distal to the lucency.

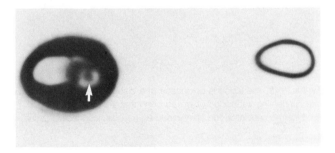

Figure 19-5. CT scan with gray-scale reversal shows that the lucent lesion is eccentrically located. The lucency contains a central, dense focus (arrow).

DIFFERENTIAL DIAGNOSIS

The differential diagnosis includes Brodie's abscess, tuberculous bone abscess, osteoid osteoma, early stages of osteosarcoma, and hemangioma.

PATHOLOGY

Curettage of the lesion was performed, and the specimen was submitted in fragments.

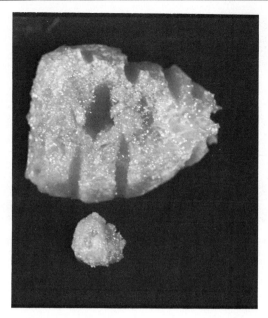

Figure 19-6. The removed portion of cortex shows a central space from which the tumor has fallen out.

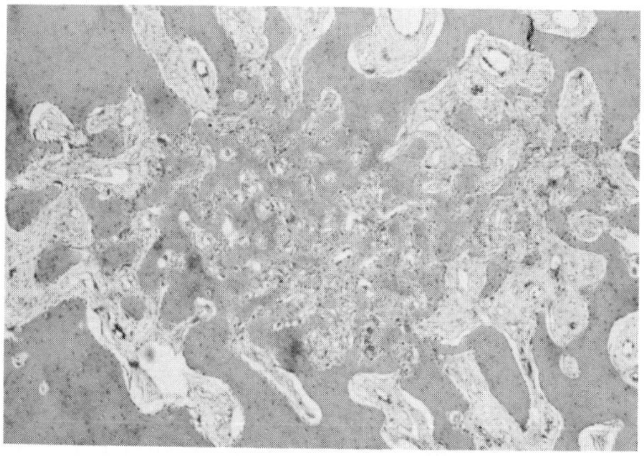

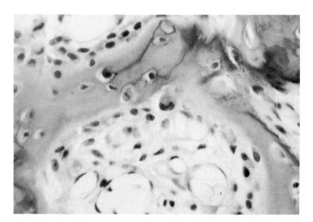

Figure 19-7. The lesion is surrounded by trabeculae of reactive bone.

Figure 19-8. The lesion is composed of a disorganized tangle of interconnecting trabeculae of woven bone that are rimmed by prominent osteoblasts and surrounded by vascular connective tissue.

DIAGNOSIS

The final pathologic diagnosis was osteoid osteoma.

[handwritten: 7-25 years]
[handwritten: pain]

DISCUSSION

Osteoid osteoma is a benign tumor of bone that was first described by Jaffe in 1935. This lesion accounts for approximately 10% of benign primary bone tumors and almost always is accompanied by pain. The pain increases at night, is relieved by salicylates, and usually occurs at the site of the tumor but can be referred to the adjacent joint.

Most osteoid osteomas occur in patients between the ages of 7 and 25 years. Common sites include the femur and tibia, which together account for 60% of the lesion sites. Twenty percent of lesions arise in the hands and feet. Osteoid osteoma occasionally occurs in the posterior elements of the spine. The precise relationship between osteoid osteoma and osteoblastoma remains unclear.

Osteoid osteoma originating in a long bone is frequently centrally located within the cortex. The tumor is most commonly diaphyseal in location, although extension to the metaphysis does occur. Epiphyseal involvement is extremely rare. Typically, a rounded or oval central lucency measuring less than 1 cm in diameter is present. This lucency, or nidus, contains variable amounts of punctate calcification. The nidus is usually single, although multiple lucent areas have been reported, and is surrounded by dense sclerosis and periosteal new bone formation. Cortical thickening is a prominent feature.

Osteoid osteoma arising in the hand is most often located in the proximal phalanx or metacarpal bone. In the foot, the talus or calcaneus is most frequently involved. Osteoid osteoma arising in a carpal bone shows a well-circumscribed, partially to completely calcified, intramedullary lesion with minimal surrounding sclerosis. A tumor arising in the vertebral column is almost always found in the posterior elements, although involvement of the vertebral body can occur. In the spine, the tumor is usually associated with scoliosis and is located at the concave surface.

[handwritten margin: hand / prox. phal / metacarpal / foot / talus / calcaneus]

Nuclear scintigraphy has been used both preoperatively and intraoperatively for identification of the tumor nidus. Osteoid osteoma typically exhibits moderate tracer uptake in the zones of sclerosis with marked uptake in the region of the nidus. The pattern of uptake is called the double-density sign. CT scan is more sensitive than plain radiographs in detecting small lucencies surrounded by cortical thickening and in defining osteoid osteomas of complex bones including the spine, pelvis, femoral neck, and calcaneus. The nidus enhances densely following intravenous contrast administration.

[handwritten margin: double density sign]

The treatment of osteoid osteoma is excision of the nidus. Prognosis is dependent on complete removal of the nidus; recurrence is frequent if excision is incomplete.

REFERENCES

Dahlin DC, Unni KK. Bone Tumors: General Aspects and Data on 8542 Cases. Springfield, IL: Charles C Thomas, 1986:88–101.

Freiberger R, et al. Osteoid osteoma: a report on 80 cases. AJR 1959; 82:194–205.

Hudson TM. Radiologic-Pathologic Correlation of Musculoskeletal Lesions. Baltimore: Williams & Wilkins, 1987:9–18.

Swee R, et al. Osteoid osteoma: detection, diagnosis, and localization. Radiology 1979; 130:117.

[handwritten: nidus enhances densely following IV.]

Case 20

HISTORY

A 28-year-old male presented with a painful, red, swollen right knee. He had undergone arthroscopic repair of an anterior cruciate ligament tear in the past.

RADIOLOGY

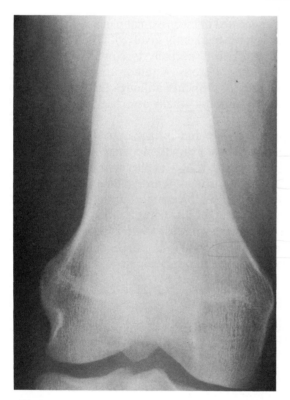

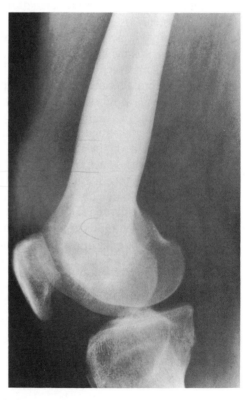

Figure 20-1. Anteroposterior (AP) radiograph shows an ill-defined zone of medullary sclerosis involving the distal metaphysis of the femur.

Figure 20-2. Lateral radiograph shows medullary sclerosis, periosteal reaction, and joint effusion.

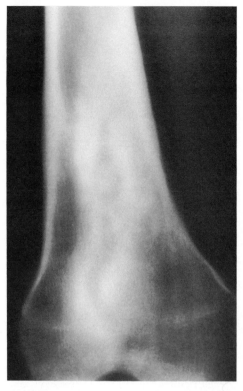

Figure 20-3. Conventional tomogram shows that the medullary sclerosis surrounds a linear lucency extending to the intercondylar notch.

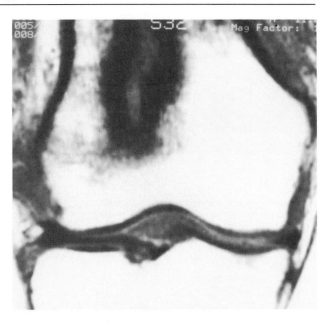

Figure 20-4. T1-weighted MR image (TR = 500, TE = 20) demonstrates the medullary sclerosis as a zone of weak signal surrounding a linear area of intermediate signal that corresponds to the lucencies seen on the tomogram.

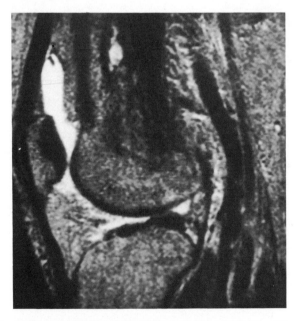

Figure 20-5. Sagittal T2-weighted MR image (TR = 2750, TE = 80) demonstrates a bright signal within the joint fluid and a small focus of bright signal within the medullary cavity of bone.

DIFFERENTIAL DIAGNOSIS

The differential diagnosis includes osteoid osteoma, eosinophilic granuloma, Brodie's abscess, acute osteomyelitis, metastasis, and fibrous dysplasia.

PATHOLOGY

The lesion was resected.

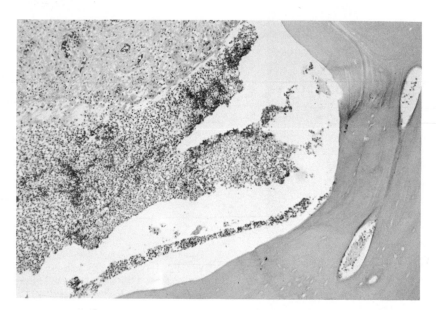

Figure 20–6. The cortex is necrotic and the haversian systems are massively enlarged and filled with inflammatory cells.

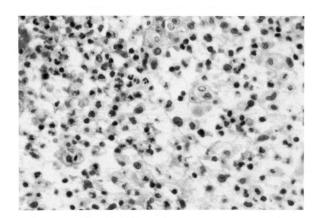

Figure 20–7. The inflammation contains neutrophils, macrophages, and lymphocytes.

DIAGNOSIS

The final pathologic diagnosis was Brodie's abscess.

[handwritten: subacute pyogenic osteo staphy]

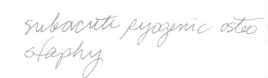

DISCUSSION

Single or multiple radiolucent abscesses may be evident during subacute or chronic stages of osteomyelitis. These abscesses were initially noted in the tibial metaphyses and described by Brodie in 1832. They are now most often seen as circumscribed lesions that show a predilection for the ends of tubular bones. They are characteristically found in subacute pyogenic osteomyelitis, usually of staphylococcal origin. It has been suggested that bone abscesses develop when an infecting organism has a reduced virulence or when the host has an increased resistance.

Although the age range is from 6 to 61 years, 75% of cases occur in patients younger than age 25 years, most commonly prior to closure of the growth plates. The male to female ratio is 2:1. Generally, there is no history of antecedent infection. The lesions characteristically appear in the metaphysis, particularly that of the tibia. Rarely, they traverse the open growth plate, affecting the epiphysis, although such extension does not commonly result in growth disturbances. In young children and infants, Brodie's abscess may occur in epiphyses and in the carpus and tarsus.

A persistent dull ache is the usual complaint. Some patients experience exacerbations and remissions of their pain. Focal tenderness, mild swelling, and erythema may be seen. Fever and an elevated white count may be present in children but are often lacking in adults. The duration of symptoms prior to diagnosis has been reported to range from 1 month to 3 years, with an average of 7 months.

The causative agent is usually *Staphylococcus aureus*, although 50% of abscesses are sterile, presumably secondary to antibiotic treatment. Abscesses vary from less than 1 cm to over 4 cm in diameter. Pathologically, granulation tissue lines the abscess cavities. A moderate fibroblastic response is present in most cases, and a fibrin layer separating bone from granulation tissue is common. Foci of necrosis may be found. The fluid in the abscess may be purulent or mucoid.

[handwritten: fluid or purulent or mucoid]

Radiographs usually demonstrate a metaphyseal radiolucency with surrounding sclerosis. The lucent region may follow a tortuous channel (see Fig. 20–3). Radiographic detection of this channel is important because it is virtually specific for osteomyelitis. Furthermore, such channels usually indicate a pyogenic process and are uncommon in tuberculosis. In the diaphysis the radiolucent abscess cavity can be located in the central or subcortical areas and may contain a central sequestrum. When an abscess is located in the cortex, the lucent lesion with a sclerotic rim and periostitis may simulate an osteoid osteoma or a stress fracture.

[handwritten: TB]

MR images are highly sensitive to acute inflammatory processes, which result in lengthened T1 and T2 relaxation times. The characteristic signal on T1 and T2-weighting of marrow fat provides excellent contrast, making MR a sensitive tool for the early detection of osteomyelitis and for following the effects of therapy. The signal intensity changes have no specificity, and the diagnosis of infection must be made by relying upon the anatomic distribution and time course.

REFERENCES

Enneking WF. Clinical Musculoskeletal Pathology (3rd rev ed). Gainesville, FL: University of Florida Press, 1990:105–123.

Hudson TM. Radiologic-Pathologic Correlation of Musculoskeletal Lesions. Baltimore: Williams & Wilkins, 1987:441–489.

Resnick D, Niwayama G. Osteomyelitis, septic arthritis, and soft tissue infection: the mechanisms and situations. *In*: Resnick D, Niwayama G (eds). Diagnosis of Bone and Joint Disorders (2nd ed). Philadelphia: Saunders, 1988:2524–2617.

Case 21

HISTORY

A 47-year-old right-handed man presented following two transient episodes of speech difficulties. The neurologic examination revealed no focal signs.

RADIOLOGY

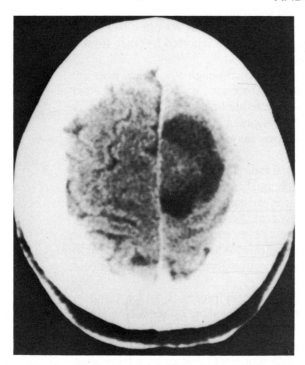

Figure 21-1. Noncontrast cranial CT scan shows an isodense mass in the high left parasagittal area. The mass abuts the falx with a relatively broad base, measures 2 cm in diameter, and is associated with an adjacent cystic component.

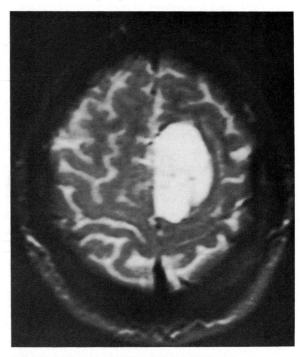

Figure 21-2. Axial T2-weighted image demonstrates heterogeneously increased signal in the mass without surrounding edema.

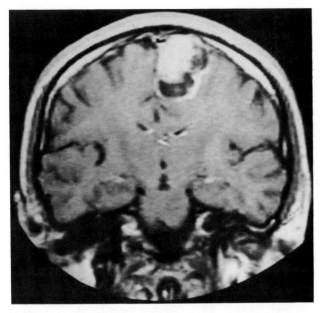

Figure 21–3. Postgadolinium T1-weighted coronal image demonstrates dense enhancement of the solid component and rim enhancement of the cystic component. The flow void in the superior sagittal sinus is preserved.

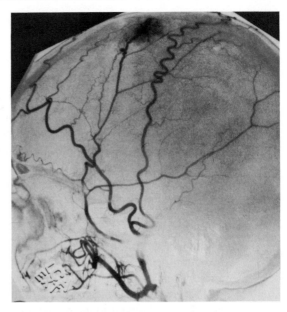

Figure 21–4. Subtraction film from a selective left external carotid arteriogram shows tumor stain in the left parasagittal region. The afferent vessel is a branch of the left middle meningeal artery.

DIFFERENTIAL DIAGNOSIS

The differential diagnosis includes cystic meningioma, cystic glioma, hemangioblastoma, and metastasis.

PATHOLOGY

The lesion was resected.

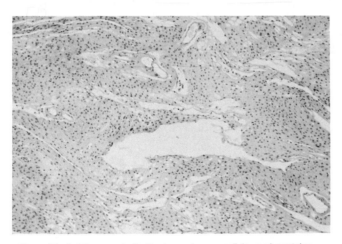

Figure 21–5. Microscopically the tumor is very cellular and contains irregular small cystic spaces.

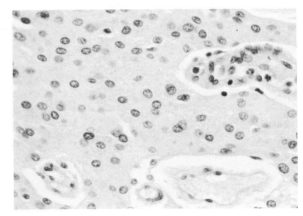

Figure 21–6. The tumor cells grow in sheets and are ovoid and contain a moderate amount of eosinophilic cytoplasm. The tumor cell nuclei lack significant pleomorphism and are relatively uniform in appearance.

DIAGNOSIS

The final pathologic diagnosis was cystic meningioma.

DISCUSSION

Cystic meningiomas account for 2% to 4% of intracranial meningiomas. Meningiomas are the most common extra-axial adult tumors, comprising 15% and 4% of all intracranial neoplasms in adults and children respectively. They arise from meningothelial cells and are divided into meningothelial, fibroblastic, and transitional (including psammomatous) types. Angioblastic "meningiomas" derive from vasoformative cells. Most commonly, meningiomas are solid, encapsulated, slow growing lobular masses that occur along a dural surface. A significant number grow in a plaquelike configuration.

Four types of cystic meningioma are recognized: (1) intratumoral cyst completely surrounded by tumor; (2) peripheral intratumoral cyst microscopically surrounded by a row of tumor cells; (3) peritumoral cyst whose wall consists partly of tumor; (4) peritumoral cyst surrounded by a distinct capsule and separate from tumor.

In a review of 166 cases of cystic meningioma, the average age at diagnosis was 45 years. Unlike conventional meningioma, males and females were affected equally. A significant number of these tumors occur in infants and children. Locations include the convexities (59%), parasagittal region (26%), and the cranial base (13%). Types 1 through 4 comprise 32%, 24%, 24%, and 21% of these tumors respectively. The majority have a meningothelial histology. Symptoms include headache, motor and visual disturbances, personality changes and seizures.

In contrast to noncystic meningiomas, the differential diagnosis of cystic meningiomas can be difficult because cysts are most often associated with glial and metastatic tumors. CT often reveals a solid mass or nodule of tumor surrounded by a cyst, which may exhibit ring enhancement. Rapid homogeneous enhancement of the solid component, a smoothly outlined cyst, and an extra-axial location along a dural margin suggest meningioma. MR imaging may show a similar enhancement pattern, and cystic tumor may be surrounded by high T2 intensity edema. The appearance of the solid component is variable. Angiography may be helpful in making the diagnosis by demonstrating the blood supply from the extracranial circulation.

Surgical resection is the primary treatment for meningioma. Incomplete resection is associated with recurrence. The use of radiation therapy by itself or as an adjunct to surgery is controversial.

REFERENCES

Fortuna A, Ferrante L, Acqui M, et al. Cystic meningiomas. Acta Neurochir (Wien) 1988; 90:23–30.

Kolluri VR, Reddy DR, Reddy PK. CT findings in cystic meningiomas. Acta Neurochir (Wien) 1987; 87:31–33.

Namba H, Sueyoshi K. Magnetic resonance imaging of a cystic meningioma. Neuroradiology 1990; 32:536.

Nauta HJW, Tucker WS, Horsey WJ, et al. Xanthochromic cysts associated with meningioma. J Neurol Neurosurg Psych 1979; 42:529–535.

Case 22

RADIOLOGY

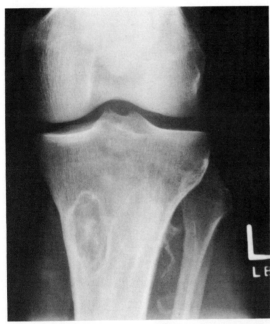 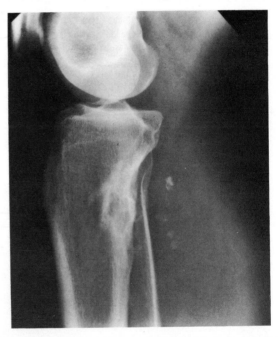

Figure 22-1. An anteroposterior (AP) radiograph of the knee reveals a lytic lesion with well-defined sclerotic margins in the proximal tibial metaphysis. Calcifications are seen extending into the soft tissues lateral to the tibia.

Figure 22-2. A lateral plain film reveals that the lytic lesion is limited to the posterior cortex of the tibia. Its shape suggests that it arose from either the surface of the tibia or the extraosseous soft tissues.

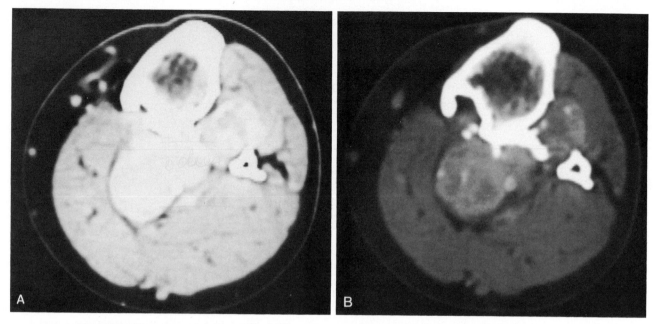

Figure 22–3. *A.* A CT scan done with intravascular contrast and displayed for soft tissues demonstrates marked enhancement of the lesion, which is anterior to the popliteal and posterior tibial vessels. The lesion has a "dumbbell" configuration extending through the intraosseous membrane. *B.* A CT scan displayed for bone demonstrates that most of the tibial changes represent periosteal new bone formation. There is relatively little evidence of active bone destruction. In areas that appear to represent tibial erosion (arrows) no tumor is seen. This suggests that the tumor has involuted from a once larger lesion.

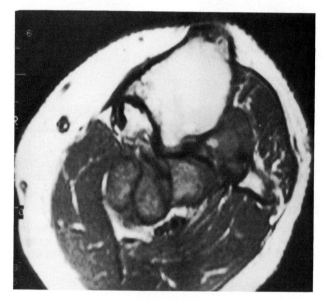

Figure 22–4. T1-weighted axial MR image shows that the lesion has a thick, well-formed capsule that appears dark on these images. This is a feature usually associated with benign lesions. The posterior tibial vessels are displaced posteriorly. Extension into the anterior compartment is demonstrated, and there is a pressure effect on the surface of the fibula.

DIFFERENTIAL DIAGNOSIS

The differential diagnosis includes parosteal osteosarcoma, periosteal chondroma or chondrosarcoma, metastatic disease, nonossifying fibroma or fibrous cortical defect, nerve sheath tumor, calcified soft tissue hematoma or myositis ossificans, and tuberculous abscess.

PATHOLOGY

The lesion was resected.

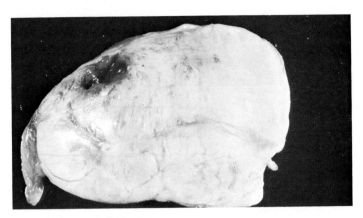

Figure 22-5. Arising from the peripheral nerve is a well-circumscribed focally hemorrhagic, tan–pale yellow glistening mass.

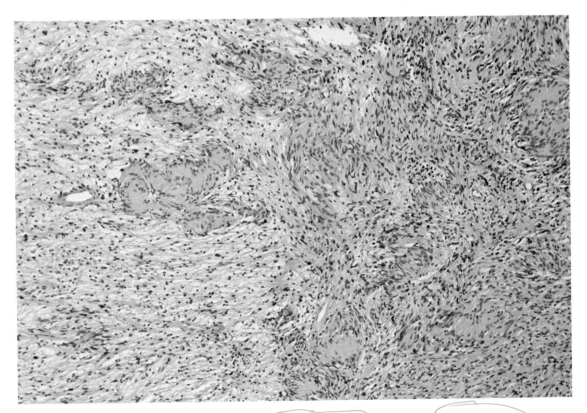

Figure 22-6. Microscopically the mass contains hypercellular (Antoni A) and relatively hypocellular (Antoni B) regions that are randomly intermixed.

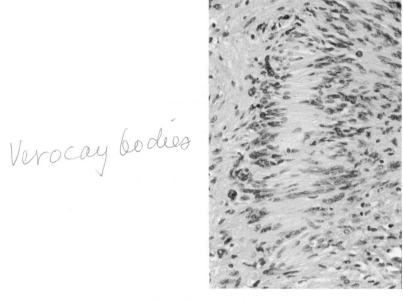

Verocay bodies

Figure 22-7. In the Antoni A regions the proliferating spindle cells are arranged in columns that are separated by eosinophilic fibrillar tissue, a structure known as a Verocay body.

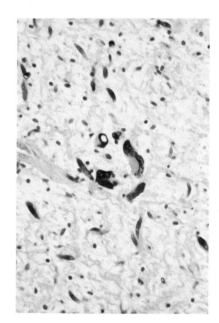

Figure 22-8. Some of the spindle cells in the Antoni B area have very large, hyperchromatic, irregular "ancient" nuclei. However, necrosis and mitotic activity are absent.

DIAGNOSIS

The final pathologic diagnosis was ancient schwannoma.

DISCUSSION

Benign schwannomas, or neurilemomas, are the most frequent benign tumors of the peripheral nerve sheath. There is some disagreement about whether these entities should be classified separately from neurofibromas. Neurilemomas are found in slightly older patients, are usually encapsulated, commonly show degeneration histologically, and are rarely seen in patients with von Recklinghausen's disease. The tumors arise in men and women equally, typically from the spinal nerve roots and the cervical, sympathetic, vagal, peroneal, and ulnar nerves. They appear most often in the head, neck, and flexor surfaces of the extremities and are most frequent in the third to fifth decades of life. The lesions are usually solitary and slow growing and are often present for several years before coming to medical attention. They may be multiple when associated with von Recklinghausen's disease. When the lesions are large, clinical manifestations are seen including pain, soft tissue mass, and neurologic findings. The tumors are freely movable except along the long axis of the nerve sheath, where attachment limits mobility. Five percent grow in a plexiform or multinodular pattern. Some patients may be vaguely aware of changes in the size of the tumors, a phenomenon related to fluctuations in the amount of cystic change occurring in the lesions. Deeper lesions are symptomatic owing to their larger size and mass effect on neighboring structures, most notably the "dumbbell" lesions arising in the posterior mediastinum, which originate from or extend into the spinal canal. Benign schwannomas rarely demonstrate malignant transformation.

Smaller tumors usually are pink, white, or yellow, but the larger lesions tend to demonstrate degenerative changes with cystification and calcification. Ancient schwannomas are usually large tumors of long duration demonstrating cyst formation, calcification, hemorrhage, and hyalinization as well as nuclear atypia, which is thought to be related to degenerative change.

Conventional radiography is helpful in detecting large lesions with calcification or those that affect adjacent structures. For example, bones may develop sclerotic, scalloped erosions or widened intervertebral foramina. CT and MR images are more effective in defining the extent of the lesions and relationships to nearby vessels, bones, or other structures. Deep, nonpalpable lesions are better demonstrated with these modalities. Schwannomas are usually well defined and smooth and have soft tissue density with areas of mixed or low attenuation values that increase slightly following intravenous contrast administration. Mixed attenuation is thought to result from the presence of hypocellular areas adjacent to regions of increased cellularity and dense collagen, cystic degeneration caused by vascular thrombosis and/or necrosis, and xanthomatous regions.

REFERENCES

Cohen LM, et al. Benign schwannomas: pathologic basis for CT inhomogeneities. AJR 1986; 147: 141–143.

Enzinger FM, Weiss SW. Benign tumors of peripheral nerves. *In*: Soft Tissue Tumors (2nd ed). St Louis: Mosby, 1983:719–735.

Ghiatas AA, Faleski EJ. Benign solitary schwannoma of the retroperitoneum: CT features. South Med J 1989; 82:801–802.

Resnick D, Niwayama G. Soft tissues. *In*: Resnick D, Niwayama G (eds). Diagnosis of Bone and Joint Disorders (2nd ed). Philadelphia: Saunders, 1988:4218–4226.

Case 23

HISTORY

A 68-year-old male presented following the incidental finding of a lung mass during hospitalization for stroke.

RADIOLOGY

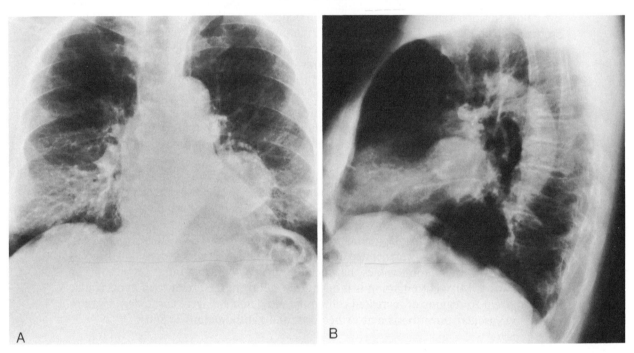

Figure 23-1. Plain film demonstrates a 7- × 6- cm left lower lobe mass abutting the take-off of the left lower lobe bronchus.

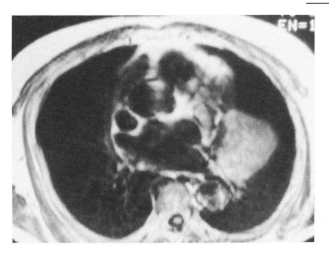

Figure 23-2. T1-weighted MR image demonstrates a large well-circumscribed left hilar mass with extrinsic compression of the lingular bronchus and left inferior pulmonary vein and without evidence of invasion. The mass is isointense to muscle and liver.

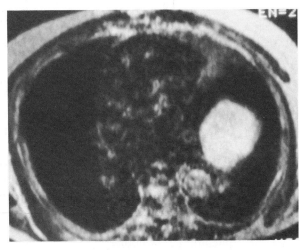

Figure 23-3. The mass becomes hyperintense on T2-weighted images.

DIFFERENTIAL DIAGNOSIS

The differential diagnosis includes primary lung carcinoma, carcinoid, fibrous mesothelioma, and hamartoma.

PATHOLOGY

The left lung mass was resected.

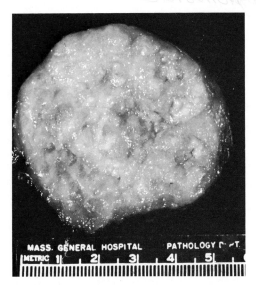

Figure 23-4. The removed lesion (8 × 6 × 4.5 cm in size) is round, well-circumscribed, firm, tan to pale yellow, a2nd glistening.

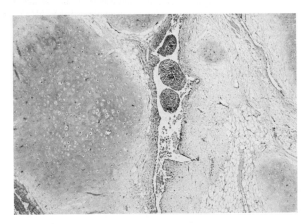

Figure 23-5. Histologically the tumor is composed of nodules of hyaline cartilage and fat that compress entrapped air spaces.

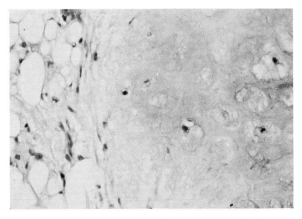

Figure 23-6. The cartilage is hypocellular and cytologically bland, and the adipocytes appear mature.

DIAGNOSIS

The final pathologic diagnosis was pulmonary hamartoma.   *most common benign*

DISCUSSION

Pulmonary hamartoma is the most common benign lung tumor, with a prevalence of 0.25% in autopsy series. A hamartoma is a disorganization of the tissues normally found in the organ. In the lung it is composed primarily of cartilage, with fibrous connective tissue, smooth muscle, fat, and rarely bone in varying amounts. True neoplasms, they have the potential for growth but apparently not for malignant degeneration. There is a slight male predominance (2:1), and the peak incidence occurs in the sixth decade. Pulmonary hamartomas are usually asymptomatic, but when they are endobronchial in location (8% to 10% of cases), patients may have atelectasis, postobstructive pneumonia, or cough.

The typical appearance on plain radiographs of a pulmonary hamartoma is a well-circumscribed, solitary, round peripheral mass less than 4 cm in size. Calcification is uncommon, but if popcorn calcification is present, the finding is pathognomonic. On CT, fat is identifiable in half the cases. Cavitation is rare.

Peripheral hamartomas require no treatment. The growth rate is slow, and the malignant potential is nonexistent. Endobronchial lesions are resected to ameliorate the complications of airway obstruction.

REFERENCES

Hamper UM, Khouri, NF, Stitik FP, et al. Pulmonary hamartoma: diagnosis by trans-thoracic needle-aspiration biopsy. Radiology 1985;155:15–18.

Sinner W. Fine needle biopsy of hamartomas of the lung. AJR 1982;138:65–69.

popcorn calcif. – pathognomonic

Case 24

HISTORY

A 20-year-old male, 2 years after resection of a left thigh mass diagnosed as "myositis ossificans," presented with a recurrent mass. Localized erythema and induration were present.

RADIOLOGY

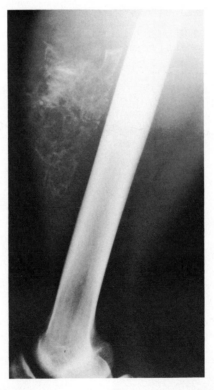

Figure 24–1. A lateral view of the left leg shows a faintly calcified mass anterior to the femur. The calcification has a linear and curvilinear pattern and appears to be peripherally distributed on the surface of the lesion.

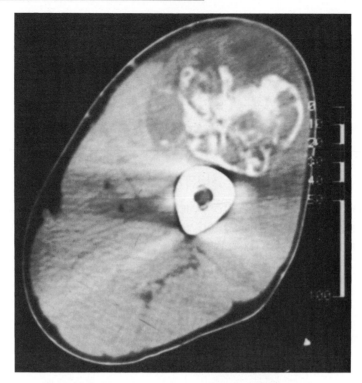

Figure 24-2. CT image reveals that some of the calcification is centrally located in the mass as well as present on the surface.

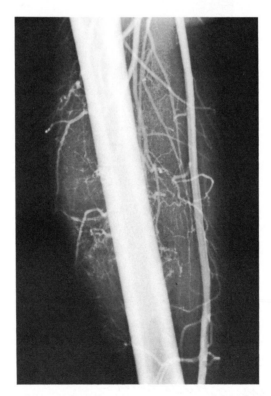

Figure 24-3. On angiography a hypervascular mass is seen to be supplied by the profunda femoris. There is arteriovenous shunting and tumor staining.

DIFFERENTIAL DIAGNOSIS

The differential diagnosis includes myositis ossificans, calcified hematoma, extraosseous osteosarcoma or chondrosarcoma, and other mesenchymal tumors (e.g., synovial sarcoma, rhabdomyosarcoma, fibrosarcoma).

PATHOLOGY

The lesion was resected.

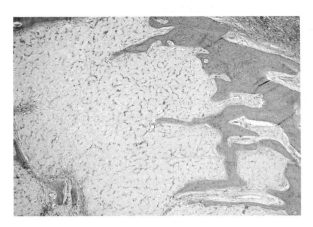

Figure 24-4. The tumor contains metaplastic trabeculae of woven bone.

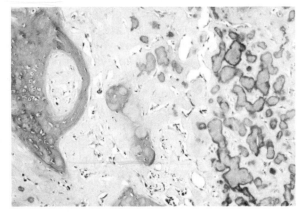

Figure 24-5. The metaplastic woven bone (right) is surrounded by pale pink stroma that is focally calcified.

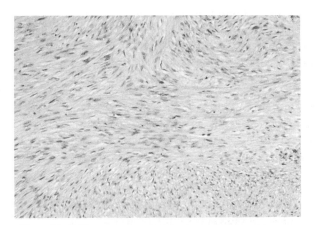

Figure 24-6. The tumor has a biphasic morphology with one component consisting of intersecting fascicles of spindle cells.

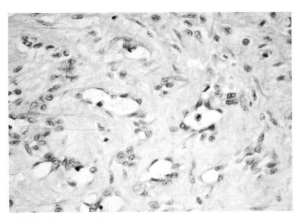

Figure 24-7. The other component consists of gland-like spaces that are delineated by cuboidal cells with epithelial features.

myositis ossificam
calcified hematoma
extraosseus osteosarcoma
or chondrosarcoma
other mesenchymal tumors
synovial sarcoma
rhabdomyosarcoma
fibrosarcoma

DIAGNOSIS

The final pathologic diagnosis was synovial sarcoma.

DISCUSSION

Synovial sarcoma (malignant synovioma) is uncommon, comprising less than 10% of soft tissue sarcomas. Most patients are 15 to 35 years old, and there is a slight male predominance. Sixty to seventy percent of lesions are located in the lower extremity. Although there is a predilection for the region of the knee and lower thigh, the tumor can occur anywhere along a limb. Interestingly, lesions are very rarely located within a joint capsule. Other unusual locations include the head, neck, chest wall, and retroperitoneum.

Patients complain of a palpable mass, often associated with deep pain and tenderness. Constitutional symptoms are unusual except with large, longstanding, poorly differentiated tumors. Because tumor growth is insidious and symptoms are vague, patients may not seek medical attention until the lesion has been present for years. This long chronicity may falsely suggest a low degree of tumor malignancy. Although many patients give a history of antecedent trauma, a causal relationship between trauma and tumor is unproved. Delay in diagnosis contributes to the frequent occurrence of metastases. The lung is most often involved (75% of metastases), followed by regional lymph nodes and bone. Synovial cell sarcoma is the most common soft tissue sarcoma to metastasize to the lymph nodes. Five-year survival rates range from 25% to 60%, and 10-year rates from 10% to 30%.

[margin handwriting: most common to metastasize to the LN.]

On plain films and CT, synovial sarcoma usually appears as a well-defined, lobulated mass of moderate density, sometimes containing cystic or necrotic regions. Thirty to fifty percent of tumors contain calcification (sometimes detectable only by CT), ranging from tiny stippling to dense sheets outlining the tumor. Although involvement of the underlying bone is uncommon, periosteal reaction occurs in 10% to 15% of cases. MR provides limited specificity in differential diagnosis but may improve anatomic delineation. Angiography usually reveals prominent neovascularity and inhomogeneous staining not only of the primary lesion but also, if present, of metastases.

Grossly, synovial sarcomas usually measure several centimeters in diameter; very large lesions are sometimes seen. Compression of adjacent structures may result in a pseudocapsule, accounting for the well-defined margins seen on imaging studies. Cyst formation may be prominent. Histologic characteristics include a biphasic pattern (as in this case), in which both synovioblastic epithelial and fibroblastic spindle cell components are present, and a monophasic pattern, in which only one of these components predominates. Calcification (thought to be a positive prognostic sign) may be dystrophic in origin or due to actual bone formation. By immunochemistry studies, tumor cells stain positive for vimentin and keratin. Although synovial sarcomas bear a resemblance to normal synovium (hence their name), there is no proof that they originate from preformed synovium or result from tissue dedifferentiation. Because of the poor outcome associated with limited local resection, treatment usually consists of radical resection or amputation in addition to radiation and chemotherapy.

Surgical excision with wide tumor-free margins and postoperative local radiation therapy is the most common treatment for these tumors. Local recurrences are common despite definitive treatment. Distant metastases may occur. Five-year disease-free survival rates are between 35% and 40%.

REFERENCES

Enzinger FM, Weiss SW. Soft Tissue Tumors. St. Louis: Mosby, 1983.

Hudson TM. Radiologic-Pathologic Correlation of Musculoskeletal Lesions. Baltimore: Williams & Wilkins, 1987:605–664.

Madewell JE, Sweet DE. Tumors and tumor-like lesions in and about joints. *In*: Resnick D, Niwayama G (eds). Diagnosis of Bone and Joint Disorders (2nd ed). Philadelphia: Saunders, 1988:3889–3943.

Case 25

HISTORY

A 70-year-old female presented with fever, right lower abdominal pain, and a palpable right lower quadrant mass.

RADIOLOGY

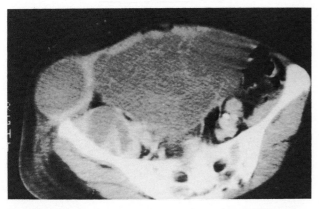

Figure 25-1. At the level of the pelvis, contrast-enhanced CT scans show a low attenuation mass containing thin, enhancing septations. The mass extends into the right iliacus muscle and through the right lateral abdominal wall.

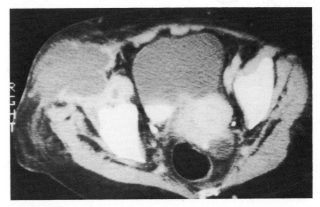

Figure 25-2. At a more caudal level, the mass shows peripheral enhancement and bulges through the right abdominal musculature into the subcutaneous fat.

DIFFERENTIAL DIAGNOSIS

The differential diagnosis includes mucinous adenocarcinoma of the colon, ovary, or appendix; abscess; and pancreatic pseudocyst.

PATHOLOGY

Multiple biopsy specimens were obtained during laparotomy from the sigmoid colon, bilateral ovaries, anterior abdominal wall, and omentum.

mucinous adenocarcinoma of colon
ovary or appendix
abscess
pancreatic pseudocyst.

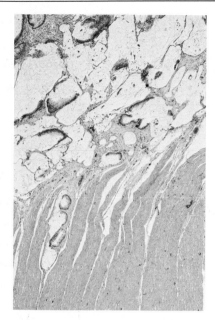

Figure 25-3. The tumor infiltrates the muscularis of the bowel wall.

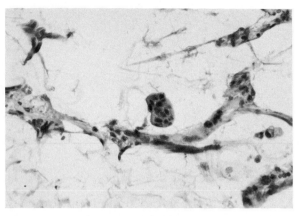

Figure 25-4. The tumor produces pools of mucin within which are small round clusters of malignant epithelial cells.

DIAGNOSIS

The final pathologic diagnosis was mucinous colonic adenocarcinoma.

assoc. with
pseudomyxoma
peritonei
villous adenoma

DISCUSSION

Colorectal carcinoma is a common disease and exceeds in number the combined total of neoplasms for the remainder of the alimentary tract. The peak age incidence is 60 to 70 years, and there is an equal sex distribution. Colon carcinoma is less prevalent in some countries, including Finland and Japan, which may be related to the low fat, high fiber diets prevalent in those countries. There is an increased risk of colon carcinoma in patients with a positive family history, ulcerative colitis, Gardner's syndrome, and familial polyposis.

increased risk
family hx
ulcerative colitis
Gardner's
familial polyposis

Adenocarcinomas are thought to arise from preexisting colonic polyps. The most common location of adenocarcinoma, the rectosigmoid colon, follows the distribution of these polyps. The size criteria for the "premalignant polyp" remain controversial, but polyps of less than 6 mm in diameter are typically benign. Polyps measuring 1 to 2 cm are malignant in 5% of cases, and lesions greater than 2 cm are malignant in 10% of patients. Villous polyps without pedunculation are more suspicious for malignancy. Typical presenting symptoms for distal lesions include rectal bleeding and obstruction. Proximal lesions tend to be more insidious, with presenting symptoms of weight loss and anemia.

benign
polyps
less 6 mm
1-2 - 5% malig
>2 - 10%

Mucinous adenocarcinoma represents approximately 15% of all colonic adenocarcinomas. This tumor is associated with villous adenoma and pseudomyxoma peritonei. Malignant peritoneal implants may generate a massive amount of mucinous ascites, which spreads throughout the peritoneal cavity, invades the omentum, and compresses the liver, spleen, and loops of bowel. The tumor may invade contiguous structures and infiltrate tissue planes. The prognosis for mucinous adenocarcinoma is relatively poor.

The malignant cells in mucinous adenocarcinoma contain the potential for secreting a gelatinous substance. If the tumor seeds the peritoneum, this gelatinous material spills into the peritoneal cavity and fills it. This condition is termed pseudomyxoma peritonei. CT attenuation of this material depends on the proportion of mucin and disseminated tumor cells that is present. Cellular pseudomyxoma peritonei demonstrates greater attenuation and, as in this case, more aggressive behavior, with invasion of mesenteric fat and development of an omental cake. Metastatic mucinous deposits often have linear and punctate calcifications on the peritoneal surface. Pseudomyxoma peritonei is more commonly due to mucinous cystadenocarcinoma of the ovary or appendix than to mucinous colon carcinoma. Although diffuse peritoneal spread is typical, extra-abdominal extension of mucinous adenocarcinoma, which has occurred in this case, is uncommon.

omental cake

Barium enema examination may be done using either a single or double contrast technique. The latter is superior in detecting smaller (1 cm or less) lesions and may be used as a screening study to detect polyps before carcinomatous change occurs. The CT appearances of benign and malignant low attenuation pseudomyxoma peritonei may be indistinguishable from each other. Diffusely disseminated mucinous material may be identical in density to ascites. Distinguishing features of pseudomyxoma peritonei include fixation and compression of bowel loops (ascites lets them float) and indentations of the hepatic or splenic margin. Contrast-enhanced CT scan, MR, and CT portography all detect liver metastases. Colonoscopy, which has become an increasingly common diagnostic modality, is more expensive, more likely to perforate the bowel, and less likely to visualize the ascending colon and cecum. However, colonoscopy remains vital in the biopsy of lesions and excision of polyps.

Figures 25–5 and 25–6 show images from the barium enema radiograph and CT scan of a 67-year-old patient with mucinous adenocarcinoma of the transverse colon and associated pseudomyxoma peritonei. In this case, the attenuation of the omental cake is greater than that in the previous case despite the abundance of mucin demonstrated by the histologic specimen (Fig. 25–7).

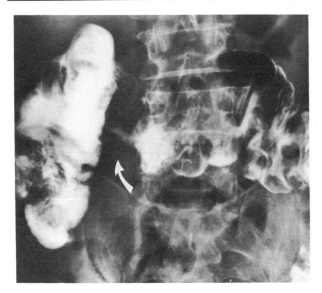

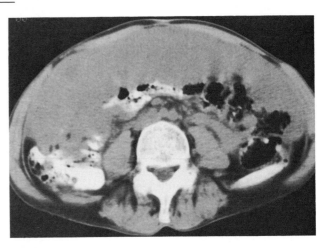

Figure 25-6. On CT scan a thick omental cake is seen to displace and compress the bowel posteriorly.

Figure 25-5. Barium enema demonstrates an apple-core lesion (arrow) involving the transverse colon.

Figure 25-8 shows an image from the CT scan of a third patient with pseudomyxoma peritonei and spread of tumor around the liver and spleen. The hepatic and splenic contours are deformed or scalloped by the pseudomyxomatous material, which shows relatively low attenuation. Decreased attenuation correlates with a greater proportion of mucin and relative hypocellularity. A scalloped hepatic contour is more frequently associated with pseudomyxoma peritonei due to benign causes including rupture of appendiceal mucocele or secretion by mucinous cystadenoma of the ovary or appendix.

Surgical resection remains the primary treatment for colorectal carcinoma in combination with hemicolectomy and low anterior or abdominoperineal resection, depending on the location and spread of the tumor. Radiation therapy is used postoperatively for transmural tumors or for palliation. Liver metastases may be treated by chemotherapy infused selectively by a hepatic arterial pump.

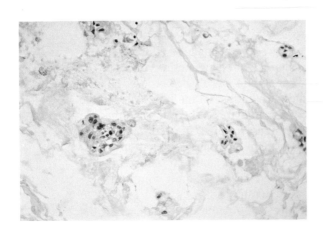

Figure 25-7. Small clusters of malignant epithelial cells are surrounded by abundant mucin.

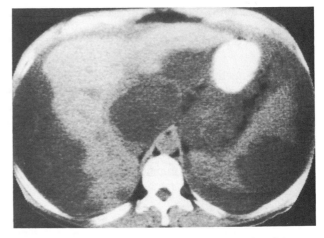

Figure 25-8. In another patient with pseudomyxoma peritonei, low attenuation material scallops the contour of the liver and spleen. This material displaces the porta hepatis and fills the lesser sac.

REFERENCES

Hulnick D, et al. Perforated colorectal neoplasms. Radiology 1987; 164:611.

Kelvin FM, et al. Colorectal carcinoma: a review. Radiology 1987; 164:1.

Case 26

HISTORY

A 6-month-old boy presented with a sudden increase in size of the right calf.

RADIOLOGY

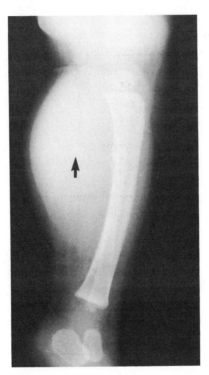

Figure 26-1. Lateral plain film shows soft tissue thickening of the calf, which contains a calcification (arrow).

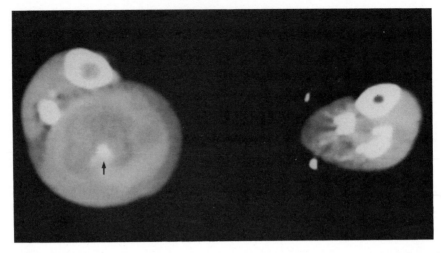

Figure 26-2. Contrast-enhanced CT scan demonstrates a heterogeneously enhancing mass that is located in the posterior compartment of the calf and contains a single calcific focus (arrow). The tibia and fibula are normal. The right calf is markedly enlarged compared with the left.

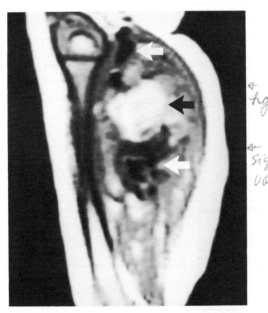

hgl

signal void

Figure 26-3. In the plane of the tibia, a sagittal T1-weighted (TR = 500, TE = 20) MR scan shows serpentine regions of signal void (white arrows) within the mass. A region of increased signal (black arrow) suggests a subacute hemorrhage.

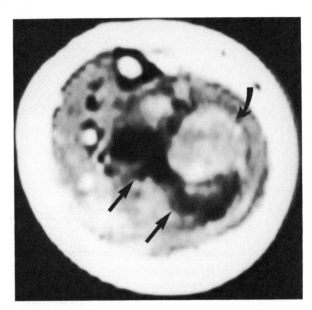

Figure 26-4. An axial T1-weighted (TR = 600, TE = 20) MR scan shows the tubular configuration (straight arrows) of the signal void as well as a high signal region (curved arrow) within the mass.

DIFFERENTIAL DIAGNOSIS

The differential diagnosis includes arteriovenous malformation, lymphangioma, and soft tissue sarcoma with hemorrhage.

PATHOLOGY

Percutaneous needle biopsy of the soft tissue mass was performed. The lesion was then resected.

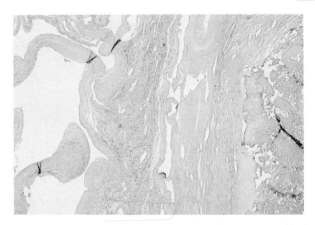

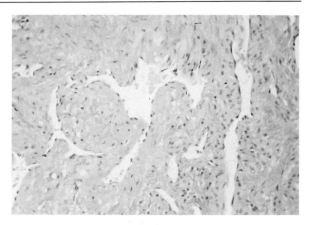

Figure 26-5. Large irregular vascular spaces surround a central region of calcification.

Figure 26-6. Vessels are lined by benign endothelial cells, and the walls contain smooth muscle cells.

DIAGNOSIS

The final pathologic diagnosis was arteriovenous malformation involving the calf.

DISCUSSION

Congenital arteriovenous malformation (AVM) is variable in presentation. Some lesions are obvious at birth because of their large size and the skin discoloration resulting from dilated tortuous subcutaneous vessels. Systemic hemodynamic effects are uncommon. Small lesions remain undetected until gradual growth causes a visible or palpable mass effect or spontaneous hemorrhage causes sudden growth and pain. Vascular lesions may be associated with a constellation of other findings and may lead to the diagnosis of Parker-Weber or Klippel-Trénaunay-Weber syndrome.

The terminology of vascular lesions reflects a spectrum of pathologic entities and includes simple and cavernous hemangiomas, angioma, angiolipoma, congenital AVM, and congenital arteriovenous fistula. In part, this complexity in terminology occurs because the majority of congenital AVMs comprise many tissue elements. Portions of the lesion may resemble cavernous hemangioma, whereas others show macroscopic communicating channels. The final pathologic diagnosis may be misleading if it reflects a sampling error.

Imaging modalities used to evaluate a possible AVM include CT, MR, angiography, and sonography with Doppler or color flow analysis. CT scan without contrast administration often shows fat within an AVM and the presence of punctate calcifications. The lesion may be entirely intramuscular with sharp margins, or it may infiltrate adjacent muscle groups and cross fascial planes in a manner similar to infection or inflammatory malignancy. During contrast administration, large vascular channels opacify densely, resembling normal vessels. Feeding arteries and draining veins may be dilated owing to rapid arteriovenous shunting.

MR imaging best demonstrates the margins of the lesion, the extent of infiltration, and the relationship to adjacent soft tissues. MR imaging may demonstrate concentric, peripheral, or central regions of decreased and increased signal intensity, indicating previous hemorrhage and blood products of differing ages. Spin-echo sequences and other "black-blood" techniques show a signal void in vessels with high flow and a variable signal in vessels with slower flow. Although MR angiography demonstrates feeding and draining vessels, the turbulent flow within the dilated vascular channels of the lesion itself results in signal loss.

Conventional angiography best shows the dynamic aspects of the AVM, the rate of opacification, the tortuous clustering of arterial branches, the premature filling of draining veins, and the degree of stasis within the AVM. Sonography shows clustered, serpentine, anechoic structures within the mass that produce Doppler signal and color enhancement, indicating turbulent blood flow.

The treatment is conservative because the lesion has a tendency to recur following surgical resection. Angiographic embolotherapy is an alternative therapy or may be used in conjunction with surgery.

REFERENCES

Widlus DM, et al. Congenital arteriovenous malformations: tailored embolotherapy. Radiology 1988; 169:511–516.

Cohen JM, Weinreb J, Redman HC. Arteriovenous malformation of the extremities: MR imaging. Radiology 1986; 158:475–479.

Musa AA, et al. Pelvic arteriovenous malformation diagnosed by color flow Doppler imaging. AJR 1989; 152:1311–1312.

Case 27

HISTORY

A 76-year-old white woman with a prior history of breast carcinoma and smoking was admitted with a stroke. She had had an intermittent history of hemoptysis for several months, and the admission chest radiograph was abnormal.

RADIOLOGY

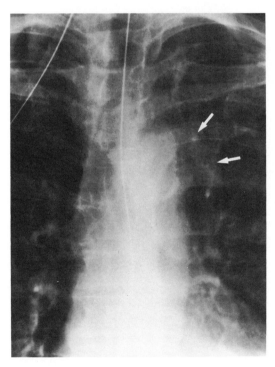

Figure 27-1. Chest radiograph demonstrates a 2- to 3-cm mass in the left suprahilar region (arrows). The mass is adjacent to the aortic arch and is not clearly separable from it on frontal or lateral views. No calcification is seen within the lesion; however, the aortic arch wall is calcified more proximally.

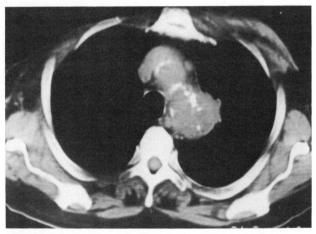

Figure 27-2. CT without contrast demonstrates that the lesion is inseparable from the arch and is noncalcified; the adjacent aortic wall is calcified, with a focal area of discontinuity in the calcified part near the mass.

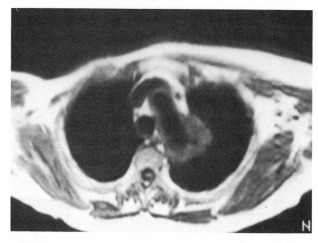

Figure 27–3. On T1-weighted MR images, a small area of signal void is seen within the mass at the boundary of the aorta; this suggests flow within the mass consistent with a pseudoaneurysm. Gradient echo images (not shown) were inconclusive for flow.

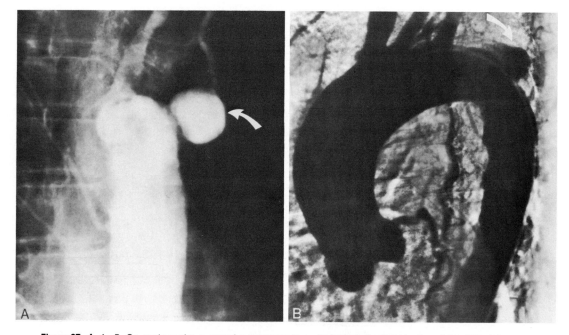

Figure 27–4. *A–B.* On angiography, a saccular aneurysm (arrow) of the aorta distal to the origin of the left subclavian artery is seen. Incidental note is made of a separate origin of the left vertebral artery from the aortic arch.

DIFFERENTIAL DIAGNOSIS

The differential diagnosis includes primary lung carcinoma, benign lung tumor, secondary lung lesion, cyst, focal lymphadenopathy (either inflammatory or neoplastic), focal pleural lesions including benign and malignant mesothelioma, an esophageal or tracheal lesion, and aneurysm of either the aorta or the pulmonary vessels.

PATHOLOGY

Repair of the thoracic aneurysm was performed, with excision of the aneurysmal sac and coverage with a Dacron graft.

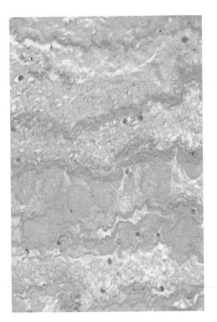

Figure 27–5. Tissue removed from the lesion shows alternating layers of red blood cells, platelets, and fibrin.

DIAGNOSIS

The final diagnosis was thoracic aortic aneurysm.

DISCUSSION

An aneurysm is a focal or diffuse dilation of an artery. Aneurysms may be classified as true aneurysms, with all three layers of the vessel wall intact; false aneurysms, with none of the three layers intact; or pseudoaneurysms, with one or two layers intact. Aneurysms may also be classified by appearance, with fusiform aneurysms involving the vessel wall circumferentially and saccular aneurysms involving a portion of the vessel wall. Generally, true aneurysms are fusiform aneurysms, and false aneurysms are saccular; however, the exceptions to this generality are too frequent for definitive application in individual cases.

Aortic aneurysms are less common in the thorax than in the abdomen. Most aneurysms are asymptomatic. Symptoms such as substernal or back pain, superior vena cava syndrome, dysphagia, dyspnea, stridor, or hoarseness usually indicate advanced disease. Arteriography remains the "gold standard" for evaluation of aneurysms; however, MR imaging may have a role in the evaluation of thoracic aneurysms.

Thoracic aortic aneurysms may be caused by or associated with many conditions, including atherosclerosis, syphilis, trauma, bacterial infection, arteritis, neoplasm, and connective tissue disorders, including Marfan's syndrome and Ehlers-Danlos syndrome. Atherosclerotic aneurysms are most common and tend to occur in the descending aorta. The majority are fusiform. Coarse calcifications are usually seen within the aneurysmal segment. Thoracic atherosclerotic aneurysms carry a worse prognosis than those in the abdomen, with a 5-year survival of less than 20% in one series. Increased size, patient age, and diastolic blood pressure are negative prognostic factors.

Syphilitic aneurysms occur in 10% to 15% of untreated syphilitics, are saccular in 75% of cases, and calcify in 15%. The calcifications are classically pencil-thin, and the aneurysm is most frequent in the ascending aorta and arch. Pulmonary arterial aneurysms may also occur.

Mycotic aneurysms were initially described by Osler in reference to aneurysms associated with bacterial endocarditis, but the term is now used to refer to any aneurysm associated with infection. Intravenous drug abuse has become a major etiologic factor. Most mycotic aneurysms are saccular. Mechanisms of seeding include septicemia with arterial wall abscess via the vasa vasorum, infection of an atheromatous plaque, trauma-induced infection (including iatrogenic infection), and contiguous infection. The proximal aorta is involved in the majority of cases. The infectious agent in mycotic aneurysms can be identified in only half the cases; when identified, *Staphylococcus*, *Streptococcus*, and *Salmonella* species are commonly involved.

Thoracic aneurysms of the aorta are treated by surgical excision and repair, additional therapy being guided by the etiology of the aneurysm.

REFERENCES

Bickerstaff LK, Pairolero PC, Hollier LH, et al. Thoracic aortic aneurysms: a population-based study. Surgery 1982; 92:1103–1108.

Dinsmore RE, Liberthson RR, Wismer GL, et al. MRI of thoracic aortic aneurysms. AJR 1986; 146:309–314.

Gonda RL, Gutierrez OH, Azodo MV. Mycotic aneurysms of the aorta: radiologic features. Radiology 1988; 168:343–346.

Johnsrude JS, Jackson DC, Dunnick NR. A Practical Approach to Angiography. Boston: Little, Brown, 1987:532–540.

Kadir S. Diagnostic Angiography. Philadelphia: Saunders, 1986:124–172.

Case 28

HISTORY

A 66-year-old male presented with bone pain, weight loss, fatigue, and headache.

RADIOLOGY

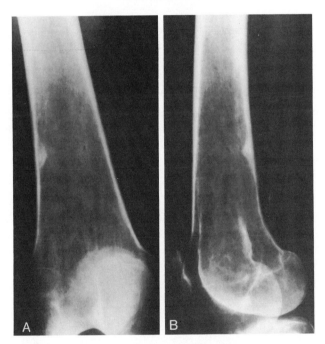

Figure 28-1. *A–B*. Plain films of the lower extremities reveal severe osteopenia, endosteal scalloping, and multiple ill-defined sclerotic areas in the distal femurs bilaterally.

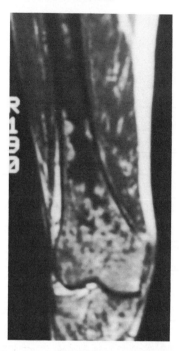

Figure 28-2. T1-weighted (TR = 700, TE = 20) images reveal large metadiaphyseal infarcts in the femur and diffusely heterogeneous marrow.

DIFFERENTIAL DIAGNOSIS

The differential diagnosis includes Gaucher's disease, hemoglobinopathies, Caisson's disease, steroids, collagen vascular disease, crystal deposition disease, radiation effect, and pancreatitis.

PATHOLOGY

A biopsy was performed. A tan-brown core of tissue was submitted for examination.

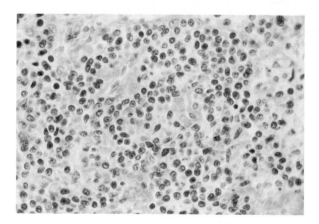

Figure 28-3. The bone marrow is approximately 95% cellular and is virtually completely replaced by a diffuse infiltrate of small lymphocytes. Scattered admixed plasmacytoid cells and plasma cells are identified. There are large aggregates of amorphous, eosinophilic material that are consistent with macroglobulin.

DIAGNOSIS

The final diagnosis was Waldenström's macroglobulinemia.

DISCUSSION

Waldenström's macroglobulinemia is a rare neoplastic disorder of the B cell lymphoid system, comprising approximately 5% of lymphoproliferative disorders. It is characterized by infiltration of the bone marrow, blood, and reticuloendothelial system by lymphocytes, plasma cells, and hybrid forms that produce a homogeneous IgM immunoglobulin that causes macroglobulinemia. Less commonly, these cells infiltrate other organs including the lungs, kidneys, central nervous system, gastrointestinal tract, and cardiovascular system.

Waldenström's macroglobulinemia typically occurs in the sixth or seventh decade of life. There is a slight male predominance. Presenting signs and symptoms result from organ infiltration as well as hyperviscosity caused by the large monoclonal IgM molecule, which has a propensity to polymerize. Hyperviscosity may cause headache, dizziness, sluggishness, visual impairment secondary to retinal venous stasis and hemorrhages, and excessive bleeding. (Inhibition of clotting factors and interference with platelet function also contribute to bleeding.) Hyperviscosity can lead to ischemia of any organ.

Marrow and reticuloendothelial infiltration lead to pancytopenia, bone pain, hepatosplenomegaly, and lymphadenopathy. Symptoms related to infiltration of other organs include dyspnea, cardiomegaly, steatorrhea, peripheral or central neuropathies, and renal failure.

Diagnosis is based on the typical bone marrow findings as well as an M protein spike on immunoelectrophoresis. Bence Jones proteinuria occurs in 20% to 30% of the cases. Associated amyloidosis is seen in 10%. An increased sedimentation rate, rouleaux formation, pancytopenia, hyperviscosity, and cryoglobulinemia are other frequent laboratory findings.

There is a spectrum of radiologic manifestations in the skeleton. These include generalized osteopenia and fractures, widening of the marrow spaces, endosteal erosion, osteolytic lesions, and osteonecrosis. Joint involvement is rare.

Radiologic evaluation of the abdomen reveals a homogeneously enlarged liver and spleen and thickening of small bowel folds with dilatation and a fine granular mucosa. Gastric involvement with multiple areas of deep ulceration has been reported. Chest films reveal a number of patterns including pleural effusions, diffuse small irregular opacities, solitary or multiple lung nodules, hilar node enlargement, and congestive heart failure. Intravenous pyelography may reveal poor renal function.

Treatment includes chemotherapy, plasmapheresis to correct hyperviscosity, and supportive therapy to control bleeding, infection, and pain. The average survival is 2 to 5 years.

REFERENCES

Carlson HC, Breen JF. Amyloidosis and plasma cell dyscrasias: gastrointestinal involvement. Semin Roentgenol 1986; 21:128–138.

Gross BH, et al. The respiratory tract in amyloidosis and the plasma cell dyscrasias. Semin Roentgenol 1986; 21:113–127.

Renner RR, et al. Roentgenologic manifestations of primary macroglobulinemia. AJR 1971; 113:499–508.

Resnick D. Plasma cell dyscrasias and dysgammaglobulinemias. In: Resnick D, Niwayama G (eds). Diagnosis of Bone and Joint Disorders (2nd ed). Philadelphia: Saunders, 1988:2358–2402.

Subbarao K, Jacobson HG. Amyloidosis and plasma cell dyscrasias of the musculoskeletal system. Semin Roentgenol 1986; 21:139–149.

Case 29

HISTORY

A 29-year-old woman presented with a 3-week history of ataxia, vertigo, and nausea.

RADIOLOGY

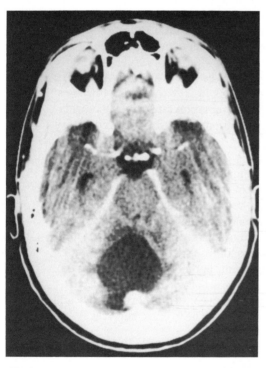

Figure 29-1. Contrast-enhanced CT scan shows a cystic mass in the posterior fossa with a densely enhancing mural nodule posteriorly.

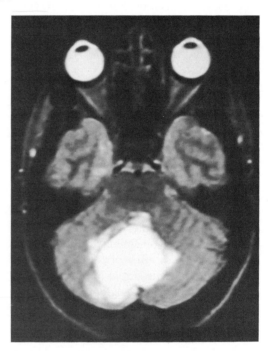

Figure 29-2. On the late echo T2-weighted MR image, both the cystic mass and mild adjacent edema are demonstrated.

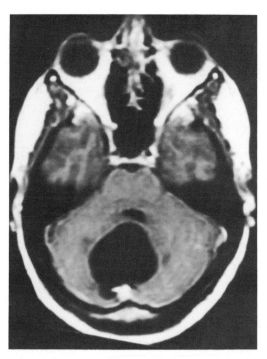

Figure 29-3. Postgadolinium T1-weighted axial image shows enhancement of the mural nodule. The cystic mass causes a mass effect upon the fourth ventricle.

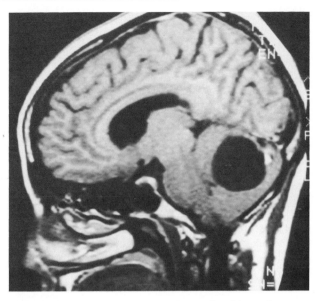

Figure 29-4. The relationship between the mural nodule, cystic mass, and surrounding mass effect is clearly demonstrated on the T1-weighted sagittal image.

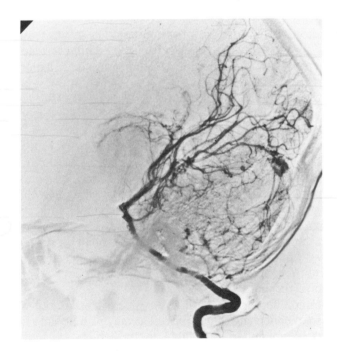

Figure 29-5. Subtraction lateral view from a left vertebral arteriogram shows hypervascularity of the posterior nodule.

PATHOLOGY

The lesion was resected.

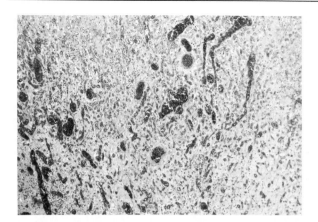

Figure 29-6. Microscopically the lesion contains numerous capillarylike blood vessels of various diameters.

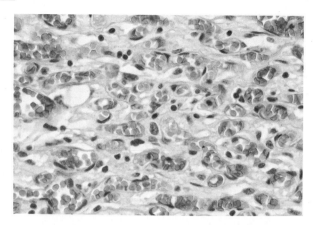

Figure 29-7. The blood vessels are filled with red blood cells and are separated by large polyhedral stromal cells that have prominent nuclei.

DIAGNOSIS

The final pathologic diagnosis was hemangioblastoma of the cerebellum.

Cyptic

most common 1° adult malignancy

DISCUSSION

Hemangioblastomas comprise 7% of all posterior fossa tumors and are the most common primary adult posterior fossa malignancy. The tumors generally occur in the cerebellum, most frequently within the paramedian hemispheric region, though they are also seen in the medulla oblongata, spinal cord, or, rarely, in the supratentorial region.

Grossly, hemangioblastoma is usually a well-demarcated cystic tumor with a small vascular mural nodule, but up to 40% of lesions are solid. Microscopically, the tumor nodule is composed of a fine mesh of capillaries along with polygonal benign-appearing stromal cells that may contain lipid or glycogen. This area can show microscopic invasion into the parenchyma, although the cyst wall is itself not neoplastic.

von Hippel-Lindau

Ten to thirty percent of patients with cerebellar hemangioblastoma meet criteria for von Hippel-Lindau syndrome, an autosomal dominant syndrome with incomplete penetrance associated with retinal angiomas, renal cell carcinoma, renal or pancreatic cysts, and pheochromocytomas. The peak incidence of tumor is during the fifth and sixth decades, although they appear earlier in von Hippel-Lindau syndrome. Ninety percent are solitary lesions. The tumors frequently appear with cerebellar signs or symptoms related to increased intracranial pressure. Some tumors produce erythropoietin and are associated with polycythemia.

The most common appearance on CT is a large cerebellar cyst with an enhancing mural nodule. A solid enhancing tumor mass that may or may not contain cysts is also seen. MR imaging is superior to CT within the posterior fossa and characteristically identifies the cyst if it is present (the cyst is usually slightly higher in signal than cerebrospinal fluid (CSF) on both T1- and T2-weighted images), an intensely enhancing mural nodule, and associated flow voids. Angiography demonstrates the nodule staining densely in a homogeneous or mottled pattern. Larger nodules may be associated with enlarged feeding arteries and arteriovenous shunting.

Successful resection of the tumor depends on complete excision of the vascular nodule. Angiography has traditionally been used to delineate the nodule, although a recent report suggests that MR may be more sensitive.

REFERENCES

Anson JA, Glick RP, Crowell RM. Use of gadolinium-enhanced magnetic resonance imaging in the diagnosis and management of posterior fossa hemangioblastomas. Surg Neurol 1991; 35(4): 300–304.

Burger PC, Scheithauer BW, Vogel FS. Surgical Pathology of the Nervous System and Its Coverings (3rd ed). New York: Churchill-Livingstone, 1991:373–386.

Lee SR, Sanches J, Mark AS, et al. Posterior fossa hemangioblastomas: MR imaging. Radiology 1989; 171:463–468.

Seeger JF, Burke DP, Knake JE, et al. Computed tomographic and angiographic evaluation of hemangioblastomas. Radiology 1981; 138:65–73.

Case 30

HISTORY

A 20-year-old female with a diagnosis of tuberous sclerosis was noted to have left flank pain and hematuria for 6 months.

RADIOLOGY

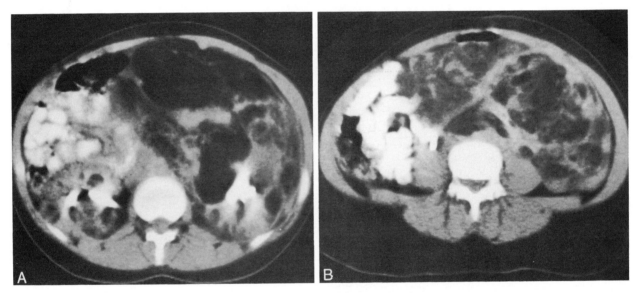

Figure 30-1. *A–B.* Two different levels from an enhanced abdominal CT scan demonstrate a 30-cm (cephalocaudal) by 20-cm (lateral) by 20-cm (anteroposterior) complex mass in the left kidney. The mass had areas of both very high and very low attenuation. The right kidney was 11 cm long and had several low attenuation areas also.

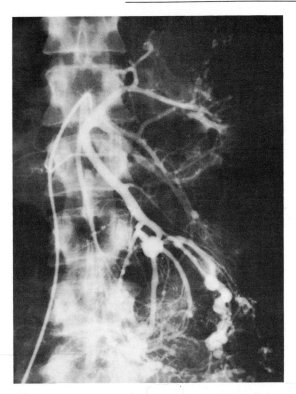

Figure 30-2. A renal angiogram shows marked enlargement of the left kidney with distorted vasculature and multiple areas of aneurysm formation. The left kidney was embolized with ethanol preoperatively.

DIFFERENTIAL DIAGNOSIS

The differential diagnosis includes angiomyolipoma, renal cell carcinoma, and liposarcoma.

PATHOLOGY

A total nephrectomy was performed.

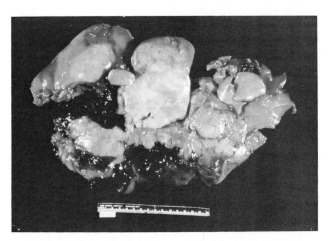

Figure 30-3. The bisected kidney is distorted by yellow-tan masses.

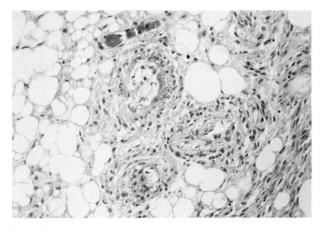

Figure 30-4. The masses are composed of a background of mature adipocytes with scattered blood vessels containing irregular coats of smooth muscle that focally form fascicles within the fat.

DIAGNOSIS

The final pathologic diagnosis was renal angiomyolipoma.

DISCUSSION

Angiomyolipomas are benign hamartomatous lesions containing varying amounts of fat, smooth muscle, and blood vessels. Histologically, these lesions are composed of normal tissues arranged in a disorganized fashion and are not true neoplasms. The lesions may arise de novo but are often seen in patients with tuberous sclerosis.

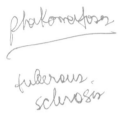

Tuberous sclerosis is one of the phakomatoses (neurocutaneous syndromes). It is characterized by autosomal dominant inheritance and clinically by seizures, mental retardation, and adenoma sebaceum of the skin. The pathogenesis of this syndrome is unknown; it is frequently associated with visceral lesions such as cardiac rhabdomyomas, renal angiomyolipoma, and pancreatic cysts. About 80% of patients with tuberous sclerosis have angiomyolipomas, which are often multiple and bilateral. The average age of onset of angiomyolipomas in these patients is 50 years, and females predominate 2:1. The lesions are typically asymptomatic unless hemorrhage occurs. More than 80% are bilateral.

Isolated angiomyolipomas arise in patients 40 to 60 years of age. There is a marked female predominance. Renal involvement is typically unilateral and solitary. Most of these lesions are symptomatic with mass effect, pain (often due to hemorrhage of necrosis), or hematuria. They may rarely rupture spontaneously into the retroperitoneum. More than half of tumors larger than 4 cm are associated with hemorrhage.

Plain films may show an area of lucency due to fat. There may also be displacement of the kidney, and 6% of lesions contain calcification. The intravenous pyelogram (IVP) may also demonstrate lucent areas, and there may be distortion of the collecting system. Ultrasound may show an echogenic mass owing to the predominant fat content. With CT, documentation of fat density can confirm the diagnosis. In the absence of fat, it may be hard to differentiate angiomyolipoma from renal cell carcinoma. On angiograms typical features are present in half the cases and include hypervascular masses with enlargement of the arteries feeding the tumor. Neovascularity and aneurysms may be seen.

Treatment for small (less than 4 cm) asymptomatic lesions is follow-up examinations. For larger, symptomatic lesions, partial nephrectomy is recommended. Complete nephrectomy may be required when the lesions are very large as in this case. Preoperative embolization is used to reduce bleeding.

REFERENCES

Arenson AM, Graham RT, Shaw P, et al. Angiomyolipoma of the kidney extending into the IVC. AJR 1988; 151:1159–1161.

Hansen GC, et al. CT diagnosis of renal angiomyolipomas. Radiology 1978; 128:789–791.

Case 31

HISTORY

A posterior mediastinal mass was discovered on a routine chest radiograph of an asymptomatic 56-year-old man.

RADIOLOGY

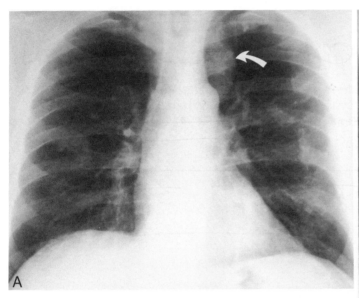

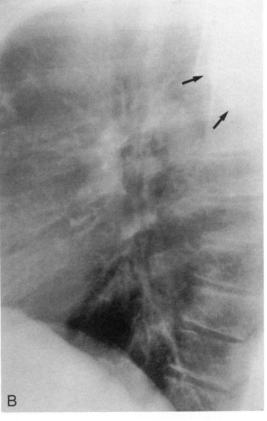

Figure 31-1. *A-B*. PA and lateral chest films demonstrate a left posterior mediastinal mass (arrows) at the T4-T5 level. There are scattered bilateral pleural abnormalities and calcified diaphragmatic pleural plaques.

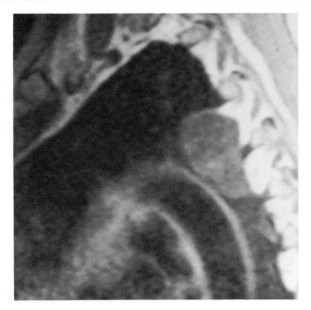

Figure 31-3. Axial T2-weighted MR scan shows that the signal of the lesion is brighter than that of CSF.

Figure 31-2. Sagittal T1-weighted MR scan shows that the paravertebral mass is lobulated. A tissue plane separates it from the proximal descending aorta. No foraminal enlargement is identified in the spine. The T1-weighted signal of the lesion is less than that of muscle.

DIFFERENTIAL DIAGNOSIS

The differential diagnosis includes neurogenic tumors, paraspinal abscess, aortic aneurysm, enteric and neurenteric cysts, lymphadenopathy, extramedullary hematopoiesis, lateral meningocele, and metastasis.

PATHOLOGY

The patient underwent excision of the mass through a left thoracotomy.

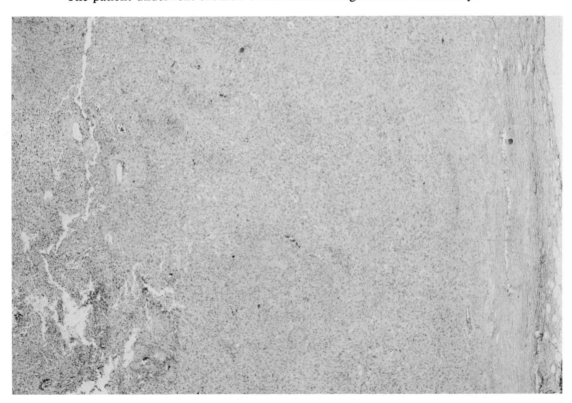

Figure 31-4. A 5- × 3- × 3-cm tan-pink rubbery nodule exuded a yellow serous fluid upon sectioning. At low power the tumor is seen to be encapsulated by a thin layer of fibrous tissue.

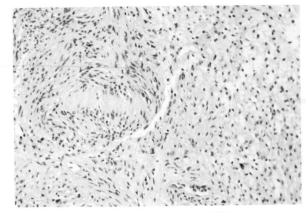

Figure 31–5. The neoplasm varies in cellularity with hypercellular portions (Antoni A) randomly distributed with the hypocellular regions (Antoni B). The tumor cells are relatively uniform in appearance and are cytologically benign.

handwritten margin notes:
neurogenic tumor
paraspinal abscess
aortic aneurysm
enteric + neurenteric cysts
lymphadenopathy
extramedullary hematopoisis
lateral meningocele
metastases

① Schwannomas
  neurilemoma
  neurofibromas
  axon, schwan & fibroblast
  malignant schwannoma
② neuroblastoma
③ paragangliomas
  (chemodectomas)

DIAGNOSIS

The final pathologic diagnosis was schwannoma.

DISCUSSION

Neurogenic posterior mediastinal tumors are of three types. Schwannomas (neurilemoma), neurofibromas, and malignant schwannomas (neurosarcoma, neurofibrosarcoma) have a neural sheath origin and constitute 31%, 10%, and less than 1% of thoracic neural tumors, respectively. Neuroblastoma, ganglioneuroblastoma, and ganglioneuroma have a sympathetic ganglia origin and constitute 14%, 14%, and 25% of thoracic neural tumors, respectively. The paragangliomas (chemodectomas) derive from the aorticopulmonary chemoreceptor bodies and aorticosympathetic paraganglia along the costovertebral sulcus and constitute 2% of the neural tumors of the thorax.

Schwannomas arise from the neural sheath Schwann cells of the cranial nerves (especially the eighth nerve), spinal nerve roots (ventral more often than dorsal), and peripheral nerves. They occur everywhere in the body and have a male to female ratio of 1:2. They account for one fourth of spinal tumors, where their location is usually intradural, but extramedullary. Schwannomas are usually asymptomatic, but large masses can cause neural compression. Spinal root tumors may extend through and enlarge the neural foramen, becoming dumbbell-shaped.

The typical schwannoma is a round mass composed histologically of both compact cellular regions (spindle cells arranged in palisades, Antoni A cells) and hypocellular regions with a watery matrix and microcystic spaces (Antoni B cells). They are hypervascular. The so-called ancient schwannoma is hypercellular, and shows nuclear atypia as well as cystic and degenerative changes, but, like all schwannomas, it is almost invariably benign. Many tumors, including bilateral acoustic neuromas, are associated with neurofibromatosis. Neurofibromas, in addition, contain all the elements of neural fibers including axons, Schwann cells, and fibroblasts.

handwritten margin notes: antoni A antoni B

The term malignant schwannoma is a misnomer because these tumors either derive from neurofibromas in patients with neurofibromatosis or arise de novo. On plain films of the chest schwannomas are discrete round masses and are rarely calcified. In contrast, the ganglion series of tumors are vertically elongated and not infrequently exhibit speckled calcification.

Mediastinal and retroperitoneal schwannomas may be quite large at the time of diagnosis because of a protracted asymptomatic period. Intercostal schwannomas may present as chest wall masses. Bone changes include enlargement of the neural foramen and erosion or sclerosis of the inferior surface of a rib or posterior aspect of a vertebral body (but not destruction).

On CT schwannomas are generally homogeneous round masses, although some may have cystic areas. Bone changes may also be evident. On MR imaging, their T1 characteristics are similar to those of muscle, but they are usually quite bright on T2-weighted images. Small intraspinal tumors may require gadolinium for detection; they enhance strongly.

Neuroblastomas usually present in infancy, ganglioneuroblastomas usually present in childhood, and ganglioneuromas usually present in late adolescence. Schwannomas have been reported from age 3 to 70 years, but most occur in the 20- to 40-year-old range. The average age of onset for a neurofibroma is 30 years. Excision is curative, and recurrence is uncommon.

REFERENCES

Harkin JC. Pathology of nerve sheath tumors. Ann NY Acad Sci 1986; 486:147–154.

Kumar AJ, Kuhajda FP, Martinez CR, et al. Computed tomography of extracranial nerve sheath tumors with pathological correlation. J Comput Assist Tomogr 1983; 7:857–865.

Reed JC, Hallet KK, Feigin DS. Neural tumors of the thorax: subject review from the AFIP. Radiology 1978; 126:9–17.

Rosai J (ed). Ackerman's Surgical Pathology (7th ed). St. Louis: Mosby, 1989:377–382, 1565–1573.

Schroth G, Thron A, Guhl L, et al. Magnetic resonance imaging of spinal meningiomas and neurinomas. Improvement of imaging by paramagnetic contrast enhancement. J Neurosurg 1987; 66: 695–700.

<h1 style="text-align:center">*Case* 32</h1>

HISTORY

A 22-year-old male presented with a recurrent mass in the sole of the right foot. Although he had been asymptomatic for approximately 15 years following a previous operation, he had noticed swelling and tenderness for several months. He was hyperphosphatemic, but serum calcium, alkaline phosphatase, and parathyroid hormone levels were normal, as was renal function.

RADIOLOGY

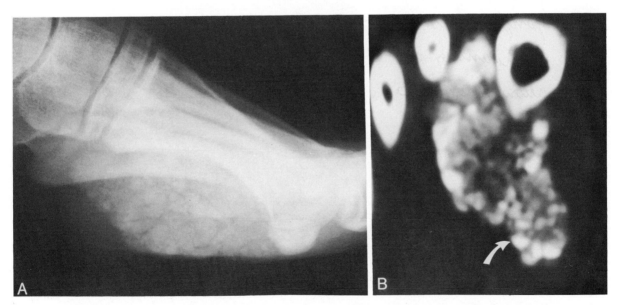

Figure 32–1. *A.* Plain film of the foot shows a 7-cm multilobular, calcified soft tissue mass on the plantar aspect of the forefoot. *B.* CT scan through the forefoot shows discrete rounded calcific foci ranging in size from 2 to 20 mm; some are homogeneous in attenuation and some have sedimentation levels. The adjacent bones are normal.

DIFFERENTIAL DIAGNOSIS

The differential diagnosis includes synovial osteochondromatosis, tumoral calcinosis, synovial cell sarcoma, and myositis ossificans.

PATHOLOGY

Local excision was performed. The lesion consisted of multiple calcific deposits surrounded by chronic foreign body reaction and fibrosis. The calcareous material had the consistency of toothpaste.

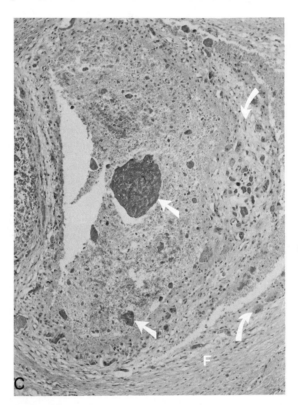

Figure 32–2. Low power photomicrograph shows calcified masses (straight arrows) with inflammatory giant cells (curved arrows) and a surrounding zone of fibrosis (F).

DIAGNOSIS

The final diagnosis was idiopathic tumoral calcinosis.

DISCUSSION

Idiopathic tumoral calcinosis is believed to result from a heritable error in phosphorus metabolism that leads to extracellular deposition of calcium hydroxyapatite crystals, most frequently in the form of periarticular soft tissue masses. Suspended calcium salts may layer out within cystic structures. The surrounding granulomatous foreign body response around the deposits results in a bright signal on T2-weighted MR images. Because the deposits are active metabolically, radionuclide bone scans are hot.

The condition is rare and appears to have autosomal dominant transmission and variable clinical expression. It is more common in blacks than other racial groups and has its most frequent age of presentation during childhood or adolescence. The lesions enlarge slowly, may attain large size, and may become symptomatic by virtue of local mechanical effects. If incompletely resected, they may recur. Other manifestations of tumoral calcinosis are elevated 1,25-dihydroxyvitamin D levels (not measured in this case), calcific myelitis, and dental abnormalities. Dietary restriction of phosphorus may be beneficial in some patients; surgical excision is reserved for symptomatic lesions. A radiologically indistinguishable condition of "secondary" tumoral calcinosis may be associated with disorders such as chronic renal failure or scleroderma.

Bone scan Hot

REFERENCES

Chew FS, Crenshaw WB. Idopathic tumoral calcinosis. AJR 1992; 158:330.

Martinez S, Vogler JB, Harrelson JM, et al. Imaging of tumoral calcinosis: new observations. Radiology 1990; 174:215–222.

Resnik CS. Radiologic vignette. Tumoral calcinosis. Arthritis Rheum 1989; 32:1484–1486.

Resnick D, Niwayama G. Soft tissues. *In*: Resnick D, Niwayama G (eds). Diagnosis of Bone and Joint Disorders (2nd ed). Philadelphia: Saunders, 1988:4242–4245.

Case 33

HISTORY

A 31-year-old female presented with chronic epigastric pain.

RADIOLOGY

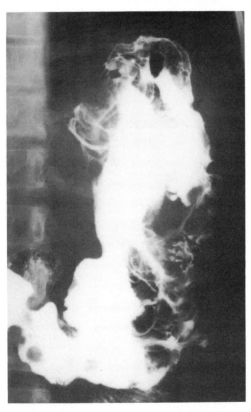

Figure 33-1. Gastrointestinal series shows thick, nodular, and tortuous rugae along the greater curvature of the stomach. The esophagus and small bowel are normal.

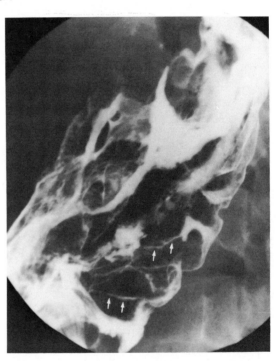

Figure 33-2. Spot image of the gastric fundus shows linear columns of barium (arrows) trapped between rugal folds.

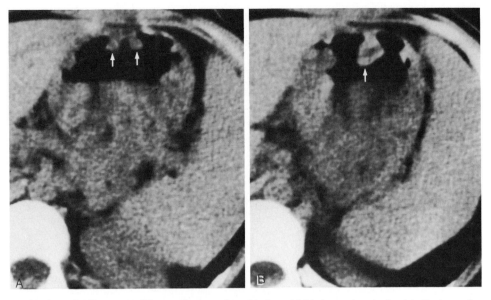

Figure 33-3. *A-B.* Noncontrast CT scan shows pedunculated rugal folds (arrows) projecting into the lumen from the anterior gastric wall, which otherwise is normal in thickness.

DIFFERENTIAL DIAGNOSIS

The differential diagnosis includes Zollinger-Ellison syndrome, eosinophilic gastritis, amyloidosis, lymphoma, infiltrative neoplasms that thicken gastric folds, and gastric varices.

PATHOLOGY

Gastrectomy was performed.

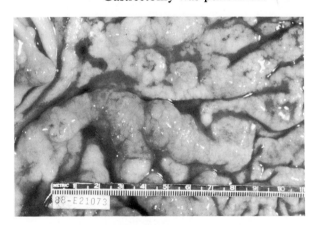

Figure 33-4. The resected stomach demonstrates enlarged cerebriform rugae measuring up to 1.5 cm in width.

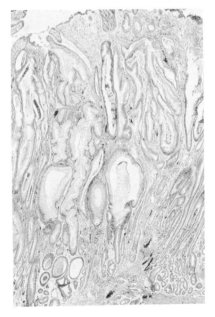

Figure 33-5. The gastric mucosa demonstrates marked hyperplasia of the gastric pits.

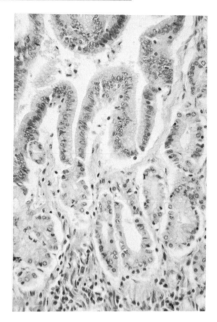

Figure 33-6. These hyperplastic gastric pits are lined by foveolar mucous cells and metaplastic epithelia.

DIAGNOSIS

The final pathologic diagnosis was Menetrier's disease.

DISCUSSION

Menetrier's disease is an uncommon idiopathic hypertrophic gastropathy characterized by hyperplasia of superficial mucosal epithelia. Hyposecretion of acid and hypersecretion of mucus can lead to excessive protein loss. Hypoalbuminemia, peripheral edema, and malnutrition complicate severe cases. Menetrier originally noted a relationship between large rugal folds, increased mucus production, and gastric cancer. Although the hyperplastic epithelia may undergo metaplastic and dysplastic changes, transformation to adenocarcinoma is uncommon. Patients present in middle age and complain of chronic, nonspecific signs and symptoms including weight loss, epigastric pain, vomiting, and gastrointestinal bleeding.

The radiographic hallmark is the presence of giant rugal folds. Normal rugae measure less than 5 mm in width and parallel the long axis of the stomach. In Menetrier's disease the rugal folds become thick, contorted, and tortuous. Gastric involvement is most prominent along the greater curvature. It usually is localized to the fundus and body but may be diffuse and include the antrum and cardia. During barium examination, enlarged, irregular folds simulate polypoid filling defects. Characteristically, barium becomes trapped in the crypts between the rugae and forms linear spicules perpendicular to the gastric contour. Hypoproteinemia may cause regular thickening of small bowel folds. On CT scan, rugal convolutions distort the mucosal surface and project into the stomach lumen. The serosal surface remains smooth, and the gastric wall, between rugae, is normal or mildly increased in thickness. Gastric varices usually involve the fundus and may simulate large rugae.

If pharmacologic therapy fails, total gastrectomy obviates the protein loss and eliminates the malignant potential.

REFERENCES

Palmer WE, Bloch SM, Chew FS. Menetrier's disease. AJR 1992; 158:62.

Sundt TM, Compton CC, Malt RA. Menetrier's disease, a trivalent gastropathy. Ann Surg 1988; 208(6):694–701.

Case 34

HISTORY

A 9-year-old girl presented with urinary tract infection.

RADIOLOGY

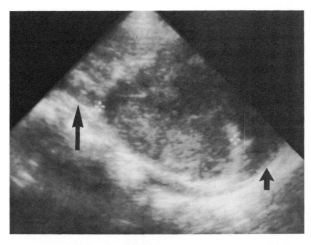

Figure 34-1. Sagittal sonography of the left kidney shows a solid upper pole mass (measuring markers). The normal midpole (long arrow) and spleen (short arrow) are identified.

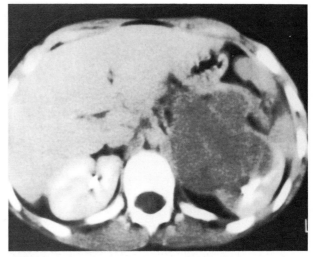

Figure 34-2. Contrast-enhanced CT scan of the abdomen demonstrates an exophytic low attenuation mass that is partially encircled by an enhancing rim. The residual renal parenchyma is displaced laterally against the abdominal wall. The left renal vein is not well visualized.

DIFFERENTIAL DIAGNOSIS

The differential diagnosis includes necrotic renal cell carcinoma, multilocular cystic nephroma, lymphoma, adrenal carcinoma, neuroblastoma, and abscess.

PATHOLOGY

Radical left nephrectomy was performed.

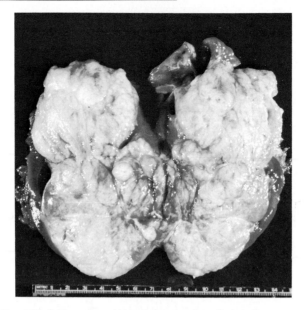

Figure 34-3. The removed kidney shows a deceptively well-circumscribed solid glistening tan-white mass.

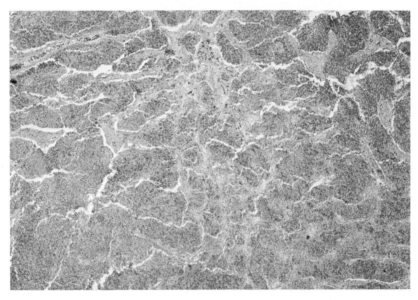

Figure 34-4. The mass is extremely cellular and is compartmentalized by fibrous septa.

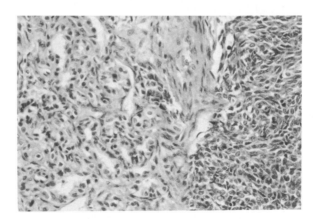

Figure 34-5. In some areas the tumor is composed of sheets of small spindle cells or blastema. In other regions, epithelial cells form tubules.

DIAGNOSIS

The final pathologic diagnosis was Wilms' tumor.

DISCUSSION

Wilms' tumor accounts for 20% of pediatric abdominal masses and is the most common primary renal tumor of childhood. The mean age of children with Wilms' tumor is 3.3 years.

Wilms' tumor affects the right and left kidneys with approximately equal frequency. No sex predilection is evident. The lesion is usually large (average diameter 11 cm) at the time of initial diagnosis. Because of its size, Wilms' tumor most often presents as a palpable abdominal mass. Less common presentations result from abdominal pain, fever, and microscopic or gross hematuria. The tumor is multifocal in 5% of cases and bilateral in 5% to 10%. Renal vein thrombosis or tumor extension into the renal vein occurs in 4% to 10% of patients. Metastases to perirenal, paracaval, and retrocrural lymph nodes are common. Distant metastases occur to the lung or, less often, to the liver.

The characteristic CT appearance of a Wilms' tumor is that of a large mass that is at least partially intrarenal and of lower density than the surrounding renal parenchyma. Extrarenal Wilms' tumor is rare. With the administration of intravenous contrast material, an enhancing pseudocapsule is frequently present. The preserved renal parenchyma is compressed into an enhancing "crescent," which surrounds the tumor in approximately 50% of cases. Calcifications are demonstrated by CT in only 16% of Wilms' tumors as opposed to neuroblastoma, in which 85% of the tumors contain calcifications. Extension of the tumor into the renal vein or inferior vena cava may be shown by CT. In addition, CT is useful in establishing the presence of metastatic disease to local lymph nodes or metastases to the liver or lung.

The prognosis for Wilms' tumor depends on the stage of the tumor at diagnosis. Stage I disease is confined to the kidney and has a 2-year survival of 95%. Extension of the tumor into the perinephric space defines stage II disease, which has a 2-year survival rate of 90%. Stage III disease is defined as involvement of local lymph nodes and stage IV disease as extension of the tumor into the renal vein or the presence of distant metastases. Stage III and IV disease have a 54% 2-year survival rate.

The treatment of Wilms' tumor is radical nephrectomy. Exploration of the inferior vena cava may be necessary to exclude vascular extension and remove tumor thrombus. Adjuvant chemotherapy is given to patients with all stages of disease. Local radiation therapy may be used.

REFERENCES

Fishman E, et al. The CT appearance of Wilms' tumor. J Comput Assist Tomogr 1983; 7:659–665.

Peretz G, Lam A. Distinguishing neuroblastoma from Wilms' tumor by computed tomography. J Comput Assist Tomogr 1985; 9:889–893.

Reiman T, et al. Wilms' tumor in children: abdominal CT and ultrasound evaluation. Radiology 1986; 160:101–105.

Case 35

HISTORY

A 29-year-old male presented with fever, weight loss, and increasing pain and swelling of the right foot.

RADIOLOGY

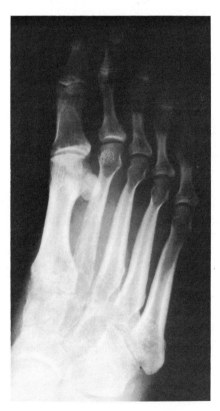

Figure 35-1. An oblique view of the right foot demonstrates permeated destruction involving the proximal two-thirds of the shaft of the second metatarsal and the second cuneiform bone. There is patchy resorption of the other cuneiform bones and probably the base of the third metatarsal as well as the tarsal navicular bone.

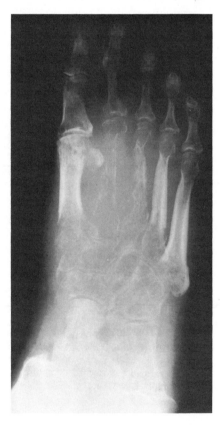

Figure 35-2. An oblique radiograph obtained three months later shows progressive destruction of the tarsus and metatarsals.

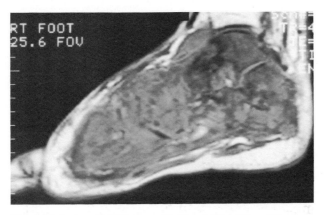

Figure 35-3. A sagittal MR scan with T1 weighting (TR = 445, TE = 20) demonstrates a huge soft tissue mass replacing all of the visualized bones of the mid and hind foot. The distal tibia appears normal.

DIFFERENTIAL DIAGNOSIS

The differential diagnosis includes primary bone sarcoma (Ewing's sarcoma, osteosarcoma), soft tissue sarcoma (rhabdomyosarcoma), metastasis, lymphoma, osteomyelitis, and Madura foot.

PATHOLOGY

A biopsy was performed.

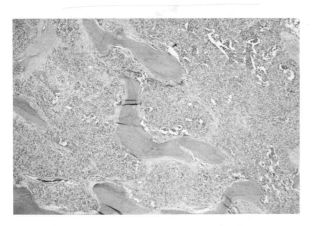

Figure 35-4. The biopsy specimen shows a very cellular neoplasm infiltrating throughout the marrow cavity.

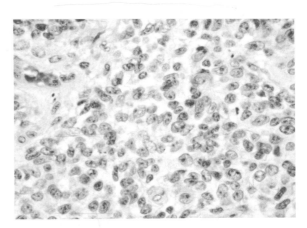

Figure 35-5. The tumor is composed of relatively small round cells that have small nucleoli and inconspicuous cytoplasm.

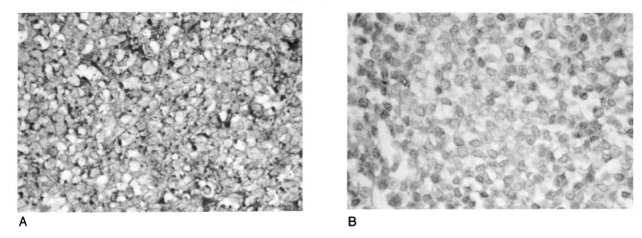

A   B

Figure 35-6. *A.* Special histochemical stains show PAS-positive magenta red granules in the cytoplasm. *B.* The tumor cells are digested by diastase. This finding confirms the presence of glycogen within the cytoplasm of the tumor cells.

DIAGNOSIS

The final pathologic diagnosis was Ewing's sarcoma.

DISCUSSION

This malignant, relatively common tumor was first described in detail by Ewing in 1921. Although the cell of origin remains unknown, Ewing's sarcoma probably is derived from either reticuloendothelial or undifferentiated mesenchymal cells of the bone marrow. Ninety percent of patients are between 5 and 30 years old at clinical presentation, and most are between 10 and 15 years old. Ewing's sarcoma also occurs rarely in infants and older patients. Males are affected more commonly than females (3:2) and whites far more commonly than blacks. Presenting complaints may simulate those of infection: fever, weight loss, anemia, leukocytosis with elevated erythrocyte sedimentation rate (ESR), and localized pain and swelling. Fifteen to thirty percent of patients have metastases at clinical presentation.

Ewing's sarcoma may develop in practically any bone, although in the majority of cases the sacrum, innominate bone, or long bones of the lower extremities are involved. Only 3% of tumors affect the hands and feet. Tumors involve the feet four times more frequently than the hands and originate in the long bones (metatarsals, phalanges) more frequently than in the tarsal bones. As in the larger tubular bones (femur, tibia, and humerus), the tumor tends to begin in a metadiaphyseal location; the classic "pure" diaphyseal location is seen in only 20% to 30% of cases. Isolated involvement of the metaphysis is uncommon, and involvement of the epiphysis is rare.

The radiographic findings of the metatarsals in Ewing's sarcoma simulate those of the larger tubular bones. These findings include poorly marginated osteolysis, cortical erosion with a permeated or "moth-eaten" appearance, periosteal reaction (laminated or sunburst pattern), and extraosseous soft tissue mass (present in 80% to 100% of patients and often far more extensive than suspected from plain films). Osteosclerosis can resemble that seen in osteosarcoma. It occurs in 10% to 40% of patients, usually in lesions of flat bones, and results from reactive bone formation and osteoid deposition around foci of necrotic bone. Pathologic fractures may be seen in a small percentage of cases. Bone scintigraphy demonstrates increased uptake by the tumor and by its bony metastases. CT and MR scanning define the extraosseous and intramedullary components of the tumor and are useful in defining radiation portals and in following response to radiation therapy and chemotherapy. On angiography, the tumor varies in vascularity but usually demonstrates at least a faint stain.

Pathologically, the diagnosis of Ewing's sarcoma is one of exclusion. The tumor cannot produce osteoid or chondroid matrix. The cells are mostly small, round, solidly packed, uniform, and undifferentiated with little cytoplasm. Their borders are indistinct.

Histologic characteristics may be nonspecific. They can be difficult to differentiate from other small cell tumors such as neuroblastoma, lymphoma, and metastatic small cell carcinoma of the lung.

Ewing's sarcoma is highly radiosensitive. Radiation and chemotherapy may be used alone or in combination with surgical excision. Considerable regression and even complete remission of the lesion may result. However, locally recurrent tumor is common, occurring in 12% to 25% of patients. Soft tissue extension is associated with increased risk of distant metastases as well as local failure. Five-year survival for patients with nonmetastatic tumor with bone-confined disease is 87% compared to 20% for those with extraosseous extension. Patients who survive for several years may eventually develop secondary radiation-induced osteosarcoma.

REFERENCES

Boyko OB, et al. MRI of osteosarcoma and Ewing's sarcoma. AJR 1987; 148:317–322.

Dahlin DC. Bone Tumors. Springfield, IL: Thomas, 1981:274–287.

Madewell JE, Sweet DE. Tumors and tumor-like lesions in and about joints. *In*: Resnick D, Niwayama G (eds). Diagnosis of Bone and Joint Disorders (2nd ed). Philadelphia: Saunders, 1988:3847–3855.

Suit HD, Mankin HJ, Kaufman SD. Sarcomas of bones and soft tissues. *In*: American Cancer Society. Cancer Manual. 1986:278–291.

Wilner D. Radiology of Bone Tumors and Allied Disorders. Philadelphia: Saunders, 1982.

Case 36

HISTORY

A 15-year-old female presented with headaches and speech difficulties.

RADIOLOGY

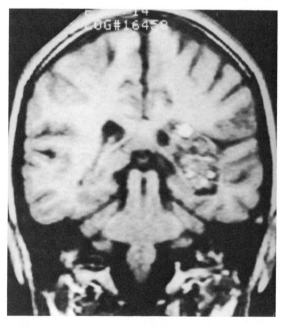 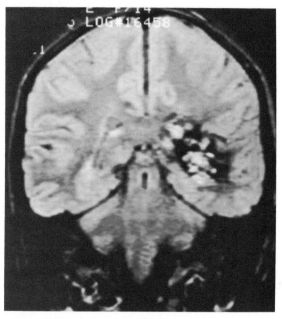

Figure 36-1. Coronal T1-weighted MR image without gadolinium shows a 3- × 2-cm heterogeneous mass. The mass is located in the left temporal lobe and exerts a minimal mass effect upon the left lateral ventricle.

Figure 36-2. Proton density coronal MR image demonstrates increased heterogeneity of the mass and enlargement of the central and peripheral low signal foci. No significant surrounding edema is present.

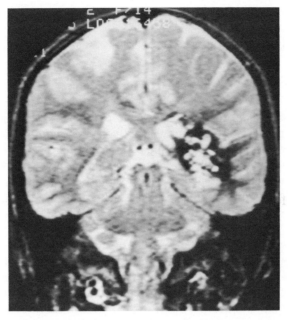

late echo T₂W presence of blood products

Figure 36–3. Progressive loss of signal on the late echo T2-weighted image suggests susceptibility effect and the presence of blood products.

DIFFERENTIAL DIAGNOSIS

The differential diagnosis includes vascular malformations, including cavernous angiomas, telangiectasias, venous angiomas, and arteriovenous malformations, metastases, and primary CNS neoplasms such as gliomas with subacute hemorrhage.

PATHOLOGY

A 2.5- × 3.0- × 1.3-cm mass was resected.

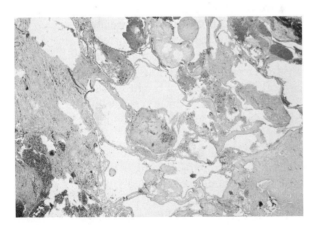

Figure 36–4. The lesion contains large round vascular spaces, some of which are filled with blood.

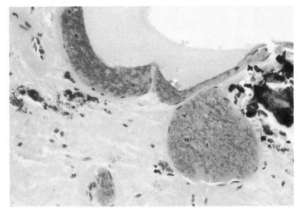

Figure 36–5. The vessels are lined by bland endothelial cells, and the intervening connective tissue contains both hemosiderin deposits and dystrophic calcification.

DIAGNOSIS

The final pathologic diagnosis was cavernous angioma.

DISCUSSION

Cerebral vascular malformations have been pathologically classified into five types: (1) arteriovenous malformations, representing abnormal communications between arteries and veins bypassing smaller conduits; (2) telangiectasias (or capillary angiomas), which are collections of thin-walled capillaries with interposed parenchyma; (3) cavernous angiomas, in which the vascular spaces are sinusoidal in appearance and lined by a single endothelial layer without intervening parenchyma; (4) venous angiomas, clusters of dilated medullary veins draining into an enlarged vein; and (5) varices, a single or small number of dilated veins with thin walls and a tortuous course.

Cavernous angiomas were diagnosed infrequently before the era of CT, but now they are an increasingly recognized CNS lesion. They represent 5% to 20% of CNS vascular malformations and most frequently occur in the third and fourth decades of life. Men and women are equally affected. Familial occurrence is rare. The lesions are usually solitary and occur with equal frequency on the right and left sides. Approximately 75% of cavernous angiomas are supratentorial and 25% are infratentorial. Supratentorial lesions often occur in the Rolandic cortex and basal ganglia, whereas in the infratentorial space the pons and cerebellar hemispheres are favored sites. Approximately 17% of lesions in one large series were intraventricular, most occurring within the third ventricle.

Once considered rare in the pediatric population, cavernous hemangiomas are being diagnosed with greater frequency because of the availability of CT. The age distribution in children is bimodal with peaks between birth and 2 years and between 13 and 16 years. The most frequent presenting symptoms are seizures, intracranial hemorrhage, signs of increased intracranial pressure, and focal neurologic deficits. The risk of hemorrhage is thought to be particularly high in neonates.

Calcification is apparent in the great majority of lesions on noncontrast CT. The lesions are usually well circumscribed and hyperdense with mild mass effect. Perilesional edema is rare. With contrast administration, there is minimal to mild enhancement.

On both T1- and T2-weighted MR sequences the lesion generally has a central area of heterogeneous bright and dark signal intensity surrounded by a peripheral region of low or absent signal. This signal-poor periphery is more prominent on T2-weighted sequences and on gradient-echo acquisitions. Pathologic investigation has correlated these areas of susceptibility effect with the presence of hemosiderin-laden macrophages immediately surrounding the angioma. Presumably these result from previous episodes of low-grade hemorrhage, which are frequently subclinical. Central areas of bright signal on both T1- and T2-weighted sequences correspond to subacute hemorrhage (extracellular methemoglobin). A surrounding bright signal due to edema is characteristically absent unless recent hemorrhage has occurred.

Angiographically, the lesions are classically manifest as avascular masses. Angiographic signs of dense venous pooling and a persistent area of capillary staining in the late venous phase are nonspecific and infrequent. Normal angiograms are seen in about one third of patients.

Surgical resection is the treatment of choice, with indications including hemorrhage, seizures, increasing size, mass effect, or elevated intracranial pressure. At surgery, severe bleeding is rarely encountered. With complete resection, 60% to 65% of patients experience complete improvement in symptoms, and the remainder have at least partial improvement. Operative mortality is less than 5%, and the lesions do not recur after total resection.

REFERENCES

Farmer JP, Cosgrove GR, Villemure J, et al. Intracerebral cavernous angiomas. Neurology 1988; 38:1699–1704.

Fortuna A, Ferrante L, Mastronardi L, et al. Cerebral cavernous angioma in children. Childs Nerv Syst 1989; 5:201–207.

Herter T, Brandt M, Szuwart U. Cavernous hemangiomas in children. Childs Nerv Syst 1988; 4:123–127.

McCormick WF. The pathology of vascular ("arteriovenous") malformations. J Neurosurg 1966; 24:807–816.

New PF, Ojemann RG, Davis KR, et al. MR and CT of occult vascular malformations of the brain. AJR 1986; 147:985–993.

Rigamonti D, Drayer BP, Johnson PC, et al. The MRI appearance of cavernous malformations (angiomas). J Neurosurg 1987; 67:518–524.

Yamasaki T, Handa H, Yamashita J, et al. Intracranial and orbital cavernous angiomas. A review of 30 cases. J Neurosurg 1989; 64:197–208.

Case 37

HISTORY

A 71-year-old female was referred for pelvic ultrasound to evaluate uterine fibroids.

RADIOLOGY

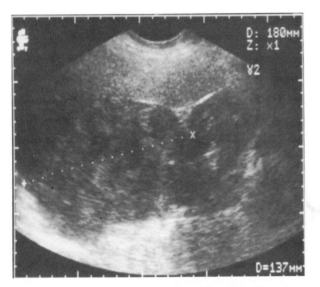

Figure 37-1. Echogenic heterogeneous mass measuring 14 cm in diameter is located between the liver and kidney.

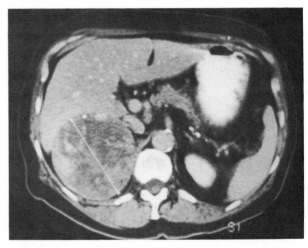

Figure 37-2. On CT scan without contrast, the lesion is smoothly marginated and separate from the liver and contains both calcification and low attenuation areas suggestive of necrosis.

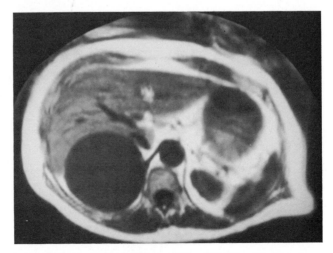

Figure 37-3. T1-weighted MR image (TR = 275, TE = 14) shows low signal intensity throughout the lesion.

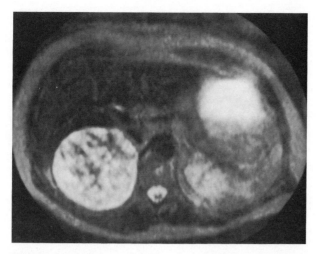

Figure 37-4. T2-weighted MR image (TR = 2360, TE = 180). Dark central signal suggests paramagnetic affect, possibly from old hemorrhage.

DIFFERENTIAL DIAGNOSIS

The differential diagnosis includes adrenocortical tumor (benign or malignant), pheochromocytoma (nonfunctioning), complex adrenal cyst (congenital or infectious), metastasis, and unilateral adrenal hemorrhage.

PATHOLOGY

Adrenalectomy was performed.

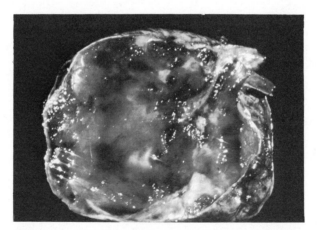

Figure 37-5. The adrenal gland is massively enlarged by a central hemorrhagic blood-stained pale tan mass that attenuates the overlying adrenal cortex.

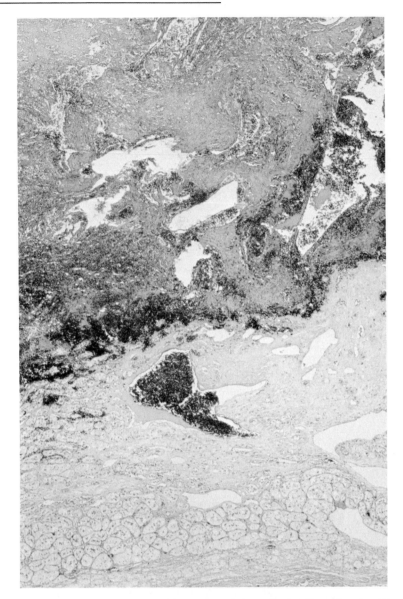

Figure 37-6. Microscopically at low power the mass is extremely hemorrhagic with small nests of identifiable tumor cells.

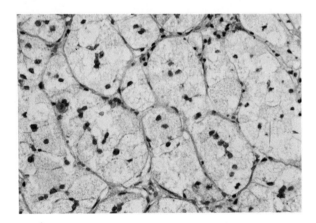

Figure 37-7. The tumor cells grow in ovoid and round clusters and have prominent vacuolated cytoplasm.

DIAGNOSIS

The final pathologic diagnosis was adrenal cortical tumor.

DISCUSSION

The normal adrenal gland possesses an outer cortex and a central medulla. The cortex has an outer zona glomerulosa, a middle zona fasciculata, and an inner zona reticularis that produce, respectively, mineralocorticoids, glucocorticoids, and sex hormones. The pheochromocytes of the medulla produce epinephrine, norepinephrine, and their metabolites. Each gland is supplied by three separate arteries arising from the aorta and the inferior phrenic and renal arteries, and each is drained by a single vein that empties into the vena cava on the right and the renal vein on the left.

Adrenal tumors may arise from both the cortex and the medulla. Functioning cortical tumors may result in hormonal overproduction syndromes: Cushing's syndrome (most common), Conn's syndrome, and adrenogenital (virilization/feminization) syndrome. Seventy-five percent of functioning tumors are benign adenomas. Nonfunctioning tumors may be incidental findings or may produce pain and symptoms owing to their mass. Regardless of whether the cortical tumor is functioning or nonfunctioning, radiologic and histologic differentiation between benign adenoma and malignant carcinoma can be difficult. Bulky tumors with distant metastases, venous invasion, bizarre nuclei, and multiple mitoses are obviously malignant. However, many carcinomas appear contained at presentation and demonstrate minimal pleomorphism and rare (or absent) mitoses.

A normal adrenal gland weighs about 4 gm; adrenal carcinomas weigh up to 4500 gm. The smallest cancer in one series weighed 33 gm. Benign adenomas can reach a size comparable to all but the largest carcinomas. Most authors agree that a patient with a tumor exceeding 100 gm (generally corresponding to a size greater than 6 cm), even with "benign" histology, should have a guarded prognosis. The most common sites of metastasis include the liver, regional lymph nodes, lungs, and peritoneal/pleural surfaces. Direct invasion of vessels and surrounding tissues, especially the kidney, also occurs.

Radiographically, CT scanning can be used to visualize both adrenal glands in more than 95% of patients. The most significant discriminators between benign and malignant adrenocortical tumors are size greater than 6.0 cm, contrast enhancement, and central hemorrhagic necrosis (these criteria do not exclude large metastases or pheochromocytomas). Contour (ie, smooth and sharply marginated as opposed to lobulated or poorly defined) and the presence of calcification are relatively inconclusive criteria. Although the success of ultrasonography in detecting smaller lesions depends on the expertise of the operator, this technique can compete in accuracy with CT only in fetuses, infants, and adults with minimal intra-abdominal fat. The major role of MR lies in its ability to differentiate larger adrenal masses from the adjacent liver and kidney by the use of multiplanar imaging. Angiography can demonstrate small adenomas (less than 1.0 cm) and can localize the side of a nonvisualized tumor by venous sampling.

Neoplasms of the adrenal medulla include tumors of chromaffin cells, pheochromocytoma (functioning or nonfunctioning, benign or malignant) and those of nonchromaffin cells, neuroblastoma, ganglioneuroblastoma, and ganglioneuroma. Myelolipoma (consisting of a mixture of fat and bone marrow elements) and mesenchymal tumors are rare. Cysts, the most common nonfunctioning adrenal mass, may be classified as congenital, infectious (echinococcal), epithelial (due to cystic degeneration of a tumor), endothelial (due to lymphangioma or hemangioma), or pseudocystic (due to organized hematoma). An inflammatory mass due to tuberculosis and histoplasmosis rarely occurs. The most common metastases to the adrenal originate from melanoma and carcinomas of the breast and lung, followed by carcinomas of the stomach, kidney, pancreas, and colon.

Because of the difficulty of discriminating between benign and malignant tumors by radiographic criteria and needle biopsy, the majority of primary adrenal neoplasms require surgical excision. The widespread use of CT has resulted in the detection of many incidental adrenal masses, resulting in the problem of how to handle these "incidentalomas." Because a carcinoma of the adrenal is unlikely to be less than 3.0 cm in size, follow-up study is usually recommended unless there is adrenal hyperfunction or a known malignancy, in which case excision or percutaneous needle biopsy is necessary.

REFERENCES

Athani VS, Mulholland SC. Primary non-functioning adrenal tumors in adults. Urology 1981; 28: 131–133.

Hussain S, et al.: Differentiation of malignant from benign adrenal masses: predictive indices based on CT. AJR 1985; 144:61–65.

Kolmannskog F, et al. CT and angiography in adrenocortical carcinoma. Acta Radiol 1992; 33:45.

Mitnick JS, et al. Non-functioning adrenal adenomas discovered incidentally on CT. Radiology 1983; 148:495–499.

Older RA, et al. Diagnosis of adrenal disorders. Radiol Clin North Am 1984; 22:433–455.

Case 38

HISTORY

A 24-year-old female presented with a chest wall mass.

RADIOLOGY

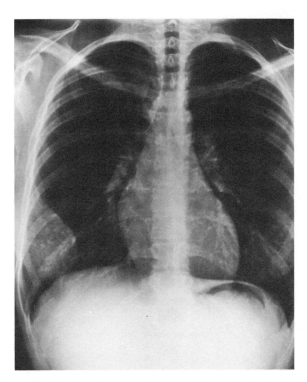

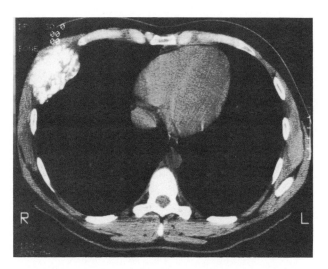

Figure 38-2. Chest CT scan demonstrates a densely calcified soft tissue mass in the right chest wall. Local rib destruction is present but no other bony abnormalities are seen. There is no parenchymal abnormality or adenopathy.

Figure 38-1. Radiograph demonstrates a well-demarcated extrapleural mass in the right chest wall associated with destruction of the right sixth posterior rib. Calcification is present within the mass; however, a specific tumor matrix cannot be identified.

DIFFERENTIAL DIAGNOSIS

The differential diagnosis includes osteosarcoma, chondrosarcoma, tumoral calcinosis, and calcium hydroxyapatite deposition and dystrophic calcified mass secondary to neoplasm, inflammation, or trauma.

PATHOLOGY

The lesion, including three rib segments, was resected.

145

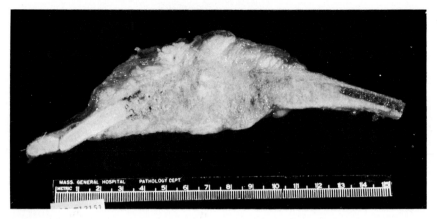

Figure 38-3. Portions of the involved rib including the costal cartilage are replaced by a large destructive tan-white mass.

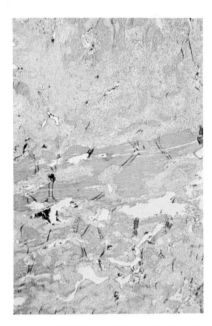

Figure 38-4. The tumor fills the medullary cavity and permeates the cortex.

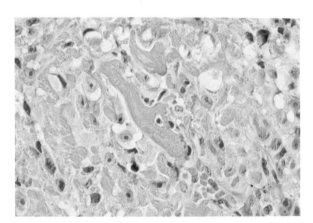

Figure 38-5. The tumor is composed of cytologically malignant ovoid cells that contain prominent nucleoli and are adjacent to neoplastic bony matrix.

DIAGNOSIS

The final pathologic diagnosis was osteosarcoma.

DISCUSSION

Chest wall lesions are uncommon. The age of the patient and the location of the tumor are important factors in determining whether a tumor is benign or malignant. Primary malignant neoplasms are significantly more common than are benign ones, and both occur twice as frequently in males as in females. Primary rib tumors more frequently arise from the anterior portion of the rib, near the costochondral junction.

Metastatic lesions are the most common malignant chest wall lesion. Generally, the margins of malignant tumors are not clearly defined. The cortex is frequently disrupted, and a soft tissue mass is common. Eighty-five percent of malignant rib tumors are symptomatic at the time of diagnosis. In children metastatic neuroblastoma is common; in males lung, kidney, and prostate tumors are common; and in females metastatic breast cancer is the most common source.

Among the primary malignant rib tumors, chondrosarcomas followed by myelomas are the most common. Chondrosarcomas typically are seen in the fourth to fifth decades of life, appearing as a large mass with rib destruction and characteristic cartilaginous calcification. Myeloma presents in patients between 50 and 70 years old, typically with painful osteolytic rib lesions.

Osteosarcomas are second only to plasma cell myeloma in frequency as a primary bone tumor. They are typically found in the second to third decades; however, they are seen in people of all ages. Males are affected more than females in a ratio of approximately 2:1. Symptoms include pain, swelling, decreased range of motion, and warmth. The skeletal location of osteosarcomas is predominantly the tubular bones of the appendicular skeleton (80%), with 50% to 75% developing in the osseous structures around the knee. Osteosarcomas of the chest wall are rare and may be indistinguishable from Ewing's sarcoma. In the ribs, osteosarcomas comprised 16 of 1274 osteosarcomas in the Mayo Clinic series.

Radiographically, typical features of osteosarcomas include a mixed osteolytic and osteosclerotic pattern, extension through the cortex with possibly a soft tissue mass, and a periosteal lesion in the form of a Codman's triangle or "sunburst" appearance.

REFERENCES

Dahlin DC, Unni KK. Bone Tumors: General Aspects and Data on 8,542 Cases. Springfield, IL: Thomas, 1986:269–307.

Gouliamos AD, Carter B, Emami B. Computed tomography of the chest wall. Radiology 1989; 134:433–436.

Hudson TM. Radiologic-Pathologic Correlation of Musculoskeletal Lesions. Baltimore: Williams & Wilkins, 1987:359–365.

Case 39

HISTORY

A 25-year-old man presented with painless winging of the scapula. He had had previous prophylactic therapeutic irradiation (approximately 20 Gy) to the lungs for Wilms' tumor in early childhood; the field included both scapulas.

RADIOLOGY

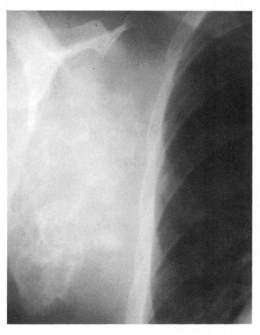

Figure 39-1. Plain films show an ossified or calcified mass involving the right scapula, displacing it away from the thoracic cage.

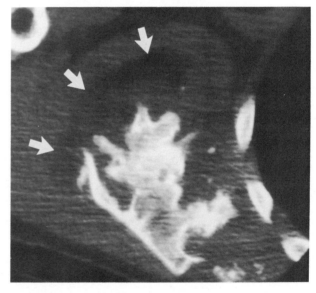

Figure 39-2. CT scan shows a broad-based exophytic lesion arising from the anterior surface of the scapula that contains mature bone and calcified cartilage but has extensive peripheral areas without mineralization (arrows). Attenuation numbers in the nonmineralized portions were consistent with cartilage.

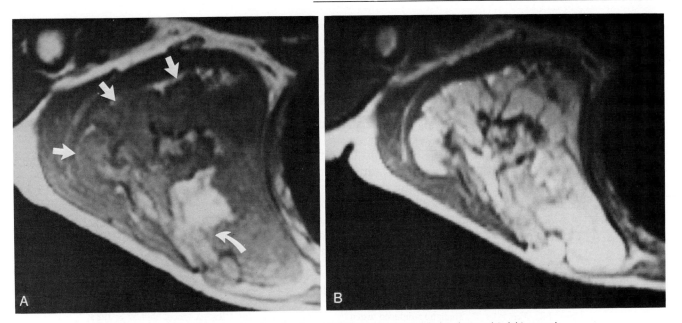

Figure 39-3*A–B.* T1-weighted and proton density axial MR images show a lobulated mass (straight arrows) extending anteriorly from the scapula. The bony stalk merges with the cortex (curved arrow). The lesion is well demarcated from the surrounding connective tissue, suggesting a noninfiltrative growth pattern.

DIFFERENTIAL DIAGNOSIS

The differential diagnosis includes chondrosarcoma, periosteal chondroma, osteo-chondroma, osteogenic sarcoma, and synovial sarcoma.

PATHOLOGY

Subtotal scapulectomy was performed. Partially calcified cartilaginous nodules were present on the anterior surface of the gross specimen.

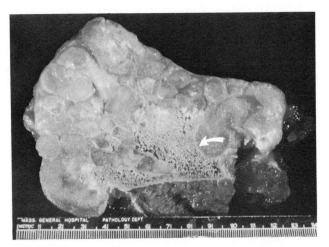

Figure 39-4. In the bisected gross specimen, a tumor containing numerous white, glistening, lobulated nodules can be seen arising from the scapula. The bony stalk merges with the cortex (curved arrow).

DIAGNOSIS

The final diagnosis was radiation-induced osteochondroma.

DISCUSSION

Osteochondromas (benign osteocartilaginous exostoses) are outgrowths of bone that are initially covered by a cartilage cap. Arising from cartilage at active epiphyseal plates, they are not considered true neoplasms but rather aberrations of normal growth. Osteochondromas may occur following a variety of traumatic insults to the perichondrial ring of the growing physis including therapeutic irradiation. Osteochondromas following radiation are identical in all respects to those occurring spontaneously and have a prevalence of approximately 6% to 12%. Malignant degeneration to chondrosarcoma in this circumstance is extremely rare. When treatment is necessary to relieve mechanical problems, surgical excision is used. The lesions do not recur.

REFERENCES

Chew FS, Weissleder R. Radiation-induced osteochondroma. AJR 1991; 157:792.

Jaffe N, Ried HL, Cohen M, et al. Radiation-induced osteochondroma in long-term survivors of childhood cancer. Int J Radiat Oncol Biol Phys 1983; 9:665–670.

Libshitz HI, Cohen MA. Radiation-induced osteochondromas. Radiology 1982; 142:643–647.

Case 40

HISTORY

A 70-year-old male with known diverticular disease presented with intermittent left lower quadrant pain.

RADIOLOGY

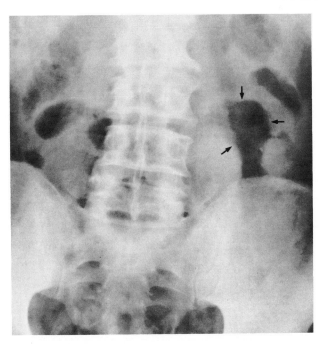

Figure 40-1. An irregular gas collection (arrows) projects over the left midabdomen.

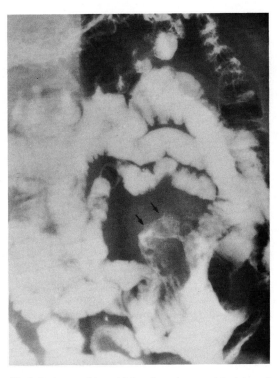

Figure 40-2. During small bowel follow-through, a persistent, irregular barium collection (arrows) is seen to be identical in configuration to the gas collection seen on KUB. Adjacent bowel loops are displaced.

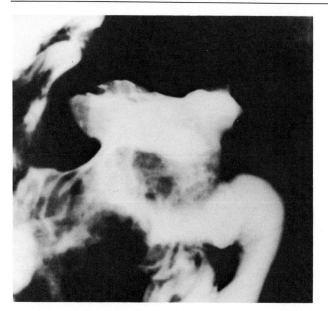

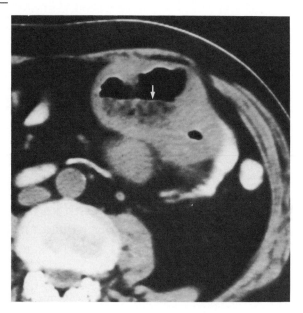

Figure 40-3. An oblique spot image shows that this collection communicates with the small bowel and represents a giant ulceration.

Figure 40-4. On noncontrast CT scan, gas-debris level (arrow) is present within this ulcerated, thick-walled mass.

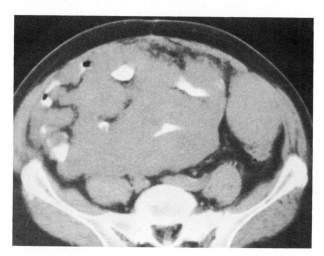

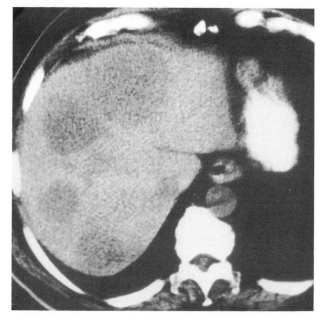

Figure 40-5. Four years following resection, noncontrast CT scan shows multiple mesenteric masses that invade the omental and mesenteric fat and compress the lumen of several bowel loops.

Figure 40-6. Multiple low attenuation focal lesions are scattered throughout the liver.

DIFFERENTIAL DIAGNOSIS

The differential diagnosis includes leiomyosarcoma, adenocarcinoma, lymphoma, neurogenic sarcoma, and malignant carcinoid.

PATHOLOGY

The lesion was resected along with contiguous portions of the bowel.

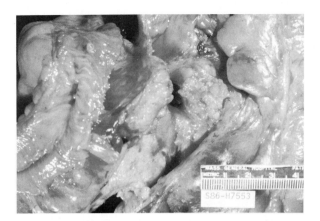

Figure 40-7. Arising in the wall of the small bowel and adhering to the colon is a solid tan-white tumor.

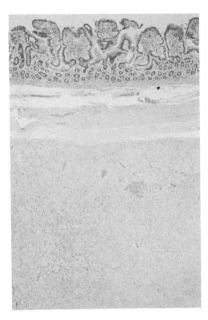

Figure 40-8. The tumor involves the muscularis of the small bowel wall.

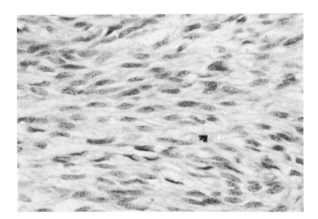

Figure 40-9. The tumor is composed of fascicles of cytologically malignant spindle cells that have blunt ends. Mitoses are numerous.

DIAGNOSIS

The final pathologic diagnosis was small bowel leiomyosarcoma.

DISCUSSION

Benign and malignant neoplasms of the small bowel are uncommon, accounting for only 2% to 5% of all gastrointestinal tract tumors. Symptoms and signs are nonspecific, absent, or intermittent and include pain, acute or chronic bleeding, partial or complete obstruction, or palpable mass. Diagnosis is often delayed owing to vague or nonspecific symptoms and the inherent limitations of the small bowel follow-through examination. Diagnosis is usually made after exclusion of abnormality in the upper GI tract and colon.

Malignant small bowel neoplasms include spindle cell tumors (leiomyosarcoma, fibrosarcoma, and liposarcoma), adenocarcinoma, malignant carcinoid, and lymphoma. Leiomyosarcoma is the most common spindle cell tumor of the small bowel and occurs, in descending order of frequency, in the ileum, jejunum, and duodenum. The tumor arises from the submucosal or subserosal wall of the small bowel. Because tumor growth is slow and exophytic to the bowel lumen, clinical signs and symptoms due to bleeding and mass effect do not occur until the neoplasm reaches enormous size and undergoes central necrosis and ulceration. Irregular intraluminal masses are unusual. Mechanical obstruction is a late manifestation.

Plain radiographs may show a soft tissue mass displacing loops of bowel. Segments of bowel may become draped over the mass and show stretching of parallel mucosal folds. Irregular collections of gas represent tumoral excavation communicating with the bowel lumen. Barium may fill mucosal ulcerations or large necrotic cavities. Fistulous tracts often develop. Although deep ulceration and fistulous tracts suggest malignancy, it is difficult to differentiate benign leiomyomas from leiomyosarcomas based on barium examination. CT demonstrates the extraluminal extent of the tumor, its relationship to intra-abdominal and retroperitoneal structures, and the presence of lymphadenopathy or metastatic disease to the liver. Cavitation is identified in addition to necrotic and hemorrhagic regions that do not communicate with the bowel lumen. Viable tumor enhances following intravenous contrast administration, maximizing the detection of central necrosis. The presence of necrosis suggests malignancy and may affect preoperative planning.

Treatment consists of complete surgical resection. Poor prognosis results from delayed diagnosis and advanced disease at the time of detection.

REFERENCE

Megibow S, et al. CT evaluation of gastrointestinal leiomyomas and leiomyosarcomas. AJR 1985; 144:727–731.

Case 41

HISTORY

A newborn presented with an abdominal mass, bilateral orbital masses, and decreased responsiveness.

RADIOLOGY

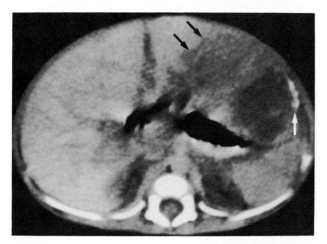

Figure 41-1. Noncontrast abdominal CT scan shows a heterogeneous mass in the left liver lobe (black arrows) with peripheral calcification (white arrow).

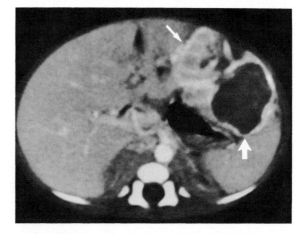

Figure 41-2. Following contrast administration, the mass demonstrates irregular enhancement (thin arrow) as well as a cystic component (thick arrow) with rim enhancement.

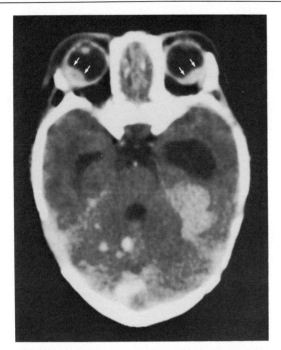

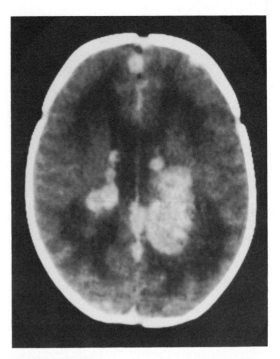

Figure 41-3. Noncontrast cranial CT scan at the level of the orbits shows bilateral retinal masses (arrows). High attenuation lesions are present in the cerebellum and left temporal lobe.

Figure 41-4. At a higher level dense masses are seen to be present in the lateral ventricles and along the falx.

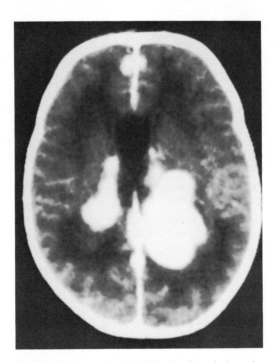

Figure 41-5. Following contrast administration these lesions show dense enhancement.

DIFFERENTIAL DIAGNOSIS

The differential diagnosis includes metastatic retinoblastoma, metastatic neuroblastoma, metastatic hepatoblastoma, and hepatocellular carcinoma.

PATHOLOGY

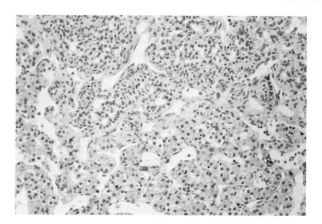

Figure 41-6. The lower portion of this histologic image demonstrates round nests of polyhedral fetal epithelial cells surrounded by prominent sinusoids. In the upper portion the embryonal component consists of cords and nests of smaller cells focally forming glandular structures.

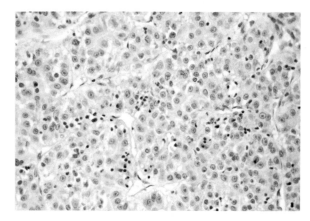

Figure 41-7. Scattered among the epithelial cells are small clusters of hematopoietic cells.

DIAGNOSIS

The final diagnosis was hepatoblastoma with central nervous system metastases.

DISCUSSION

Hepatoblastoma is the most common hepatic malignancy in children and accounts for 50% of pediatric liver tumors. This tumor is third in frequency among abdominal neoplasms, behind Wilms' tumor and neuroblastoma. Hepatoblastoma usually is detected during the first 3 years of life and rarely occurs after age 6. There is a slight female predominance. The tumor typically presents as an asymptomatic upper abdominal mass during routine physical examination. When symptoms occur, they include fever, weight loss, nausea, vomiting, and pain. Hepatoblastoma may be associated with congenital abnormalities such as tetralogy of Fallot, persistent ductus arteriosus, extrahepatic biliary atresia, Beckwith-Wiedemann syndrome, and diaphragmatic or umbilical hernia. Depending on tumor grade, local lymphatic spread or distant hematogenous metastases are common.

Laboratory studies show marked elevation of the serum alphafetoprotein level. Anemia, leukocytosis, and abnormal liver function test results are also common. Histologically, hepatoblastoma is similar to immature liver tissue with varying degrees of differentiation. Embryonal, fetal, and anaplastic subtypes may occur. The tumor is classified as pure epithelial or mixed depending on the presence and proportion of epithelial and mesenchymal tissue. Complex mesenchymal elements may include osteoid, cartilage, muscle, hematopoietic tissue, and primitive mesenchyme.

Hepatoblastoma can be difficult to differentiate from hepatocellular carcinoma. Presenting symptoms and clinical features of both tumors are nonspecific. Hepatocellular carcinoma tends to occur in an older age group unless the child has a risk factor such as cirrhosis. Hemangioendothelioma is usually detected in patients less than 6 months old and must also be differentiated from hepatoblastoma. Hemangioendothelioma is associated with high-output congestive heart failure as well as cutaneous cavernous hemangiomas and usually has a characteristic radionuclide appearance. Early tracer activity occurs in the liver owing to increased blood flow followed by delayed clearance due to arteriovenous shunting and blood pooling. Ultrasound shows multiple sonolucent regions, and angiography shows contrast collections in sinusoidal lakes that persist into the venous phase.

Hepatoblastoma is evaluated by plain film, sonography, CT, MR imaging, or angiography. Plain films show displacement of bowel from the right upper abdomen, suggesting hepatomegaly or mass lesion. Calcification is detected in 30% to 50% of cases and usually represents mineralization of osteoid. On sonography, the mass is hyperechoic and heterogeneous, although hypoechoic or anechoic regions may result from cyst formation or tumor necrosis.

CT delineates tumor location and segmental liver involvement. Hepatoblastoma may be a solitary liver mass or multicentric. Without intravenous contrast the tumor is lower in attenuation than normal liver. Following contrast administration, enhancement is heterogeneous and demonstrates sharply marginated lobulations and internal nodularity. The appearance is nonspecific on MR imaging, which shows hypointense signal on T1-weighted sequences and hyperintense signal on T2-weighted sequences. The tumor is hypervascular on angiography. Metastases to the central nervous system show imaging characteristics similar to those of the primary tumor.

Prognosis is related to histologic subtype. Epithelial cell and fetal subtypes are most favorable if the tumor is confined to the liver. Although hepatoblastoma can be resected in the majority of cases, only half of these patients are cured. The prognosis is poor in patients with multifocal involvement, unresectable tumor, recurrent disease, or metastases.

REFERENCES

Boechat MI, et al. Primary liver tumors in children: comparison of CT and MR imaging. Radiology 1988; 169;727–732.

Dachman AH, et al. Hepatoblastoma: radiologic-pathologic correlation in 50 cases. Radiology 1987; 164:15–19.

Gauthier F, et al. Hepatoblastoma and hepatocarcinoma in children: analysis of a series of 29 cases. J Pediatr Surg 1986; 27(5):424–429.

Case 42

HISTORY

A 42-year-old male presented with a nontender left posterior thigh mass.

RADIOLOGY

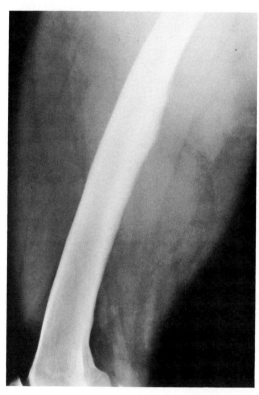

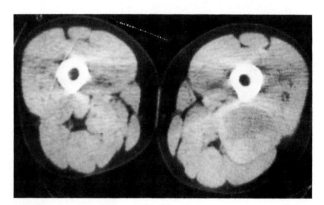

Figure 42-2. The central portions of the lesion are lucent on CT scans after intravenous contrast.

Figure 42-1. There is a rounded soft tissue mass posterior to the femur that has produced a pressure effect and a small amount of solid periosteal response on the underlying bone.

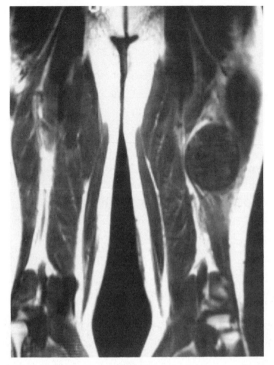

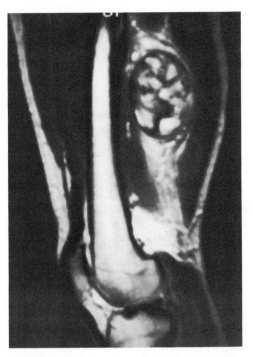

Figure 42-3. On T1-weighted (TR = 600, TE = 16) images the lesion has a well-formed margin and exhibits low signal intensity with multiple internal septations.

Figure 42-4. On T2-weighted (TR = 2000, TE = 40) images the multilocular appearance is enhanced.

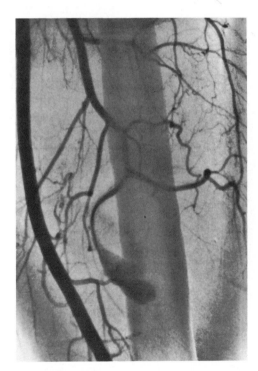

Figure 42-5. A branch of the left profunda femoris artery terminates in an abnormal lobulated collection of contrast material. Most of the mass is avascular.

DIFFERENTIAL DIAGNOSIS

The differential diagnosis includes soft tissue neoplasm (benign or malignant), false aneurysm (traumatic, iatrogenic, or mycotic), and hematoma.

PATHOLOGY

The lesion was resected.

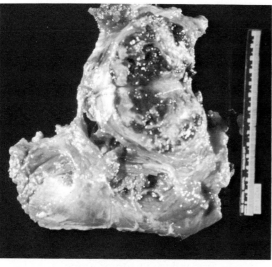

Figure 42-6. The ovoid hemorrhagic, focally tan mass is well circumscribed from the adjacent skeletal muscle.

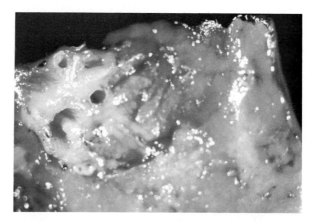

Figure 42-7. The mass is in continuity with a medium-sized muscular artery.

Figure 42-8. Microscopically the mass consists of organizing hemorrhage surrounded by a pseudocapsule.

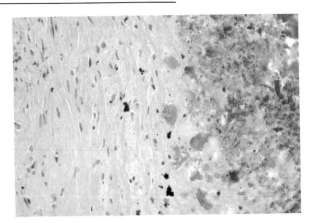

Figure 42–9. The pseudocapsule contains fibroblasts, collagen, and scattered red blood cells.

DIAGNOSIS

The final diagnosis was pseudoaneurysm of the profunda femoris.

DISCUSSION

An aneurysm is a localized arterial dilatation. In true aneurysms the internal elastic lamina remains intact, and there is dilatation of all layers of the arterial wall. True aneurysms may be fusiform or saccular. Ninety percent are due to atherosclerosis. Other types of aneurysms include mycotic, syphilitic, neoplastic (secondary to tumor emboli), and vasculitic aneurysms.

Dissecting aneurysms are associated with lues, polyarteritis nodosa, fibromuscular dysplasia, mucoid degeneration of the media, trauma, and surgery. Histologically, they demonstrate separation of the media from the internal elastic lamina. The detached intima is often displaced against the opposite wall by intramural hematoma. Frequently, all that is left of the true lumen is a thin slit.

False aneurysms (pseudoaneurysms) are saclike structures that communicate with the true arterial lumen. They result from disruption of all layers of the arterial wall and are contained by the periarterial connective tissue. The most common causes include trauma (penetrating missile, knife, or percutaneous biopsy needle), a previous vascular procedure (angiography or anastomotic surgery), and rupture of a true (mycotic, vasculitic) aneurysm. Rarely, a false aneurysm may result from blunt trauma. The size of a false aneurysm depends on the nature of the contiguous connective tissue, the age of the aneurysm, and the amount of intraluminal clot. If the perivascular connective tissue is able to contain the extravasated blood, the aneurysm will tamponade itself when its pressure equals the mean arterial pressure. If the connective tissue is weak and the lumen remains patent, blood will continue to enter during systole and exit during diastole, leading to formation of a "pulsatile hematoma." As the false aneurysm ages, a sharply marginated fibrous wall forms and encapsulates the aneurysm. Contained hematoma may organize and even become endothelialized.

In differentiating pseudoaneurysms from other mass lesions, ultrasound plays an important role by demonstrating the relationship of the lesion to other vessels, the presence of a fluid component, and, if Doppler ultrasound is available, the presence of blood flow. If the aneurysm is pulsatile and adjacent to bone (usually in the extremities), plain films may demonstrate pressure erosion. A hyperostotic bony response is unusual. If the lumen remains patent, angiography may demonstrate an irregular collection of contrast material as well as a local mass effect with displacement of adjacent vessels, depending on the size of the associated hematoma.

Some pseudoaneurysms are amenable to treatment by embolization. Usually, however, surgical repair is necessary in order to prevent further pulsatile dilatation and potential rupture.

REFERENCES

Abrams HL (ed.). Angiography, Vascular and Interventional Radiology (3rd ed). Boston: Little, Brown, 1983.

Kadir S. Diagnostic Angiography. Philadelphia: Saunders, 1986.

Case 43

HISTORY

A 2-month-old male presented with a bulging anterior fontanelle and a 3-day history of lethargy.

RADIOLOGY

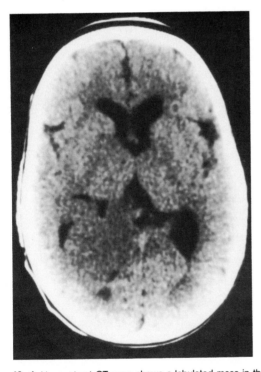

Figure 43-1. Noncontrast CT scan shows a lobulated mass in the trigone of the right lateral ventricle. The mass is slightly hypodense compared to normal brain.

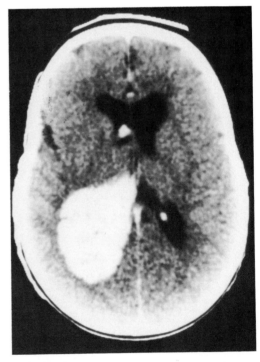

Figure 43-2. Following intravenous contrast injection, the right trigonal mass enhances homogeneously. There is an enhancing focus in the frontal horn of the right lateral ventricle.

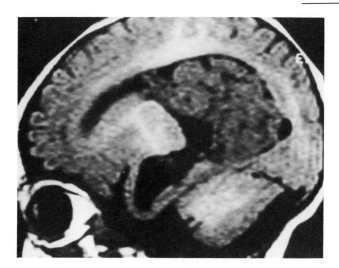

Figure 43-3. The mass is papillary in character on this T1-weighted sagittal MR image.

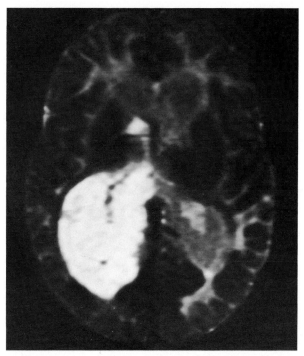

Figure 43-4. Late echo T2-weighted axial image of the intraventricular right trigone and frontal horn components shows a hyperintense signal and a central linear low signal region suggestive of a flow void.

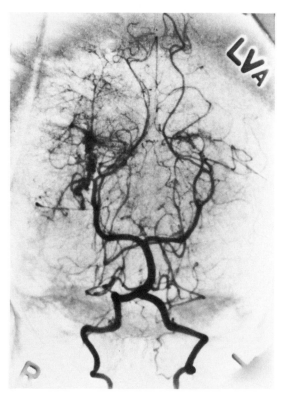

Figure 43-5. Subtraction anteroposterior view from a left vertebral arteriogram shows hypervascular tumor.

DIFFERENTIAL DIAGNOSIS

The differential diagnosis includes choroid plexus papilloma, choroid plexus carcinoma, meningioma, ependymoma, subependymoma, subependymal giant cell astrocytoma, glioma, and metastatic carcinoma.

PATHOLOGY

A 4.0- × 4.0- × 2.5-cm mass was resected.

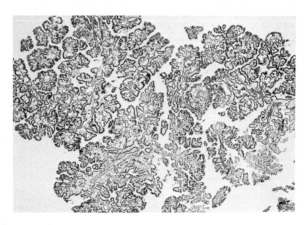

Figure 43-6. At low power the lesion has a very prominent papillary configuration.

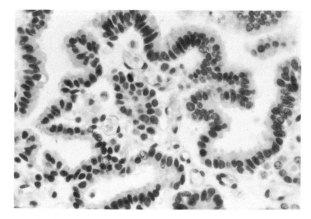

Figure 43-7. The papillae are lined by cuboidal to columnar type epithelium. The nuclei are located at the base of the cells and do not demonstrate cytologic atypia. The central portions of the papillae contain blood vessels and loose connective tissue.

DIAGNOSIS

The final pathologic diagnosis was choroid plexus papilloma.

DISCUSSION

Choroid plexus papillomas are uncommon, comprising 0.3% to 0.7% of all intracranial tumors and 3% of intracranial tumors in children. Choroid plexus papillomas in children are generally seen before the age of 16, with 70% of cases occurring in children 2 years of age or less. Although they can arise anywhere along the distribution of the choroid plexus, these tumors are found most frequently in the lateral ventricles in children (67% to 75% of cases) and in the fourth ventricle in adults. Microscopically, they have a papillary structure composed of vascularized connective tissue stalks lined by a single layer of cuboidal or columnar epithelial cells.

Hydrocephalus is seen almost invariably and has been attributed either to increased cerebrospinal fluid (CSF) production or to adhesions from tumoral hemorrhage causing either interventricular or extraventricular obstruction. Symptoms and signs are typically those of increased intracranial pressure: headache, vomiting, and increasing head circumference.

On unenhanced CT scans an isodense to hyperdense, well-defined, lobular intraventricular mass is typically demonstrated. Intense contrast enhancement is noted. Inhomogeneous calcifications are present in 20% to 30% of tumors. On T1-weighted MR images the mass is generally isointense or mildly hypointense to gray matter, and there is corresponding hyperintensity on T2-weighted images. Large blood vessels within the tumor, prior hemorrhage, and areas of calcification or cystic change frequently result in a heterogeneous appearance on MR imaging. The ventricular system is enlarged.

A minority of choroid plexus papillomas undergo malignant transformation into choroid plexus carcinomas. Both choroid plexus papillomas and choroid plexus carcinomas can metastasize to CSF pathways, although this type of spread is more common with carcinomas. Carcinomas may extend through the ventricular wall into the parenchyma; patients are less likely to present with hydrocephalus. Given the risk of malignant transformation, the recommended treatment for choroid plexus papilloma is complete surgical resection.

REFERENCES

Boyd MC, Steinbok P. Choroid plexus tumors: problems in diagnosis and management. J Neurosurg 1987; 66:800–805.

Hawkins J. Treatment of choroid plexus papillomas in children: a brief analysis of twenty years' experience. Neurosurgery 1980; 6:380–384.

Jelinek J, Smirniotopoulos JG, Parisi JE, et al. Lateral ventricular neoplasms of the brain: differential diagnosis based on clinical, CT and MR findings. AJR 1990; 155:365–372.

Spallone A, Pastore FS, Giuffre R, et al. Choroid plexus papillomas in infancy and childhood. Childs Nerv Syst 1990; 6:71–74.

Case 44

HISTORY

A 56-year-old female presented with a mass in the right upper quadrant.

RADIOLOGY

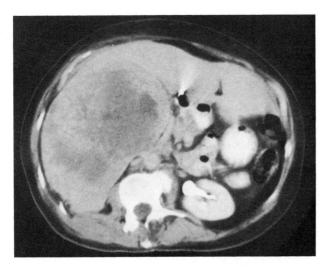

Figure 44–1. CT scan shows a heterogeneous right upper quadrant mass with central low density. The origin is not clear from this image.

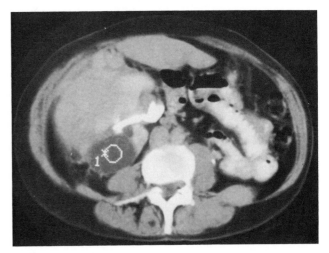

Figure 44–2. Caudally the mass blends imperceptibly with the right kidney.

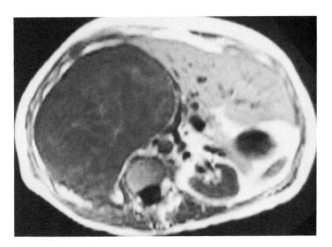

Figure 44–3. T1-weighted (TR = 275, TE = 14) MR image at the same level as the CT.

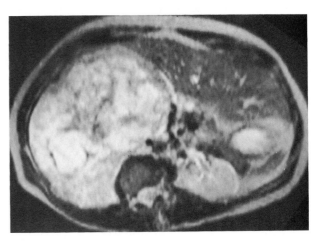

Figure 44–4. T2-weighted (TR = 2350, TE = 120) image.

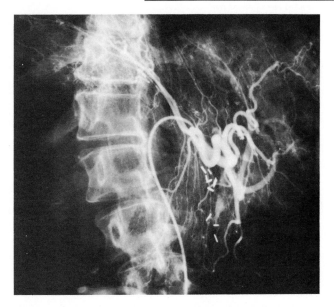

Figure 44–5. A hypovascular mass with faint neovascularity at its periphery displaces the right hepatic artery medially.

DIFFERENTIAL DIAGNOSIS

The differential diagnosis includes metastasis, renal or adrenal mass, and retroperitoneal soft tissue sarcoma.

PATHOLOGY

The lesion was resected.

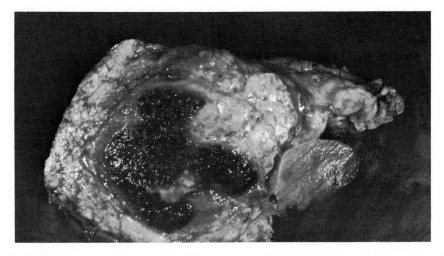

Figure 44–6. The large, centrally hemorrhagic, solid tan mass is well demarcated but abuts the renal capsule.

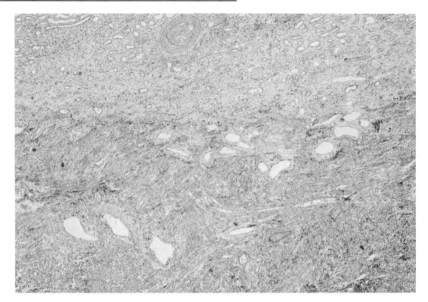

Figure 44–7. The tumor appears to arise from the capsule but does not invade the renal parenchyma.

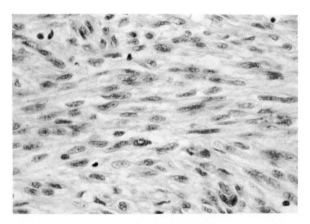

Figure 44–8. The tumor is composed of cytologically malignant hyperchromatic spindle cells. The nuclei of the spindle cells have prominent blunt ends.

DIAGNOSIS

The final pathologic diagnosis was leiomyosarcoma of the renal capsule.

DISCUSSION

Leiomyosarcoma (LMS) is a malignant tumor of smooth muscle origin. It can arise from blood vessel walls and visceral smooth muscle and thus may be found anywhere in the body. It accounts for a small number of gastric, small bowel, colorectal, and retroperitoneal malignancies. It is the third most common retroperitoneal sarcoma behind liposarcoma and malignant fibrous histiocytoma.

Sarcomas comprise 3% of renal malignancies, the most common of which is leiomyosarcoma. Eighty-five cases of renal LMS were reported through 1986. The tumor usually arises from capsular or pericapsular tissue but can also originate from the renal pelvis, renal vessels, or parenchymal muscle rests. The lesions vary from fully encapsulated to nonencapsulated. Prognosis is most dependent on histologic grade, but size and encapsulation are also significant. Retroperitoneal LMS of nonrenal origin are typically large at the time of discovery and carry a poor prognosis. Their behavior is similar to that of renal LMS. The age range for renal LMS is 10 to 83 years, with most patients in the fifth to seventh decades. The male to female ratio is 1:1.4. The lesions commonly produce flank pain with or without hematuria. Gastrointestinal symptoms and weight loss may occur. A firm, sometimes tender, palpable mass is a common finding.

Following nephrectomy, local recurrences are common and usually present within 3 years. Hematogenous metastases are found in the lungs, bone, liver, and mesentery. Regional lymph node involvement is unusual. Most patients die within 2 years despite aggressive therapy.

LMS in all sites commonly exhibit necrosis, cystic change, and hemorrhage. CT often reveals large masses with extensive cystic and necrotic areas. Metastatic foci frequently exhibit central necrosis. Calcification is said to be a common finding in renal LMS but is distinctly unusual in other locations.

Ultrasound generally reveals a complex mass with cystic components. The appearance of renal LMS on intraventricular pyelograms (IVP) is nonspecific and may consist of calyceal displacement, hydronephrosis, or nonfunction. Arteriography reveals that LMS in all sites are hypovascular. Renal capsular tumors are frequently supplied by capsular vessels.

Most renal LMS are treated by nephrectomy alone. Combination chemotherapy is effective in some cases. Retroperitoneal tumors are treated by excision of all gross tumor and postoperative radiation therapy. Recurrences are common at all sites.

REFERENCES

Granmayeh M, et al. Sarcoma of the kidney: angiographic features. AJR 1977; 129:107–112.

Hartman DS, et al. Leiomyosarcoma of the retroperitoneum and inferior vena cava. Radiological-pathological correlation from the archives of the Armed Forces Institute of Pathology (AFIP). Radiographics 1992; 12:1203.

McLeod AJ, et al. Leiomyosarcoma: computed tomographic findings. Radiology 1984; 152:133–136.

Pucci B, et al. The radiology of sarcomas and sarcomatoid carcinomas of the kidney. Clin Radiol 1987; 38:249–254.

Rakowsky E, et al. Leiomyosarcoma of the kidney. Urology 1987; 29:68–70.

Case 45

HISTORY

A 45-year-old male presented with fever, night sweats, and mild dry cough.

RADIOLOGY

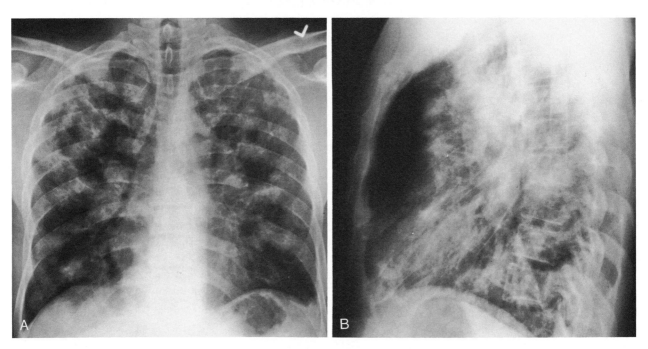

Figure 45-1. *A–B.* Chest x-ray revealed diffuse 1- to 3-cm nodular opacities with hilar and mediastinal adenopathy.

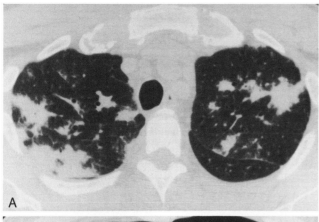

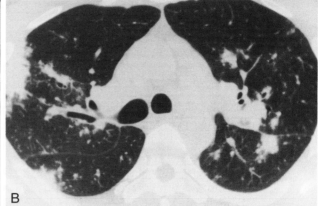

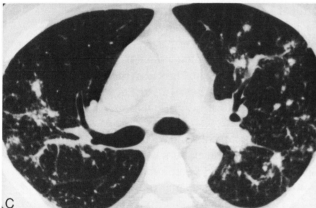

Figure 45-2. Conventional CT (*A–B*) and high resolution CT (*C*) confirmed adenopathy and showed air bronchograms in several of the nodules. In addition, multiple small 1- to 3-cm nodular and linear opacities were distributed along bronchovascular bundles and in subpleural areas.

DIFFERENTIAL DIAGNOSIS

The differential diagnosis includes tuberculosis, sarcoidosis, atypical mycobacterial infection, and lymphoma.

PATHOLOGY

Right paratracheal node biopsy was performed.

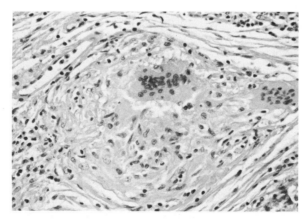

Figure 45-3. A large multinucleated giant cell is demonstrated in one of numerous well-formed noncaseating granulomas.

DIAGNOSIS

The final diagnosis was sarcoidosis.

DISCUSSION

Sarcoidosis is a multisystem disease of unknown etiology characterized by non-caseating granuloma formation. Although most patients are asymptomatic at initial diagnosis, 20% to 50% have pulmonary symptoms, most frequently dyspnea or dry cough. Virtually all patients have roentgenographically visible parenchymal disease or hilar adenopathy at some time during the course of the disease. Constitutional symptoms are also common; fever is present in approximately 17% of cases. Pulmonary manifestations result in the greatest morbidity and mortality. Twenty to twenty-five percent of patients develop permanent pulmonary functional impairment.

Sarcoidosis in the chest is manifest first as hilar and mediastinal adenopathy. Diffuse pulmonary disease frequently appears simultaneously with hilar nodal regression, but parenchymal lung disease does not precede adenopathy. The earliest parenchymal lung lesion of sarcoidosis is an idiopathic alveolitis associated with an increased number of activated T lymphocytes and macrophages. This alveolitis may result in alveolar filling with inflammatory cells, leading to a radiographic appearance of consolidation or air-space abnormality.

Granuloma formation is thought to evolve from the alveolitis. The most frequent radiologic appearance of pulmonary sarcoid is a reticulonodular pattern of parenchymal lung abnormality. Pathologically, this corresponds to interstitial granulomas distributed along the lymphatics of the bronchovascular bundles. As the granulomas mature, there is an increase in fibroblasts and epithelioid cells with a decrease in lymphocytes and macrophages. In some cases the granulomas may resolve completely whereas in others progressive fibrosis and replacement with hyaline material may ensue, sometimes leading to end-stage pulmonary fibrosis. Granuloma formation within the lungs appears to be a relatively late occurrence.

In approximately 2% to 4% of cases pulmonary sarcoid presents as multiple parenchymal nodules. Typically, the nodules are greater than 1 cm in size and simulate the appearance of metastatic disease. Rarely, the presentation may be that of an isolated pulmonary nodule. It has been suggested that the nodular form of pulmonary sarcoid has a better prognosis than the reticulonodular form and that it represents an earlier stage of disease.

On plain films it may be difficult to differentiate active and potentially reversible granulomatous nodularity and alveolitis from irreversible end-stage fibrosis. CT and high-resolution CT have become increasingly important. CT can delineate the distribution of granulomas along the lymphatics in the bronchovascular sheath and to a lesser extent along the interlobular septa, the major fissures, and the subpleural regions. CT may also demonstrate unsuspected cystic changes, areas of fibrosis, and complications of sarcoid such as cavitation and mycetoma formation, blebs, bullae, pneumothorax, and bronchiectasis. However, like plain films, CT cannot exclude or "rule out" sarcoidosis; granulomas may be discovered in biopsy specimens from patients whose plain films or CT scans are normal.

The radiologic, pathologic, and physiologic parameters of disease activity do not always correlate with each other. Pulmonary function testing may be the best predictive index of disease. Remission of pulmonary disease may be either spontaneous or steroid induced. The overall mortality is 5% to 10% and is most commonly secondary to fibrosis and cor pulmonale. However, approximately 65% of patients recover completely with minimal or no residual pulmonary disease. In 70% to 80% of patients there is resolution of chest x-ray abnormalities.

REFERENCES

Hamper UM, Fishman EK, Khouri NF, et al. Typical and atypical CT manifestations of pulmonary sarcoidosis. J Comput Assist Tomogr 1986; 10:928–936.

Hunninghake GW, Garrett KC, Richardson HB, et al. Pathogenesis of the granulomatous lung diseases. Am Rev Resp Dis 1984; 130:476–496.

Lynch DA, Webb RW, Gamsu G, et al. Computed tomography in pulmonary sarcoidosis. J Comput Assist Tomogr 1989; 13:405–410.

Muller NL, Kullnig P, Miller RR. The CT findings of pulmonary sarcoidosis: analysis of 25 patients. AJR 1989; 152:1179–1182.

Onal E, Lopata M, Lourenco RV. Nodular pulmonary sarcoidosis: clinical, roentgenographic and physiologic course in 5 patients. Chest 1977; 72(3):296–300.

Rose RM, Lee RG, Costello P. Solitary nodular sarcoidosis. Clin Radiol 1985; 36:589–592.

Case 46

HISTORY

A 6-year-old boy presented with an expanding ecchymotic, soft, tender calf mass and inguinal adenopathy.

RADIOLOGY

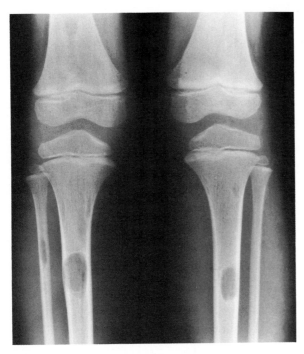

Figure 46-1. An AP plain film of both knees reveals multifocal lytic lesions of both tibias, the right fibula, and the right femur. The lesions are well marginated and have thin, faintly sclerotic boundaries.

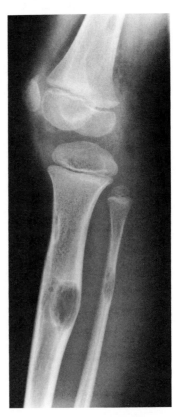

Figure 46-2. A lateral view of the right distal femur and proximal tibia shows that the lesions have expanded the posterior tibial cortex. The soft tissues in front of the tibia appear thickened. Additional skeletal lesions were observed in the right proximal femur, the wing of the right ilium, and the left humerus.

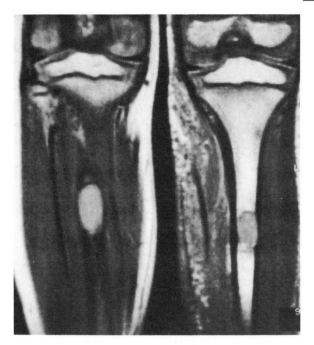

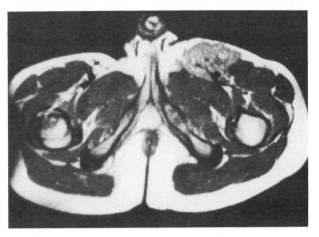

Figure 46–4. An axial MR image through the level of the lesser trochanter (TR = 1000, TE = 40) shows similar soft tissue findings surrounding the femoral artery.

Figure 46–3. An MR scan done with proton-density technique (TR = 1000, TE = 40) demonstrates the right tibial lesion as an area of uniform intermediate signal intensity demarcated by a well-formed margin. The soft tissue process on the left is seen as an extensively infiltrating pattern of serpiginous lines involving both muscle and subcutaneous tissues.

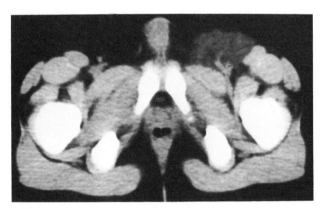

Figure 46–5. A CT scan through the same area shows that the lesion is of low attenuation, suggesting water density.

DIFFERENTIAL DIAGNOSIS

The differential diagnosis includes hemangiomas, multiple eosinophilic granulomas, metastases, and multiple enchondromas.

PATHOLOGY

A biopsy was performed.

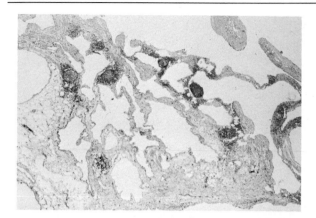

Figure 46–6. The lesion consists of numerous irregular lymphatic spaces separated by loose connective tissue and containing lymphoid follicles.

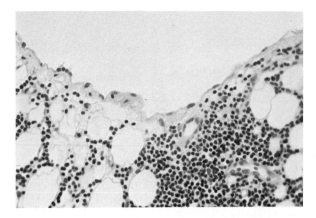

Figure 46–7. The irregular lymphatic spaces are lined by bland endothelial cells. Many of the lumens are empty or contain a proteinaceous exudate.

DIAGNOSIS

The final pathologic diagnosis was lymphangiomatosis of bone and soft tissue.

DISCUSSION

Lymphangiomas are congenital lesions that probably develop from sequestered lymphatic sacs, although some think that they may be related to incompetent valves in normal lymphatic channels. Seventy-five percent occur as cervical masses in children, 20% as axillary masses, and the remaining 5% in other locations such as the mediastinum, retroperitoneum, and bones. These lesions can grow aggressively and can cause difficult management problems. There is a wide spectrum of appearance of lymphangioma of bone, ranging from one or more isolated lesions to widespread cystic angiomatosis and Gorham's disease (massive osteolysis or vanishing bone disease). Lymphangioma of bone is much less common than hemangioma. The absence of red blood cells in the vascular channels is the finding that allows the diagnosis to be made pathologically. However, hemangioma from which the blood has escaped can mimic a lymphangioma, and conversely, if blood is introduced into the spaces of a lymphangioma it can resemble a hemangioma.

Cystic lymphangiomatosis is characterized by multicentric angiomatous tumors arising in bone. Hemangiomas may be mixed with lymphangiomas. Unlike solitary lymphangiomas, which are seen in middle life, these occur mainly in children and adolescents with a male predominance. Involvement can be regional or widespread. Soft tissue or visceral lesions are frequently associated, and other clinical findings include chylothorax, hepatosplenomegaly, and lymphedema. Medical attention is sought because of complications resulting from mass effect. Bony lesions most commonly affect the skull, pelvis, ribs, scapula, humerus, tibia, and fibula. Bony changes include erosive or "soap bubble" (osteolytic with septations) lesions or ill-defined radiolucencies. Although in some patients symptoms can be mild, in others the progression of osteolysis can be relentless. Sequelae can include pathologic fractures with severe pain and swelling.

Although indistinguishable from hemangiomas on plain films, specific diagnosis of lymphangiomas can be made by lymphangiography if contrast accumulates within the lesions. MR imaging generally shows a signal intensity equal to that of fat on T1 images and greater than fat on T2-weighted images, though this varies slightly owing to the variable content (debris, blood, lymph) of the cystic spaces. MR is useful in evaluating the extent of disease and may be helpful in distinguishing lymphangiomas from other similar appearing lesions.

Pathologically, the lesions vary greatly in size and may involve an entire bone. Unilocular or multilocular cystic spaces, separated by trabeculae, are seen. When sectioned, they are poorly defined and may ooze turbid, milky, or clear fluid. Histology reveals widely patent, thin-walled vascular spaces lined by flat endothelial cells. These spaces are filled with eosinophilic, granular, proteinaceous fluid. The clinical course is related to osteolysis and the extent of disease.

REFERENCES

Siegel MJ, et al. Lymphangiomas in children: MR imaging. Radiology 1989; 170:467–470.

Resnick D, Kyriakus M, Greenway GD. Tumors and tumor-like lesions of bone: imaging and pathology of specific lesions. *In*: Resnick D, Niwayama G (eds). Diagnosis of Bone and Joint Disorders (2nd ed). Philadelphia: Saunders, 1988:3799–3801.

Case 47

HISTORY

A 40-year-old man presented with increasing abdominal girth.

RADIOLOGY

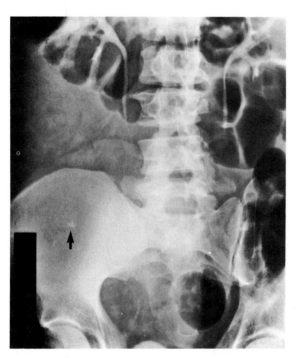

Figure 47-1. Kidney, ureter, bladder (KUB) film obtained during an intravenous pyelogram (IVP) demonstrates displacement of bowel by a large soft tissue mass that contains a calcific focus (arrow) as well as a diffusely mottled lucency (best seen superior to the right ilium).

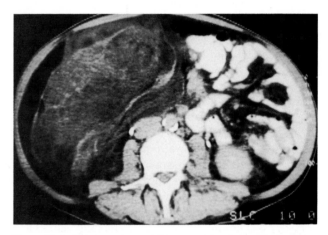

Figure 47-2. Contrast-enhanced CT scan of the abdomen shows a large, fatty mass with linear and nodular soft tissue stranding. Bowel is displaced to the left.

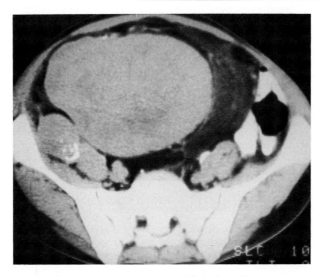

Figure 47-3. At the level of the pelvis, a bilobed, nonfatty component demonstrates sharp margination and increased attenuation. Punctate calcifications involve the posterior component.

DIFFERENTIAL DIAGNOSIS

The differential diagnosis includes lipoma, liposarcoma, diffuse infiltrative lipomatosis, retroperitoneal lipomatosis, angiomyolipoma, adrenal myelolipoma, and cystic teratoma.

PATHOLOGY

A 30- × 20- × 7-cm soft tissue mass was resected.

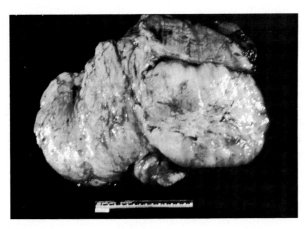

Figure 47-4. The multinodular tumor has different components that range from pale yellow to tan-white.

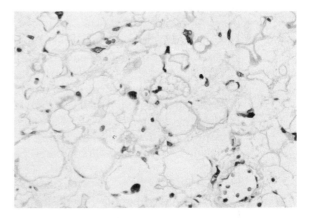

Figure 47-5. The pale yellow component is composed of mature adipocytes with scattered atypical cells that have vacuolated cytoplasm. These vacuolated cells are lipoblasts and scallop the tumor cell nuclei.

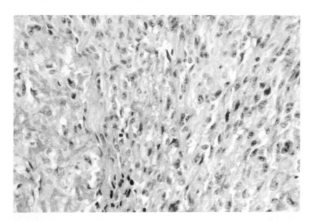

Figure 47-6. The tan or nonfatty portion of the tumor is much more cellular and is composed of cytologically malignant spindle cells that produce extracellular matrix that represents tumor bone.

DIAGNOSIS

The final pathologic diagnosis was retroperitoneal liposarcoma.

DISCUSSION

Soft tissue sarcomas account for less than 1% of all malignancies. Liposarcoma accounts for 5% to 25% of soft tissue sarcomas. The most common site of liposarcoma is the extremities, particularly the inner thigh. Other locations include the trunk and, rarely, the breast, genitalia, and GI tract. Liposarcoma occurs most frequently during the fifth and sixth decades with a slight male predominance.

Retroperitoneal liposarcoma may remain asymptomatic for months to years. Patients often present with increasing abdominal girth. The tumor grows to massive proportions, occasionally weighing more than 60 pounds. It enlarges slowly and displaces rather than invades adjacent organs. Pain is a late symptom. Mass effect may obstruct the inferior vena cava, ureters, and GI tract. Bulky tumors occasionally cause hypoglycemia by secreting an insulinlike polypeptide.

Liposarcomas have a spectrum of histologic variations. Several classification systems have been devised. One common system recognizes three classes. Lipogenic liposarcoma contains abundant lipid and scarce myxoid matrix. This tumor is usually low grade with an 80% 5-year survival. Myxoid liposarcoma contains abundant mucin and scarce lipid. This tumor is most common and is of intermediate grade. Survival is correspondingly decreased. Pleomorphic liposarcoma contains immature cells and a smaller proportion of adipocytes and myxoid matrix. This is a high-grade tumor that has a 20% 5-year survival rate.

The most important prognostic factor is tumor grade, which is determined by the degree of differentiation of malignant lipoblasts. Well-differentiated, low-grade tumors are slow growing, displace adjacent structures, and metastasize uncommonly. Poorly differentiated tumors are aggressive, infiltrate the surrounding tissue, and frequently metastasize by the time of diagnosis. Hematogenous metastases are most common and typically involve the lung, bone, and liver. Regional lymph node metastases and direct vascular invasion are rare. A retroperitoneal location results in a worse prognosis than a location on the extremities, possibly because of their greater size and proximity to vital structures at diagnosis. Treatment consists of surgical resection and, if excision is incomplete, postoperative radiation.

Once a retroperitoneal neoplasm becomes large, practically any imaging modality can detect it. Plain abdominal radiographs of lipogenic liposarcoma show bowel displacement by a radiolucent mass. Intravenous pyelography can show renal, ureteral, or bladder displacement and hydronephrosis. On ultrasound, hyperechogenicity suggests the presence of fat. Myxoid tumors sometimes have complex cystic regions.

CT scans of benign lipomas demonstrate an encapsulated, nonenhancing mass of homogeneous fat density. Thin linear strands sometimes occur. The appearance of liposarcoma depends on the proportion and complexity of fatty tissue. Lipogenic tumors are predominantly of fat density and have more numerous, thicker soft tissue strands than expected in benign lipomas. Myxoid liposarcoma shows, as in this case, heterogeneous attenuation greater than that of water but less than that of muscle. The tumor extends along anatomic planes parallel to muscle bundles, vessels, and nerves and may grow from the retroperitoneum into the spinal canal through neural foramina. Focal calcifications are common. The pattern and degree of contrast enhancement depend on fat content and necrosis.

MR signal intensity of benign lipoma is identical to that of normal subcutaneous fat. As with CT, lipogenic liposarcoma may be difficult to differentiate from its benign counterpart, but usually it demonstrates regions of linear or nodular T1-weighted low and T2-weighted high signal intensity.

In this case, no part of the tumor suggests benign lipoma. Figures 47-7 and 47-8 show images from the CT scan of a 40-year-old patient with liposarcoma. At the level of the kidneys, the homogeneously fatty appearance suggests benign lipoma. There is no linear or nodular stranding and no dominant region of higher attenuation. At the level of the pelvis, however, the mass shows lobulated nodules of higher attenuation and irregular margins that indicate malignancy.

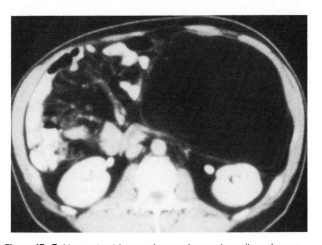

Figure 47-7. Noncontrast image shows a large retroperitoneal mass that is homogeneously low in attenuation and identical to fat. The appearance is typical for a benign lipoma. The bowel and mesentery are displaced to the right.

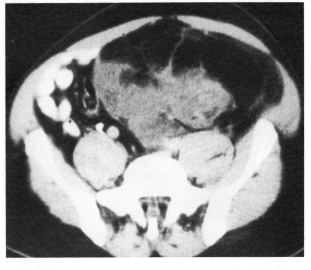

Figure 47-8. At the level of the pelvis, however, a solid component shows irregular margins and suggests malignancy.

REFERENCES

Dooms GC, et al. Lipomatous tumors and tumors with fatty component: MR imaging potential and comparison of MR and CT results. Radiology 1985; 157:479–483.

Fitzgerald BJ, Lyons K. Fatty retroperitoneal tumors: plain film and computed tomographic appearances. Postgrad Med J 1987; 63:847–850.

Waligore MP, et al. Lipomatous tumors of the abdominal cavity: CT appearance and pathologic correlation. AJR 1981; 137:539–545.

Case 48

HISTORY

A 10-year-old girl presented with a history of intermittent constipation for 1 year and occasional abdominal pain. Both symptoms had become worse during the past 8 days.

RADIOLOGY

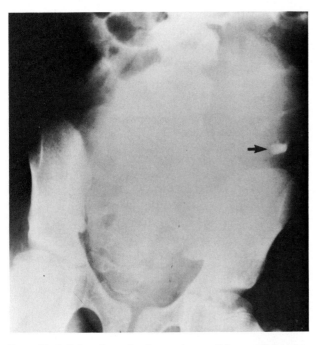

Figure 48–1. Plain radiography shows a large soft tissue mass arising from the pelvis and extending into the abdomen. There is a dense area of calcification (arrow).

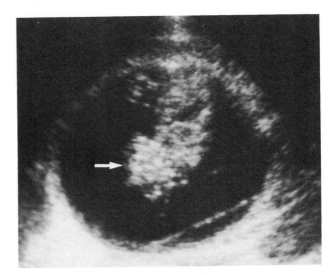

Figure 48–2. Transverse sonogram of the pelvis shows a 7- × 6-cm complex mass superior to the bladder. An internal echogenic region (arrow) appears to dangle from the anterior wall of the mass and is surrounded by hypoechoic material. A normal left ovary is not identified.

DIFFERENTIAL DIAGNOSIS

The differential diagnosis includes abscess, hematoma, hemorrhagic ovarian cyst, dermoid cyst, and ectopic pregnancy.

PATHOLOGY

The surgically resected mass measured 6.5 × 6.0 × 3.0 cm.

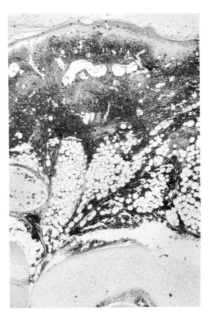

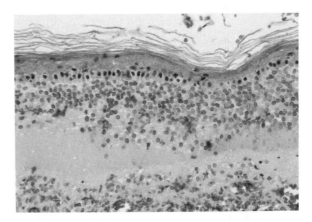

Figure 48–4. The squamous epithelium is multilayered and keratinizing, and there is underlying hemorrhage.

Figure 48–3. The ovary is largely replaced by a cystic mass. The cyst wall is focally lined by squamous epithelium and also contains cartilage and fat.

DIAGNOSIS

The final pathologic diagnosis was benign teratoma.

DISCUSSION

Ovarian neoplasms are uncommon in children and account for less than 1% of all pediatric tumors. Teratoma is the most common ovarian tumor in children. Less frequent ovarian neoplasms in the pediatric population include granulosa-theca cell tumors, adrenal rest tumors, and gonadoblastomas.

Teratomas are congenital tumors derived from the pluripotential cells of all three germ layers. The tumors often contain fat. Bone and tooth are present in 18% and 7%, respectively. The tumors are usually mature and benign, although approximately 1% degenerate into malignant squamous cell carcinoma.

The ovary is the second most common site for teratoma formation in the pediatric population. A sacrococcygeal location is most frequent. Cystic ovarian teratomas usually arise in adolescent girls; neonatal and early childhood presentations are less common. Teratomas may be bilateral in 20% of cases. Ovarian teratomas may be discovered as a palpable abdominal mass but frequently occur with signs of an acute abdominal condition caused by torsion of the involved ovary, rupture of the cyst, or infection of the cyst.

On plain radiographs of the abdomen, teratomas appear as soft tissue masses. Fat-fluid levels may be present on upright films. Teratomas in children typically contain less fat than those in adults. Calcifications may also be present in the form of teeth or bone fragments.

Sonographically, teratomas have a varied appearance ranging from purely cystic to mixed cystic and solid lesions, to solid masses. The fatty component of the tumor also varies in appearance. The mass may be echogenic if fat is intermixed with hair, or it may be echolucent if pure fat is present. The echolucency is presumed to be secondary to the lack of interfaces within a homogeneously fatty mass. The dermoid plug, an echogenic focus containing hair follicles, frequently arises from the cyst wall as in this case. Calcifications may also be identified by ultrasound, although CT detects them with greater sensitivity.

Cystic ovarian teratomas are treated by surgical excision. Asymptomatic tumors are resected to obviate the possibility of malignant degeneration.

REFERENCES

Fearnow E, Deluca S. Dermoid cyst of the ovary. Am Fam Prac 1988; 37:109–110.

Sandler M, et al. Gray-scale ultrasonographic features of ovarian teratomas. Radiology 1979; 131:705–709.

Sheth S, et al. The variable sonographic appearance of ovarian teratomas: correlation with CT. AJR 1988; 151:331–334.

Case 49

HISTORY

A 71-year-old Chinese immigrant complained of back pain. He denied having fevers, sweats, or neurologic symptoms.

RADIOLOGY

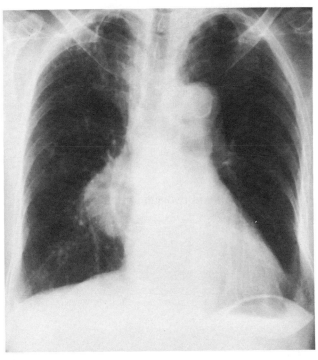

Figure 49–1. AP radiograph of the chest demonstrates biapical nodular densities and scarring. There is volume loss in both lung apices and pleural thickening. Bilateral paraspinal masses are present at the level of the left atrium.

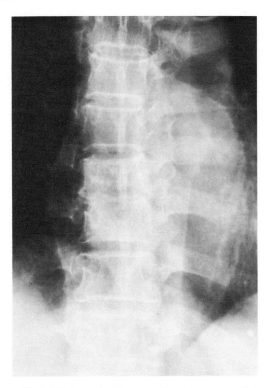

Figure 49–2. AP view of the thoracic spine demonstrates destruction of the disc between T8 and T9. A soft tissue mass surrounds the T8 and T9 vertebrae.

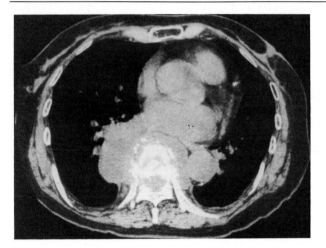

Figure 49-3. A CT scan through the level of the destroyed disc demonstrates a large paraspinal mass.

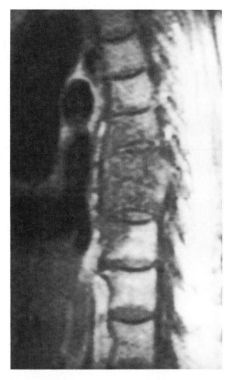

Figure 49-4. A sagittal MR scan done with T1 weighting (TR = 400, TE = 22) demonstrates complete obliteration of the disc space between T8 and T9. A soft tissue mass extends posteriorly into the spinal canal, displacing the spinal cord. The process has extended along the anterior spinal margins both caudally to involve the superior portion of T10 and superiorly to involve the T7 vertebral body. There is no gibbus deformity.

DIFFERENTIAL DIAGNOSIS

The differential diagnosis includes tuberculous spondylitis and pyogenic osteomyelitis. Metastasis and primary bone tumor are much less likely.

PATHOLOGY

A biopsy was performed.

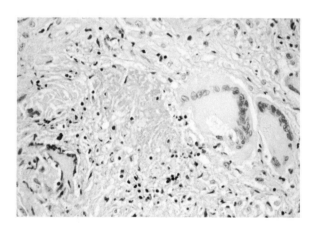

Figure 49-5. The biopsy specimen contains clusters of histiocytes of varying sizes. Many histiocytes have epithelioid characteristics, and some are multinucleated with the nuclei oriented toward the periphery of the cell (Langhans' giant cell). In the center of the clusters of histiocytes is eosinophilic necrotic tissue.

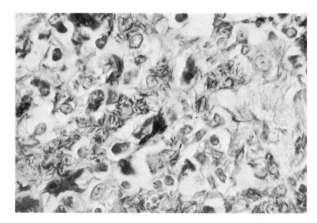

Figure 49-6. An acid-fast stain shows numerous rod-shaped red organisms within the cytoplasm of some of the histiocytes.

DIAGNOSIS

The final pathologic diagnosis was tuberculous spondylitis.

DISCUSSION

In the United States the yearly incidence of tuberculosis per 100,000 population had decreased from 200 cases in 1920 to 55 in 1950 to 14 in 1977. The prevalence of disease is much higher than these numbers suggest because only a small number of persons infected by *Mycobacterium tuberculosis* become clinically ill. Extrapulmonary sites are involved in 15% of cases and osteoarticular sites in 2% to 5%. Spondylitis comprises about half of the osteoarticular cases.

Tuberculous spondylitis is the result of hematogenous spread of organisms from a primary pulmonary source or from any source following reactivation. Infection destroys the end plate, invades the disc cartilage, and spreads to the neighboring vertebral body. Once beneath the longitudinal ligament, tuberculous exudate extends caudally and cranially, eroding the anterior aspect of many vertebral bodies. Compression fractures and angular kyphosis (gibbus deformity) result from bone destruction.

Paravertebral abscess occurs in 95% of patients and often calcifies. Unlike the more inflammatory abscesses due to pyogenic organisms, tuberculous abscesses provoke relatively little warmth and erythema. This "cold" abscess may extend into the pleural space, mediastinum, psoas muscle, or retropharyngeal space, depending on its location. Pus can burrow for an extraordinary distance and perforate the skin or penetrate into a body cavity or organ. A burrowing psoas abscess may drain from the groin. Inflammatory tissue can penetrate the posterior longitudinal ligament, resulting in an epidural abscess with eventual neurologic symptoms. Cord compression with paraplegia, once called "Pott's paralysis," occurs most frequently in the thoracic spine (presumably because the upper and middle thoracic spinal canal is narrowest). This epidural abscess can rupture the dura and infect the subarachnoid space.

Plain film findings may not be evident for weeks to months. The earliest signs include disc space narrowing, osteopenia, and paravertebral mass. CT scanning defines bone destruction, the relationship of the abscess to adjacent structures, and the presence of soft tissue calcification. MR imaging demonstrates prolonged T1 and T2 signals from involved vertebral bodies and provides valuable information about the thecal sac and spinal cord.

One of the distinguishing features of tuberculous spondylitis is the involvement of several vertebral bodies, unlike pyogenic infection, which usually destroys only two contiguous vertebral bodies. Paraspinal abscess is much less marked in patients with pyogenic infection, and the tendency of the lesion to involve the anterior parts of the vertebral bodies is lacking. Bony sclerosis, uncommon with tuberculosis, occurs within weeks to months after bacterial infection.

REFERENCES

Glassroth J, Robins AG, Snider ED. Tuberculosis in the 1980's. N Engl J Med 1980; 302(26): 1441–1449.

Jaffe HL. Metabolic, Degenerative and Inflammatory Diseases of Bones and Joints. Philadelphia: Lea & Febiger, Philadelphia, 1972.

Petersdorf FG, et al (eds). Harrison's Principles of Internal Medicine (10th ed). New York: McGraw-Hill, 1983.

Resnick D, Niwayama G. Ankylosing spondylitis. *In*: Resnick D, Niwayama G (eds). Diagnosis of Bone and Joint Disorders (2nd ed). Philadelphia: Saunders, 1988:1103–1170.

Case 50

HISTORY

A 68-year-old woman experienced acute mental status changes during long-term hospitalization in the intensive care unit.

RADIOLOGY

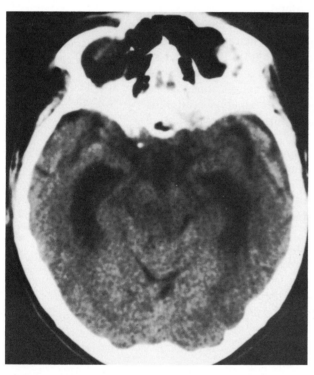

Figure 50-1. Noncontrast cranial CT scan obtained at the level of the sylvian aqueduct demonstrates a low density lesion located in the right tectal midbrain. Dilatation of both temporal horns suggests compression of the aqueduct and obstructive hydrocephalus.

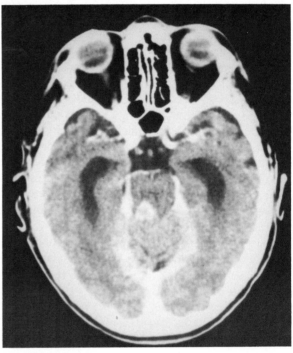

Figure 50-2. Contrast-enhanced CT scan shows a 1-cm ring-enhancing lesion in the right tectum. There is low attenuation edema in the brainstem. The aqueduct is compressed.

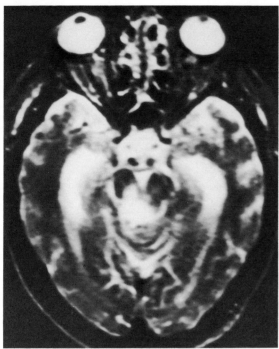

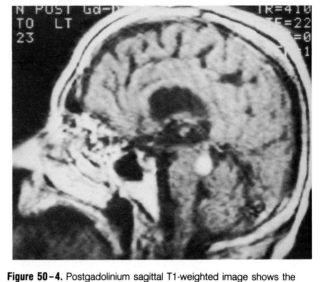

Figure 50–4. Postgadolinium sagittal T1-weighted image shows the tectal location of the lesion and its relationship to the cerebral aqueduct and fourth ventricle.

Figure 50–3. The late echo T2-weighted MR image demonstrates both the hyperintense lesion and the adjacent edema.

DIFFERENTIAL DIAGNOSIS

The differential diagnosis includes metastasis, glioma, abscess, tuberculoma, and lymphoma.

PATHOLOGY

The patient died. An autopsy was performed.

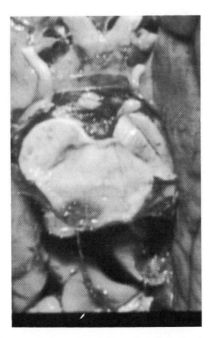

Figure 50–5. The gross specimen shows that the lesion is eccentrically located in the right tectum. The lesion is well circumscribed and hemorrhagic.

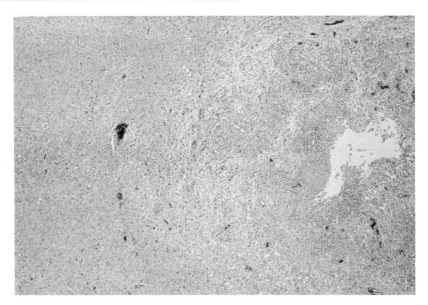

Figure 50-6. Microscopically the lesion is cavitated, and the lumen is surrounded by numerous inflammatory cells.

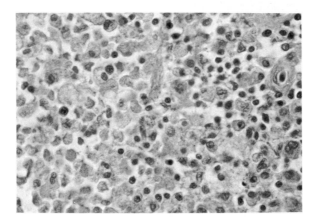

Figure 50-7. The inflammatory cells are focally necrotic and consist mainly of lymphocytes, plasma cells, and macrophages.

DIAGNOSIS

The final pathologic diagnosis was nocardial tectal abscess.

DISCUSSION

Nocardia is a ubiquitous, aerobic, gram-positive, weakly acid-fast bacterium. Clinical infections are typically seen in immunocompromised hosts, particularly patients with lymphoreticular malignancies, severe alcoholism, chronic steroid use, or acquired immune deficiency syndrome (AIDS). The primary focus of infection is the lungs. Multiorgan dissemination is present in 40% of patients. The most common site of secondary infection is the brain, which is involved in 27% of patients with systemic infection. *Nocardia* meningitis and single or multiple brain abscesses are seen. The *Nocardia asteroides* species accounts for 90% of these infections. No typical location or appearance of *Nocardia* brain abscess has been noted.

The differential diagnosis for ring-enhancing lesions in the brain includes abscess, primary neoplasm, metastasis, infarction, and noninfectious inflammatory lesions. The typical CT appearance of an abscess is a low-density lesion with an enhancing rim and surrounding edema. The rim is usually thin and uniform in appearance with a smooth inner margin. The enhancing rim is sometimes thinner on its medial or ventricular margin, possibly because of inhibition of fibroblast migration within the less well perfused deep white matter.

On MR imaging, abscesses appear as regions of low T1-weighted signal and increased T2-weighted signal. A thin encapsulating rim of increased T1 and decreased T2 signal is often present, which is attributed to the paramagnetic effects of either free radicals within macrophages or hemorrhage at the periphery of the lesion. As in the findings on CT, a ring of smooth, thin-walled gadolinium enhancement is typically seen.

Nocardial abscesses present diagnostic difficulties because of their nonspecific appearance. The diagnosis is sometimes not made before autopsy. The primary treatment is open or stereotactic surgical drainage in combination with trimethoprim-sulfamethoxazole antibiotics. Even with treatment, the mortality of patients with central nervous system involvement is about 40%.

REFERENCES

Bertoldi RV, Sperling MR. *Nocardia* brain stem abscess: diagnosis and response to medical therapy. Bull Clin Neurosci 1984; 49:99–104.

Haimes AB, Zimmerman RD, Morgello S, et al. MR imaging of brain abscesses. AJR 1989; 152: 1073–1085.

Hall WA, Martinez AJ, Dummer JS, et al. Nocardial brain abscess: diagnostic and therapeutic use of stereotactic aspiration. Surg Neurol 1987; 28: 114–118.

Hershewe GL, Davis LE, Bicknell JM. Primary cerebellar brain abscess from nocardiosis in a heroin addict. Neurology 1988; 38:1655–1656.

Talvar P, Chakrabarti A, Ayyagari A, et al. Brain abscess due to *Nocardia*. Mycopathologica 1989; 108:21–23.

Case 51

HISTORY

A 77-year-old male presented with left-sided abdominal pain.

RADIOLOGY

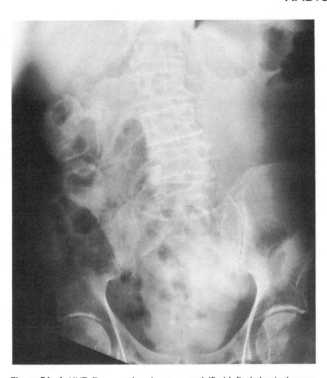

Figure 51-1. KUB film reveals a large noncalcified left abdominal mass displacing bowel to the right.

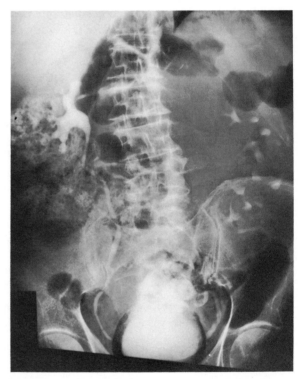

Figure 51-2. Intravenous pyelogram (IVP) demonstrates enlargement of the left kidney with stretching and distortion of the calices but preservation of the reniform shape.

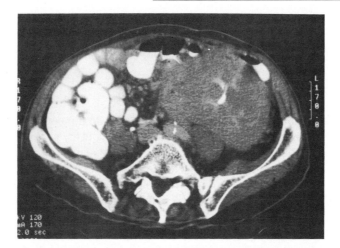

Figure 51-3. Abdominal CT scan shows a mass infiltrating and engulfing the right kidney. A faint outline of enhancing renal parenchyma can be identified, but the infiltrating mass is otherwise nonenhancing.

PATHOLOGY

A biopsy of the mass was obtained.

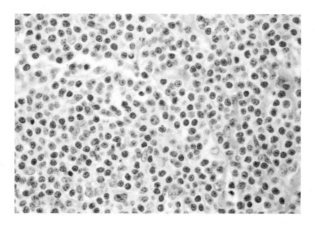

Figure 51-4. The lesion is composed of sheets of small lymphoid cells. Some of the cells demonstrate plasmacytoid features, with eccentric purple cytoplasm and nuclear chromatin distributed in a clock-face pattern.

DIAGNOSIS

The final pathologic diagnosis was primary lymphoma of the kidney.

DISCUSSION

Primary renal lymphoma is rare because the kidneys do not contain lymphoid tissue. Metastatic involvement of the kidney by lymphoma, however, is common. In autopsy series one third of lymphoma patients have renal involvement. Typically, multiple nodules involving both kidneys are found. Other presentations of metastatic lymphoma include solitary nodules, renal invasion from contiguous nodal disease, and diffuse involvement of a kidney, as in this patient. The nodular morphology common among B cell lymphomas is thought to reflect a degree of differentiation toward forming lymph nodelike elements. Renal involvement is more common in non-Hodgkin's lymphoma than in Hodgkin's disease. Burkitt's lymphoma and AIDS-related lymphomas have the greatest affinity for the kidneys.

The highly infiltrative nature of lymphoma allows it to grow without disrupting the renal structure or function until it is far advanced. Thus, renal lymphoma is detected late in its course, the most common presentation being abdominal pain or an abdominal mass, often with microscopic hematuria. Some patients have proteinuria and develop the nephrotic syndrome. Uremia is rare even though renal lymphoma is bilateral in 61% of cases. Hydronephrosis occurs when retroperitoneal adenopathy compresses the ureters or when renal stones form from the excess uric acid caused by the high rate of nucleic acid turnover. Hypertension may occur when the kidney becomes ischemic as a result of the tumor compressing the renal artery.

Diagnosis can often be made by fine-needle aspiration, as in this patient, thereby avoiding nephrectomy. Although renal involvement indicates disease, the prognosis may still be favorable owing to effective chemotherapy.

REFERENCES

Cotran RS, Kumar V, Robbins SL. Pathologic Basis of Disease (4th ed). Philadelphia: Saunders, 1989.
Davidson AJ. Radiology of the Kidney. Philadelphia: Saunders, 1985:307–314.
DeVita VT, Longo DL, Hubbard SM, et al. The lymphomas: biologic implications of therapy and therapeutic implications of the new biology. In: Berard CW, Dorfman RF, Kaufman N (eds). Malignant Lymphoma. Baltimore: Williams & Wilkins, 1987.
Harris GJ, Lager DJ. Primary renal lymphoma. J Surg Oncol 1991; 46:273–277.
Jafri SZH, et al. CT of renal and perirenal non-Hodgkin lymphoma. AJR 1982; 138:1101–1105.

Case 52

HISTORY

A 54-year-old male presented with a chronic pulmonary disease and recent complaints of blood-streaked sputum.

RADIOLOGY

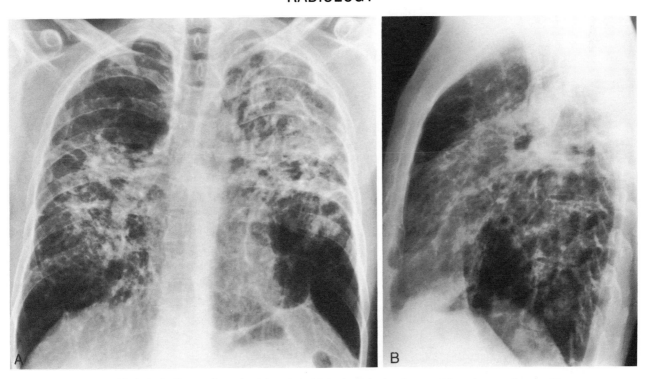

Figure 52-1. *A – B.* Chest radiographs demonstrate bilateral, predominantly upper lobe pulmonary fibrosis with retraction of the hila and apical bullous changes. No definite adenopathy is seen, but calcified left hilar nodes are present. There is a suggestion of a left upper lobe cavitating nodule with pleural thickening.

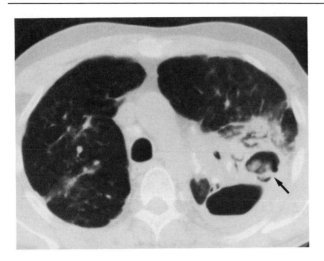

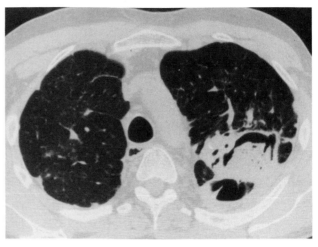

Figure 52-2. CT scan demonstrates right paratracheal and bilateral hilar calcified adenopathy (not shown). There is dense bilateral upper lobe fibrosis and a cavitating mass (arrow) in the left upper lobe. CT in the prone position (not shown) demonstrated a mobile component.

Figure 52-3. High resolution CT scans with 1.5-mm thick slices show the fibrosis and the cavitated mass.

DIFFERENTIAL DIAGNOSIS

The differential diagnosis includes mycetoma in chronic fibrotic lung disease such as sarcoidosis, tuberculosis, or occupational lung disease.

PATHOLOGY

Serologic studies performed during the current admission were positive for *Aspergillus fumigatus*. An open lung biopsy had been performed during a previous hospitalization.

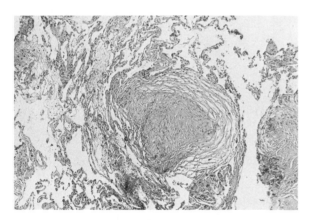

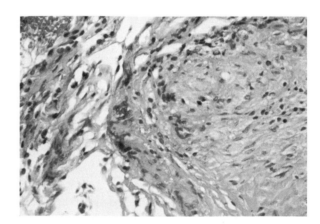

Figure 52-4. Lung biopsy specimen obtained during previous hospitalization shows small well-formed granulomas within the interstitium.

Figure 52-5. The granulomas are epithelioid and contain histiocytes with scattered multinucleated giant cells. Surrounding these cellular aggregates is a small amount of interstitial fibrosis.

DIAGNOSIS

The final diagnosis was chronic sarcoidosis with mycetoma.

DISCUSSION

Mycetomas are saprophytic fungus balls composed of a mass of septated mycelia plus cellular debris from the host. They invariably occupy preexisting cavities, cysts, or bullae within the lung. Fibrocystic pulmonary sarcoidosis, with its bronchiectatic and bullous cavities, is second only to tuberculosis as the most common antecedent lung disease associated with mycetomas. Aspergillomas are the most common type. An aspergilloma may present with hemoptysis; fatal hemorrhage from an aspergilloma is the second most common cause of death in patients with sarcoidosis.

The diagnosis of pulmonary aspergilloma is often made because of the characteristic radiographic appearance of a mobile opacity within a cavity surrounded by a crescent of air. Pleural thickening overlying cavities containing a fungus ball or preceding the appearance of a fungus ball has been described.

REFERENCES

Fajman W, Greenwald L, Staton G, et al. Assessing the activity of sarcoidosis: quantitative 67-Ga-citrate imaging. AJR 1984; 142:683–688.

Pare JAP, Fraser RG. Synopsis of Diseases of the Chest. Philadelphia: Saunders, 1983.

Rockoff SD, Rohatgi PK. Unusual manifestations of thoracic sarcoidosis. AJR 1985; 144:513–528.

Case 53

HISTORY

A 40-year-old woman complained of dysphagia for 2 months.

RADIOLOGY

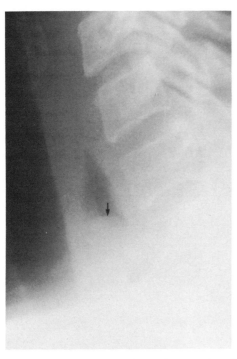

Figure 53–1. Lateral neck radiograph shows the apex of a soft tissue mass (arrow) in the esophagus.

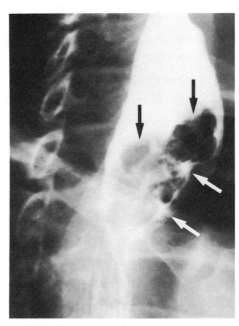

Figure 53–2. Barium esophagram shows an intraluminal polypoid lesion (black arrows) with deep ulceration (white arrows).

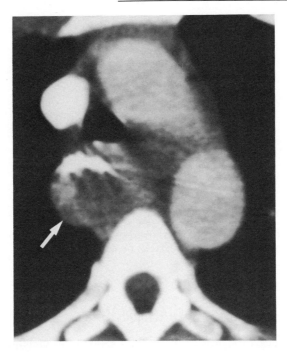

Figure 53-3. Contrast-enhanced CT scan at the level of the transverse aortic arch shows a mass (arrow) involving the posterior esophageal wall. Oral contrast is present in the esophageal lumen.

DIFFERENTIAL DIAGNOSIS

The differential diagnosis includes esophageal carcinoma, inflammatory polyp, and impacted food bolus.

PATHOLOGY

Esophagectomy was performed.

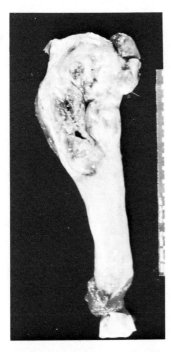

Figure 53-4. The resected esophagus demonstrates a large ulcerated mass with heaped borders.

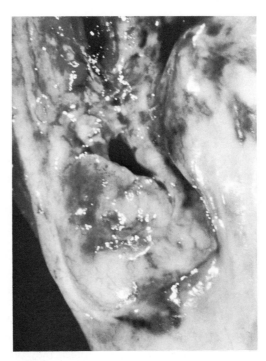

Figure 53-5. The superficial portions of the mass are hemorrhagic and focally pigmented.

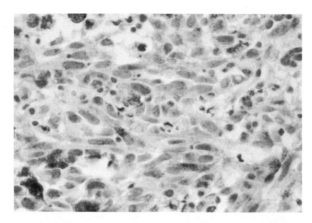

Figure 53-6. The mass consists of elongated malignant cells, many of which contain intracytoplasmic brown pigment.

DIAGNOSIS

The final pathologic diagnosis was primary esophageal melanoma.

DISCUSSION

Primary malignant melanoma of the esophagus is rare, accounting for 0.1% to 0.2% of esophageal malignancies and 0.5% of noncutaneous melanomas; melanoma metastatic to the esophagus may be even less common. The lesion is thought to arise from benign melanocytes found in the normal esophageal epithelium. The tumors spread horizontally along the epithelium but also grow vertically to form polypoid masses that are usually covered by intact mucosa. Adjacent satellite nodules may exist. Symptoms of dysphagia are related to mass effect, by which time the lesions are clinically advanced. The biologic behavior is aggressive, with hematogenous metastases to many organs and tissues and lymphatic metastases to the mediastinal and supraclavicular nodes.

On barium esophagram, primary melanoma usually appears as a polypoid intraluminal filling defect within a dilated esophageal segment. The surface is usually smooth except for focal ulcerations. CT is unlikely to demonstrate the depth of invasion into the esophageal wall, but this knowledge probably has no effect on outcome.

Figures 53-7 through 53-10 show images from the barium swallow, noncontrast enhanced CT scan, and MR image of a 33-year-old patient with benign esophageal leiomyoma. The pathology is shown in Figures 53-11 through 53-13. In contrast to neoplasms originating from the mucosal layer of the bowel wall, such as the common adenocarcinoma or uncommon primary melanoma, the great majority of leiomyomas arise intramurally. Leiomyoma is the most common benign esophageal neoplasm and involves the distal esophagus in more than 50% of cases. Six percent of all gastrointestinal leiomyomas are located in the esophagus. Whereas esophageal adenocarcinoma or primary melanoma requires wide surgical resection, patients with benign leiomyoma may be followed if there are no symptoms.

When a leiomyoma is viewed in profile, a barium swallow shows a smooth intramural defect and margins that form an obtuse angle with the wall of the esophagus. There is no undercutting of the margins. The mucosal surface remains intact unless the tumor becomes necrotic with ulceration of the overlying mucosal layer. Cavitation is uncommon. As the leiomyoma grows slowly, the esophageal lumen becomes draped over the intramural mass, which causes an eccentric mass effect without infiltration or direct invasion. On CT the tumor may project into the mediastinum or displace the adjacent lung and simulate a pulmonary mass. Leiomyoma is the most common of all esophageal neoplasms to present as a mediastinal mass.

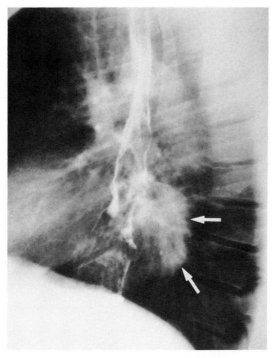

Figure 53-7. Lateral chest film obtained after a barium swallow shows a middle mediastinal mass (arrows) causing extrinsic deformity of the esophageal lumen.

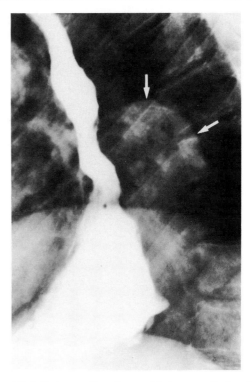

Figure 53-8. Barium swallow shows extrinsic mass effect on the esophagus at the level of the lesion (arrows). The mucosa is intact.

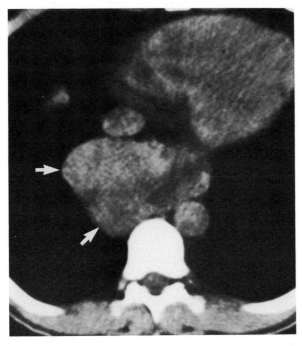

Figure 53-9. On noncontrast CT scan the subcarinal mass (arrows) displaces the inferior vena cava anteriorly and is not separate from the esophagus.

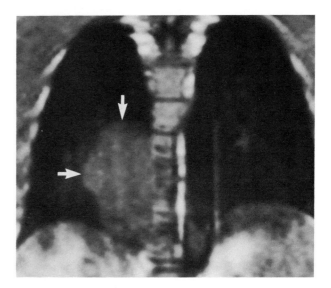

Figure 53-10. On T1-weighted coronal MR image (TR = 430, TE = 20), the signal intensity of the mass (arrows) appears isointense with muscle.

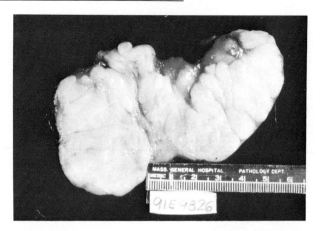

Figure 53–11. The bisected well-circumscribed mass is firm and tan-white.

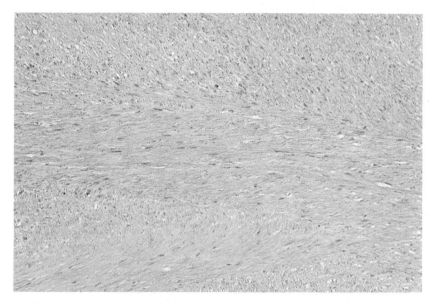

Figure 53–12. The hypocellular lesion consists of broad fascicles of spindle cells.

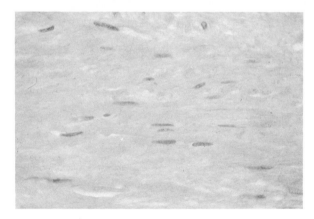

Figure 53–13. The spindle cells have elongated blunt-ended nuclei and tapered eosinophilic cytoplasmic processes.

REFERENCES

Isaacs JL, Quirke P. Two cases of primary malignant melanoma of the oesophagus. Clin Radiol 1988; 39:455–457.

Sabanathan S, Eng J, Pradam GN. Primary malignant melanoma of the esophagus. Am J Gastroenterol 1989; 84:1475–1481.

Case 54

HISTORY

A 7-year-old girl presented with progressive abdominal distention.

RADIOLOGY

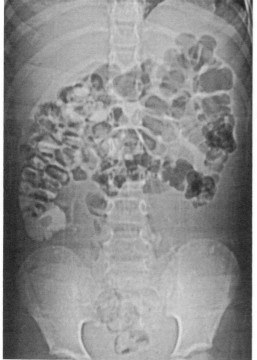

Figure 54-1. CT scout view of the abdomen shows superior displacement of bowel out of the pelvis.

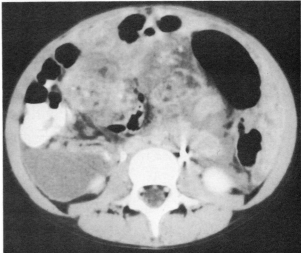

Figure 54-2. Contrast-enhanced CT scan demonstrates heterogeneous enhancement of a central mass lesion containing regions of fat, fluid, and soft tissue attenuation. Peritoneal fluid is present in the right paracolic gutter.

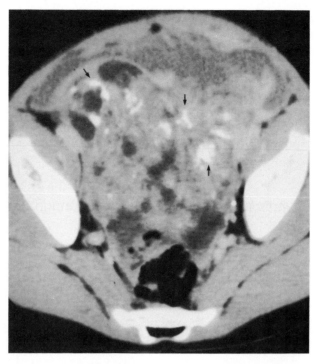

Figure 54-3. At the level of the pelvis the heterogeneous mass contains calcifications (arrows). Neither uterus nor ovaries can be identified separate from the mass.

DIFFERENTIAL DIAGNOSIS

The differential diagnosis includes malignant teratoma, neuroblastoma, rhabdomyosarcoma, and lymphoma.

PATHOLOGY

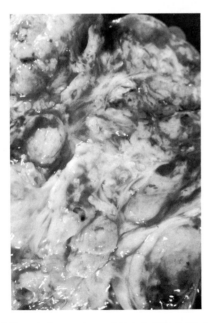

Figure 54-4. Resected ovary demonstrates multiple focally hemorrhagic solid nodules.

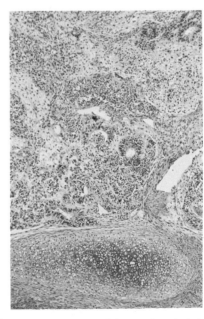

Figure 54-5. Various components of the neoplasm include cartilage and epithelial elements.

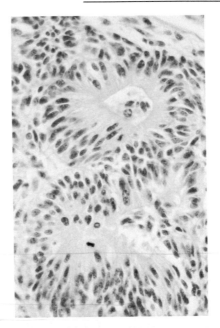

Figure 54–6. Portions of the tumor demonstrate rosettes formed by malignant elongated cells with eosinophilic cytoplasmic extensions oriented around a central lumen.

DIAGNOSIS

The final pathologic diagnosis was malignant ovarian teratoma.

DISCUSSION

Teratomas arise from totipotential cells, which differentiate into ectodermal, meso-dermal, and endodermal elements. Benign teratoma contains well-differentiated cells and organoid elements. Most of these benign lesions are complex cystic structures containing a preponderance of ectodermal elements. Malignant teratomas contain immature cells that are incompletely differentiated and not organized into organoid structures. These malignant lesions are typically solid. The most anaplastic of malignant teratomas contain abundant neuroepithelial elements and demonstrate local invasion and distant metas-tases.

Teratomas occurring in childhood most commonly arise from the sacrococcygeal region. Most congenital teratomas are benign and are detected at birth because of mass effect on the perineum. The older the patient at the time of detection, the greater the likelihood that the tumor is malignant. Ovarian teratomas are bilateral in 10% of patients. The majority of ovarian teratomas occur after the age of 6, predominantly during adolescence. Like sacrococcygeal tumors, malignant degeneration occurs with increasing age. Two thirds of patients with ovarian teratoma eventually present with a palpable pelvic or abdominal mass. Another common presentation is pain, nausea, and vomiting due to torsion of the mass or spontaneous hemorrhage. Patients with malignant teratoma may develop constitutional symptoms including malaise and weight loss.

Plain films show a pelvic or abdominal mass with bowel displacement. Calcifications are present in the majority of cases and sometimes look like teeth. Radiolucent collec-tions of fat occur less frequently in younger patients and typically indicate a benign tumor. Fat is uncommon in malignant lesions because of the lack of cellular differentia-tion. Whereas sonography shows a cystic component in benign teratoma, malignant lesions are usually solid and homogeneously heterogeneous. Sonography also shows obstructive hydronephrosis when the lesion compresses the ureters. Because these lesions are often large, CT better delineates the relationship of the tumor to the pelvic and abdominal organs. CT is more sensitive in identifying small collections of fat and calcific foci as well as infiltration of adjacent organs and the peritoneal cavity.

Resection of a benign teratoma alone or in combination with the ovary results in cure. Both sacrococcygeal and ovarian tumors are resected as soon as feasible because of their potential for malignant transformation. Malignant teratomas have usually pene-trated the ovarian capsule by the time of surgery and have invaded the surrounding structures. Most are unresectable at the time of diagnosis. These patients undergo de-bulking followed by radiation or chemotherapy.

REFERENCES

Billmire DF, Grosfeld JL. Teratomas in childhood: analysis of 142 cases. J Pediatr Surg 1986; 21:548–551.

Shith S, et al. The variable sonographic appearances of ovarian teratomas: comparison with CT. AJR 1988; 151:331–334.

Siegel MJ, et al. Radiographic findings in ovarian teratomas in children. AJR 1978; 131:139–141.

Case 55

HISTORY

An 18-year-old male presented with a painless mass involving the right upper tibia.

RADIOLOGY

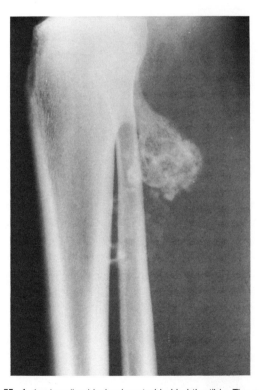

Figure 55-1. A mineralized lesion is noted behind the tibia. The more cranial portions of the lesion are more densely mineralized and appear to be in continuity with the tibial cortex. The point of attachment between the lesion and the tibia is a classic "chimney sign." Proximally the lesion is densely mineralized and ossified. The more distal parts of the lesion appear more lucent, flocculent, and curvilinear.

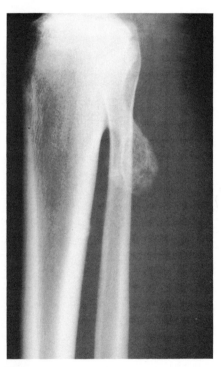

Figure 55-2. On a similar film obtained 1 year earlier much less mineralization was present.

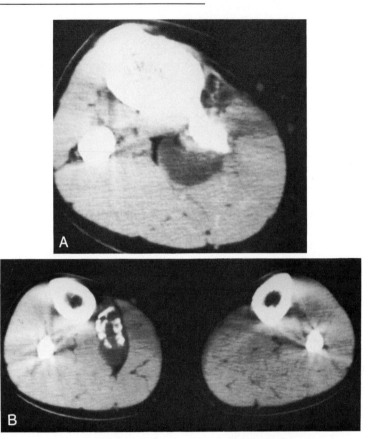

Figure 55–3. *A.* CT scan shows cortical continuity of the lesion with the tibia. A low attenuation soft tissue mass is present. *B.* More distally, the low attenuation soft tissue mass contains calcifications within it.

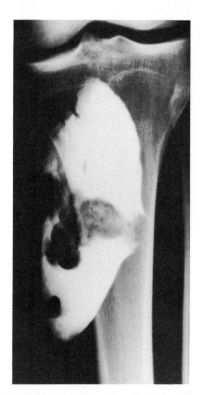

Figure 55–4. Fluid was aspirated from the lesion. After contrast injection, multiple filling defects can be seen.

DIFFERENTIAL DIAGNOSIS

The differential diagnosis includes malignant transformation of an osteochondroma, bursa formation with or without secondary osteochondromatosis, and previously fractured osteochondroma.

PATHOLOGY

The lesion was resected.

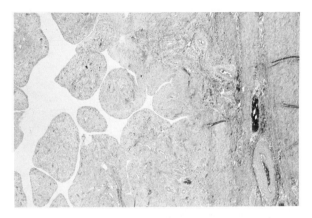

Figure 55-5. A portion of the specimen consists of a cystic structure into which protrude broad fronds of synovium. The fronds are lined by synovial cells.

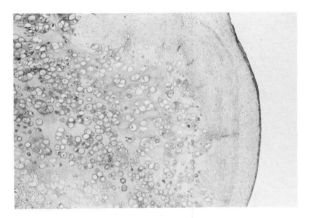

Figure 55-6. Within the wall of the synovial tissue is hypocellular cytologically bland hyaline cartilage.

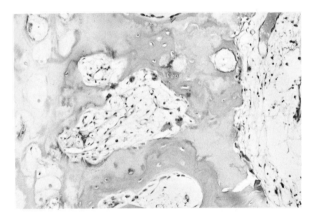

Figure 55-7. The base of the cartilage is undergoing enchondral ossification.

DIAGNOSIS

The final diagnosis was bursal osteochondromatosis complicating an osteochondroma.

DISCUSSION

In this patient a bursa formed as a complication of an adjacent ostechondroma. Synovial osteochondromatosis, in turn, formed within the bursa. For other complications of osteochondromas, see Case 7. Synovial chondromatosis (SC) or osteochondromatosis is a rare benign monoarticular condition in which cartilaginous nodules form through metaplastic transformation of the connective tissue of synovial membranes. It can affect joints, bursae, or tendon sheaths. The cause of primary synovial chondromatosis is unknown, but it is most likely a reactive response of the synovial membrane rather than a neoplastic change. As the cartilaginous nodules continue to grow they may remain attached to the synovium by a vascular pedicle, or they may become detached, forming a loose body. These loose bodies may continue to increase in size as the cartilage receives nourishment from the synovial fluid. The nodule may even reestablish its vascular supply by implanting itself within the hyperplastic synovium at a different location.

The most common joints affected by synovial chondromatosis are the knee, hip, and elbow. Primary SC may affect only a portion of the synovium or the entire synovium of a particular joint. The disorder is more common in men and usually is diagnosed in the third to fifth decades. The patient presents with joint pain, swelling, and possibly limitation of motion or locking. Mineralized loose bodies can be visualized on plain films as multiple juxta-articular densities of varying size and shape. The involved joint may become widened and eroded, eventually leading to secondary osteoarthritis.

Secondary osteochondromatosis is a separate entity in which loose bodies are formed as a result of trauma to the articular surface and subarticular bone. Processes that can result in secondary synovial (osteo)chondromatosis include osteoarthritis, neuropathic arthropathy, osteochondritis dissecans, rheumatoid arthritis, tuberculosis of the joint, and osteochondral fractures. Primary and secondary synovial chondromatosis can be differentiated histologically because the latter contains fragments of the articular surface. Furthermore, in primary SC the synovial membrane is hyperplastic, and larger numbers of cartilaginous nodules are seen. It is not always possible to distinguish primary from secondary synovial chondromatosis radiographically, especially primary SC, in which many of the cartilaginous nodules are radiolucent. Jaffe (1958) diagnosed primary synovial chondromatosis only when there was cartilage metaplasia in the subsynovial tissue. Since then, Milgram (1977) and Schajowicz (1981) have extended Jaffe's criteria to include patients with four or more osteocartilaginous loose bodies in a joint in the absence of synovial metaplasia when no other cause can be found.

The traditional treatment for synovial chondromatosis is surgical removal of the loose bodies and synovectomy. It may be technically impossible to remove all synovial tissue. Some practitioners advocate synovectomy only for patients who have an "active" or proliferative synovium on histologic examination. Removal of the loose bodies alone may be adequate in patients with late-stage or quiescent disease.

REFERENCES

Casselman J, et al. CT findings in synovial chondromatosis of the temporomandibular joint. J Comput Assist Tomogr 1987; 11(5):898–900.

Jaffe HL. *Tumors and Tumorous Conditions of the Bones and Joints.* Philadelphia: Lea and Febiger, 1958.

Lagier R. Case report 451. Skel Radiol 1987; 16:660–665.

Maurice H, et al. Synovial chondromatosis. J Bone Joint Surg 1988; 70B(5):807–811.

Milgram J, Keagy R. Bursal osteochondromatosis: a case report. Clin Orthop 1989; 144:269–271.

Milgram JW. The classification of loose bodies in human joints. Clin Orthop Rel Res 1977; 124:282–302.

Peterson H. Multiple hereditary osteochondromata. Clin Orthop 1989; 239:222–230.

Schajowicz F. *Tumor and Tumorlike Lesions of Bone Joints.* New York: Springer Verlag, 1981.

Case 56

HISTORY

A 17-year-old boy presented with ataxia.

RADIOLOGY

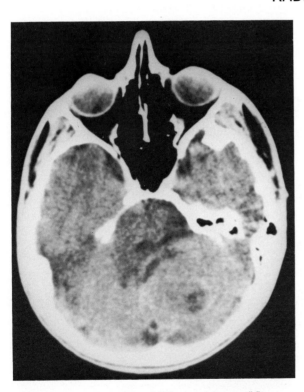

Figure 56-1. Noncontrast-enhanced CT scan shows a mildly hyperdense mass involving the superior vermis and left cerebellum. There is a linear low attenuation area anteromedially and a rounded low attenuation area centrally with no calcification. The mass measures approximately 5 cm in diameter.

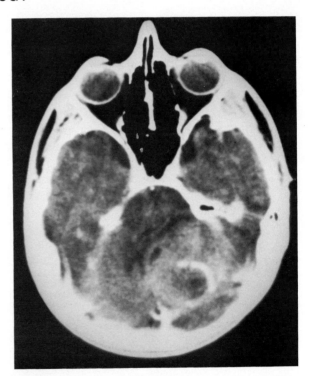

Figure 56-2. Following contrast administration the mass enhances heterogeneously, and the low attenuation regions persist. Another linear region enhances densely and suggests a vessel. The fourth ventricle is compressed anteriorly.

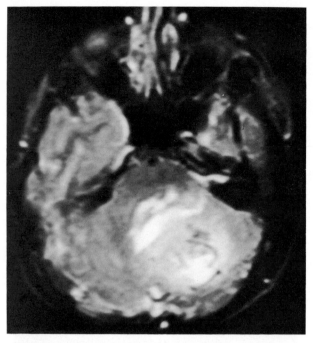

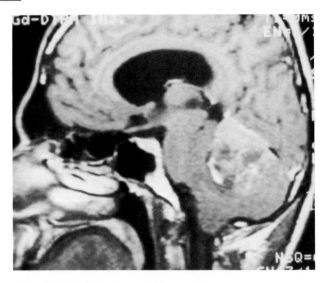

Figure 56–4. Patchy enhancement surrounds hypointense foci within the mass on the sagittal postgadolinium T1-weighted image. The cerebral aqueduct is compressed.

Figure 56–3. Late echo T2-weighted axial MR image shows that the mass is heterogeneous and only mildly hyperintense.

DIFFERENTIAL DIAGNOSIS

The differential diagnosis includes ependymoma, medulloblastoma, astrocytoma, meningioma, and choroid plexus papilloma.

PATHOLOGY

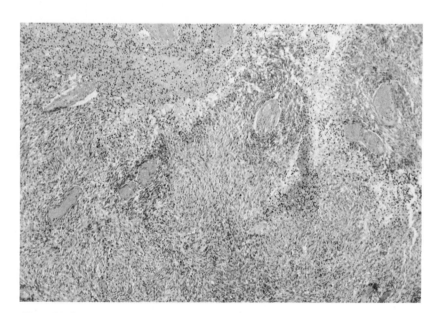

Figure 56–5. The tumor is very cellular and contains irregular areas of hemorrhagic necrosis.

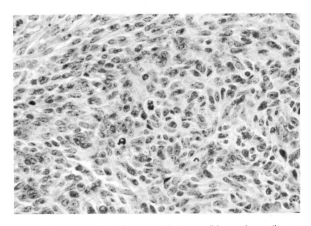

Figure 56-6. The tumor cells are relatively small hyperchromatic areas and are round to elongated. Mitoses are numerous.

DIAGNOSIS

The final pathologic diagnosis was medulloblastoma.

DISCUSSION

Medulloblastoma is the second most frequent posterior fossa neoplasm in children after cerebellar astrocytoma. The tumors are part of the spectrum of primitive neuroectodermal tumor (PNET) and generally originate at the roof of the fourth ventricle. Histologically, the lesion is hypercellular, composed of poorly differentiated hyperchromatic cells with scant cytoplasm. The lesions commonly occur in the midline and fill the fourth ventricle, although they can extend laterally into the cerebellar hemisphere, particularly in older patients. There is a male to female ratio of 3:2, and peak incidence occurs between the ages of 3 and 5. Clinical manifestations are similar to those of other posterior fossa tumors, including signs and symptoms of increasing intracranial pressure, such as headache, vomiting, papilledema, ataxia, and nystagmus. However, the onset of symptoms in patients with medulloblastoma is typically acute, with hydrocephalus and ataxia occurring early. The tumor is highly malignant and has a marked propensity for invasion of the leptomeninges and spread through the cerebrospinal fluid pathways. Distant metastases, most often to bone but also to the liver and lungs, usually occur late in the disease.

The typical appearance of medulloblastoma on CT is a well-marginated, solid, high density, homogeneously enhancing mass located within the fourth ventricle and associated with hydrocephalus. On MR imaging the tumor is generally hypointense on T1-weighted images and nearly isointense with brain parenchyma on T2-weighted images, probably because of its high cell density. Gadolinium enhancement is usually marked. However, up to 47% of medulloblastomas demonstrate atypical features including cystic or necrotic change, calcification, hemorrhage, lack of contrast enhancement, eccentric location, or supratentorial extension. This characteristic may be reflected in an atypical or heterogeneous appearance on both MR and CT, making differentiation from ependymoma or astrocytoma difficult.

Both gadolinium-enhanced MR and myelography are used to detect drop metastases along the spinal subarachnoid space. Enhanced MR is also helpful for detecting subependymal seeding in the brain. Treatment consists of surgical resection in combination with radiation therapy.

REFERENCES

Altman N, Fitz CR, Chuang S, et al. Radiologic characteristics of primitive neuroectodermal tumors in children. Am J Neuroradiol 1985; 6:15–18.

Ganti SR, Silver AJ, Diefenbach P, et al. Computed tomography of primitive neuroectodermal tumors. Am J Neuroradiol 1983; 4:819–821.

Kleinman GH, Hochberg FH, Richardson EP. Systemic metastases from medulloblastoma: report of two cases and review of the literature. Cancer 1981; 48:2296–2309.

Zee CS, Segall HD, Miller C, et al. Less common CT features of medulloblastoma. Radiology 1982; 144:97–102.

Case 57

HISTORY

A 53-year-old female presented following the incidental finding of a renal mass on an ultrasound examination performed to evaluate a 3-day history of jaundice.

RADIOLOGY

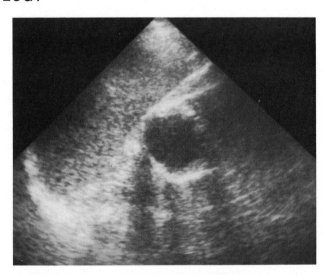

Figure 57-2. Ultrasound demonstrates that the mass is cystic. Acoustic shadowing is evident owing to the calcification of the wall.

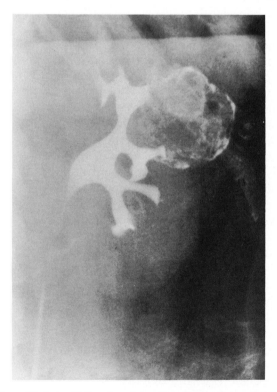

Figure 57-1. An AP film of a retrograde pyelogram demonstrates a 4-cm mass with a calcified wall in the upper pole of the left kidney.

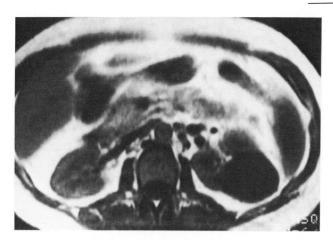

Figure 57-3. T1-weighted axial MR images (TR = 400, TE = 15). The mass has a smooth well-demarcated border and is of uniform low attenuation.

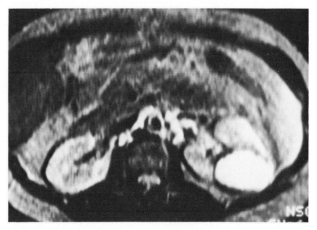

Figure 57-4. T2-weighted axial image (TR = 2000, TE = 96). The mass is of uniform brightness. The calcification in the wall is evident from a thin rim of absent signal, particularly on the medial aspect of the mass.

DIFFERENTIAL DIAGNOSIS

The differential diagnosis includes echinococcosis, malakoplakia, segmental xanthogranulomatous pyelonephritis, abscess, hematoma, and tuberculoma.

PATHOLOGY

Nephrectomy was performed.

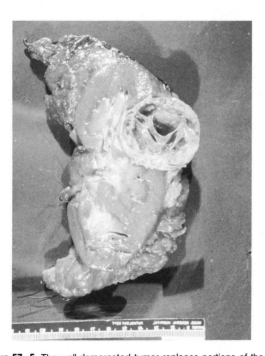

Figure 57-5. The well-demarcated tumor replaces portions of the renal cortex and bulges into the overlying capsule. The tumor is markedly cystic.

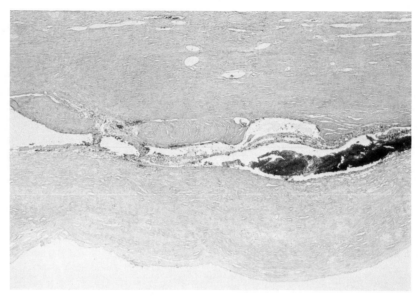

Figure 57-6. Histologically the cyst lumen contains red blood cells and within the wall are small groups of atypical epithelial cells.

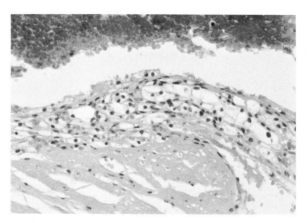

Figure 57-7. The tumor cells have prominent clear cytoplasm.

DIAGNOSIS

The final pathologic diagnosis was renal cell carcinoma (cystic variant).

DISCUSSION

Renal cell carcinoma, also termed renal adenocarcinoma or hypernephroma, comprises 85% of all renal neoplasms but less than 3% of adult malignancies. Renal cell carcinoma is a neoplasm of the tubular epithelium, probably arising in the proximal convoluted tubules. The peak incidence occurs in the sixth and seventh decades, and there is a male to female ratio of 2:1. Presenting signs and symptoms include hematuria, flank pain, flank mass, fever, weight loss, varicoceles, and paraneoplastic syndromes. There appears to be some association with tobacco and phenacetin use.

Most lesions are readily diagnosable by their imaging characteristics. On noncontrast-enhanced CT scans, the lesions are isodense or hyperdense with respect to the kidney; following contrast administration there is variable enhancement (usually less than that of the normal renal parenchyma), depending on vascularity and injection technique. Typical CT findings include a thick irregular wall, a lobulated contour, and irregular calcifications. A calcified renal mass is carcinoma until proven otherwise; peripheral rim calcifications may be seen in a significant number of lesions, causing confusion with simple cysts. Urographically, the neoplastic kidney has normal function in most cases. On angiography the lesions are predominantly hypervascular (5% hypovascular). Prominent neovascularity and arteriovenous fistulas are often present.

Cystic renal cell carcinomas represent a subgroup of renal cell carcinomas that may be difficult to differentiate from benign renal cysts. Specific CT and sonographic criteria have been established for the diagnosis of a simple renal cyst. On CT, a simple renal cyst should have uniform low density (0 to 20 HU), no enhancement following intravenous contrast administration, an imperceptible wall when the cyst projects beyond the renal outline, and a smooth interface with the renal parenchyma. No internal calcifications should be present. On ultrasound, simple renal cysts should be anechoic, have smooth, sharply defined walls, and have posterior acoustic enhancement.

Approximately 95% of all renal cysts fulfill the above criteria and can be confidently diagnosed as simple renal cysts without further evaluation. The remaining 5% of renal cysts are indeterminate. A significant percentage (31%) of indeterminate lesions are shown pathologically to be malignant.

Recently, MR has been used to evaluate those cysts that cannot be diagnosed by CT and sonography. Proposed MR criteria for simple cysts are similar to those applying to sonography and CT with additional requirements for the behavior of the cyst fluid. Simple renal cysts are generally filled with a fluid that is similar in composition to serum. This composition leads to a T1 signal intensity that is less than that of the renal medulla and comparable to that of urine. On T2-weighted sequences, the lesions show a markedly increased signal relative to renal parenchyma. By contrast, the fluid in cystic renal cell carcinoma is usually hemorrhagic and contains increased lipid and lactic acid dehydrogenase levels leading to a T1 signal intensity that varies from intermediate to high intensity. These lesions also show increased intensity on T2-weighted images.

About 25% of patients with renal cell carcinoma have metastases at presentation. The most common sites of metastases are the lungs, lymph nodes, liver, bone, adrenal gland, and contralateral kidney.

The primary treatment for renal cell carcinoma is radical nephrectomy (curative only for early disease). In patients in whom the tumor has extended to the vena cava, radical nephrectomy and total removal of thrombus from the vena cava can also be curative. Adjuvant chemotherapy is also given when metastases are present. The prognosis for both cystic and solid renal cell carcinoma ranges from a 5-year survival rate of 68% for stage I disease to a 5-year survival of 9% for stage IV disease.

In the case presented, the imaging is suggestive of malignancy because of the low-level echoes demonstrable on ultrasound and the peripheral calcifications visible on plain film and MR images. Interestingly, however, the fluid within the cyst behaves like that of a benign cyst with a T1 signal intensity lower than that of the renal medulla.

REFERENCES

Curry N, et al. An evaluation of the effectiveness of CT versus other imaging modalities in the diagnosis of atypical renal masses. Invest Radiol 1984; 19:447–452.

Davidson A. Diagnostic set—large, unifocal, unilateral. *In*: Davidson A (ed). Radiology of the Kidney. Philadelphia: Saunders, 1985.

Hartman D, et al. Cystic renal cell carcinoma. Urology 1986; 28:145–153.

Johnson C, et al. Renal adenocarcinoma—CT staging of 100 tumors. AJR 1987; 148:59–63.

Lang E. An algorithmic approach to the diagnosis and staging of renal neoplasms. Radiol Clin North Am 1986; 24:683–694.

Lee J, Sagel S, Stuart R. Computed Body Tomography with MRI Correlation (2nd ed). New York: Raven Press, 1989.

Marotti M, et al. Complex and simple renal cysts: comparative evaluation with MR imaging. Radiology 1987; 162:679–684.

Case 58

HISTORY

A 55-year-old female resident of a sanitorium, who was receiving antituberculosis therapy, presented with persistent fevers, cough, and night sweats.

RADIOLOGY

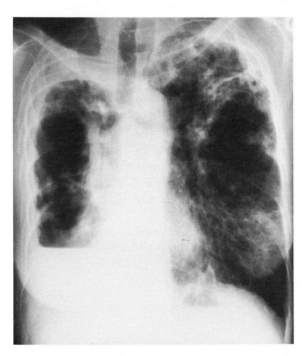

Figure 58-1. Chest radiograph demonstrates marked destruction of normal pulmonary architecture on the right, with little tissue resembling lung parenchyma. There is extensive cavitation and an air-fluid level within a dominant cavity. There is volume loss. On the left patchy areas of consolidation are superimposed upon extensive fibroapical changes. Prominent bilateral pleural thickening is present.

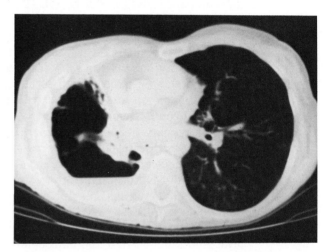

Figure 58-2. CT scan demonstrates a thick pleural rind surrounding parenchymal destruction on the right, with right hilar calcification. Scarring and cavitation in the left upper lung are present, with relative sparing of the lower lobe.

DIFFERENTIAL DIAGNOSIS

The differential diagnosis includes tuberculosis, atypical mycobacterial infections, necrotizing bacterial pneumonia (including organisms such as *Klebsiella*, *Staphylococcus*, and *Streptococcus*), fungal infections, and nocardiosis or actinomycosis.

PATHOLOGY

A right pneumonectomy was performed.

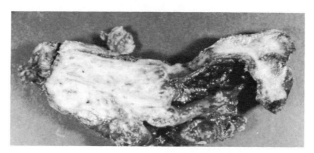

Figure 58-3. The gross specimen shows consolidated anthracotic pulmonary parenchyma with areas of pale yellow discoloration.

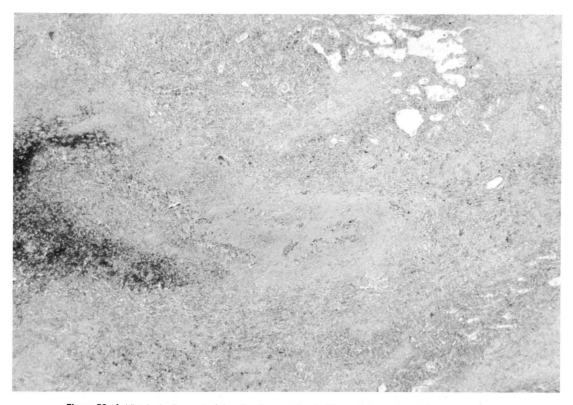

Figure 58-4. Histologically most of the alveoli are obliterated by an inflammatory infiltrate and fibrosis.

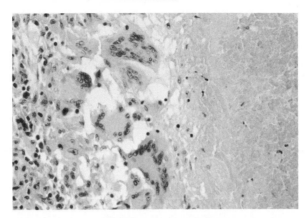

Figure 58-5. The inflammation is characterized by regions of necrosis surrounded by multinucleated giant cells and epithelioid histiocytes. Acid-fast stains were positive, and culture was positive for an atypical mycobacterium, *Mycobacterium avium-intracellulare.*

DIAGNOSIS

The final pathologic diagnosis was atypical mycobacterial pneumonia.

DISCUSSION

In 1900 tuberculosis was the leading cause of death in the United States. With improved sanitation and the advent of effective antibiotics, the death rate decreased markedly. In the last 20 years there has been a mild resurgence in the incidence of tuberculosis and a larger increase in the incidence of atypical mycobacterial infections. Although infection with nontuberculous mycobacteria most common among immunocompromised patients (particularly those with acquired immune deficiency syndrome [AIDS]), the prevalence of nontuberculous mycobacteria among immunocompetent patients may be greater than the prevalence of tuberculosis.

Mycobacteria are classified into tuberculous and nontuberculous forms. Nontuberculous forms are able to grow in culture at both 25 and 37°C, whereas *Mycobacterium tuberculosis* grows only at 37°C. Nontuberculous mycobacteria are further subcategorized by culture characteristics such as morphology, rate of growth, and pigmentation. Clinically important organisms include *M. avium* and *M. intracellulare* (commonly grouped together owing to their similar culture appearance), *M. xenopi*, and *M. kansasii.* However, the clinical treatment, prognosis, and radiographic appearance are the same for all species.

Infection with nontuberculous mycobacteria in immunocompetent patients is similar to secondary tuberculosis. The typical patient is 60 to 65 years old, and there is an equal sex distribution. Whites are more commonly afflicted than other racial groups, and the disease often occurs in patients with chronic obstructive pulmonary disease or other long-standing pulmonary disease. Radiographically, approximately 50% of patients may have an upper lobe–dominated parenchymal pattern of nodular or alveolar opacities like that seen in tuberculosis, but the others have equal or greater involvement of the middle and lower lobes. Pleural effusions and adenopathy are infrequent in nontuberculous mycobacterial infections of immunocompetent patients. Cavitation occurs in 43% to 90% of patients and is commonly associated with thin cavity walls.

The clinical appearance of nontuberculous mycobacterial infection in AIDS patients is distinct from that seen in immunocompetent hosts. Ten to twenty percent of AIDS patients are diagnosed with nontuberculous mycobacteria during life, and autopsy studies indicate that more than 50% of patients are infected. The patients are younger, and there is a male predominance. Unlike immunocompetent patients, AIDS patients invariably have extrapulmonary infections. On chest radiography, patchy, often bilateral and coalescing alveolar densities are typical, and adenopathy may be present. Cavitation and pleural effusions are not uncommon.

Nontuberculous mycobacterial infection in immunocompetent patients is a potentially curable disease, and multidrug regimens of antimycobacterial drugs are used.

REFERENCES

Albelda SM, Kern JA, Marinelli DL, et al. Expanded spectrum of pulmonary disease caused by nontuberculous mycobacteria. Radiology 1985; 157: 289–296.

Marinelli DC. Non-tuberculous mycobacteria infection in AIDS: clinical, pathologic and radiographic features. Radiology 1986; 160:77–82.

Pare JAP, Fraser RG. Synopsis of Diseases of the Chest. Philadelphia: Saunders, 1983:287–321.

Woodring JH, Vandiviere HM, Fried AM, et al. Update: the radiographic features of pulmonary tuberculosis. AJR 1986; 146:497–506.

Case 59

A 58-year-old physician with stable angina presented with a 1-month complaint of epigastric pain.

RADIOLOGY

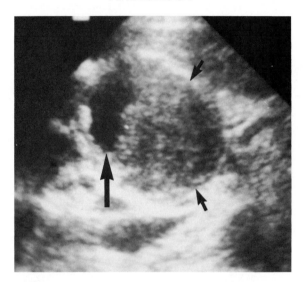

Figure 59-1. Transverse sonogram of the pancreas shows a heterogeneous mass (small black arrows) located in the region of the pancreatic head. The mass contains an anechoic region (large black arrow).

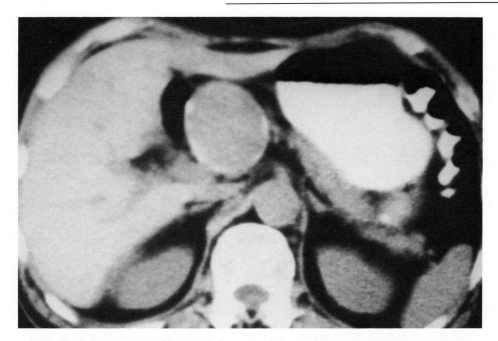

Figure 59-2. On noncontrast CT scan this 5-cm mass is homogeneous with peripheral calcifications.

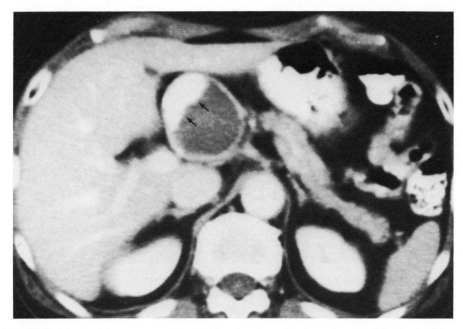

Figure 59-3. Following intravenous contrast administration, the mass shows dense, peripheral enhancement (arrows) identical to that of the aorta.

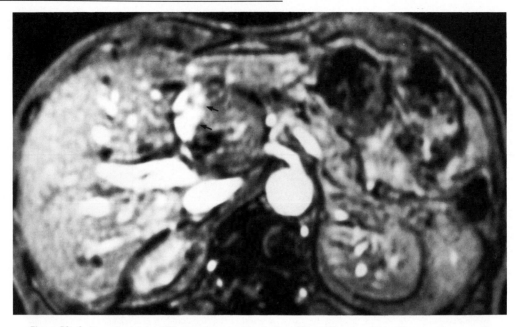

Figure 59-4. A gradient echo MR sequence sensitive to flow (TR = 22 msec, TE = 13 msec, flip angle 30 degrees) shows an elliptical region of heterogeneously increased signal (arrows) representing turbulent flow.

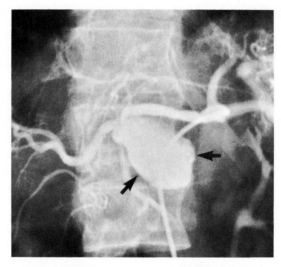

Figure 59-5. Selective celiac arteriography demonstrates an elliptical contrast collection (arrows) at the bifurcation of the common hepatic artery into the proper hepatic and gastroduodenal arteries.

DIFFERENTIAL DIAGNOSIS

The differential diagnosis includes cystic neoplasm of the pancreas, pancreatic pseudocyst, pancreatic abscess, choledochal cyst, and aneurysm.

PATHOLOGY

The patient underwent exploratory laparotomy with resection of a 9- × 4- × 4-cm mass lesion. The cut surface (not shown) demonstrated laminated thrombosis with focal areas of calcification.

Figure 59-6. Attached to the wall are intermixed layers of fibrin, red blood cells, and platelets.

DIAGNOSIS

The final diagnosis was hepatic artery aneurysm.

DISCUSSION

Hepatic artery aneurysm often causes vague symptoms until leaking blood progresses to rupture and catastrophic hemorrhage. Increased use of ultrasound and cross-sectional imaging has resulted in diagnosis of asymptomatic aneurysms followed by elective therapy such as surgical resection or percutaneous catheter embolization. Hepatic artery aneurysms are the second most common aneurysm of the splanchnic arteries. Splenic artery aneurysms occur with greater frequency. Before the antibiotic era, most hepatic artery aneurysms had a mycotic etiology. Atherosclerosis is now the most common cause, and infection accounts for only 10% of hepatic artery aneurysms. Other causes include penetrating trauma, cystic medial necrosis, and polyarteritis.

Hepatic artery aneurysms are extrahepatic in 80% of cases and intrahepatic in 20%. Aneurysms of the hepatic artery occur more frequently in men, and those of the splenic artery occur more frequently in women. Hepatic artery aneurysms may result in a triad of symptoms and signs including abdominal pain radiating to the right shoulder, hemobilia, and obstructive jaundice. The complete triad is seen in less than one third of patients. Up to 80% of hepatic artery aneurysms first come to medical attention owing to symptoms caused by leak or rupture. Rupture can occur into the peritoneal cavity, biliary tree, or gastrointestinal tract.

Imaging methods include plain radiographs, sonography, CT, MR imaging, and angiography. Curvilinear calcifications in the wall of the aneurysm are sometimes detected in the right upper quadrant. On ultrasound, the aneurysm is indistinguishable from a cystic mass, depending on the size of the residual lumen, and may be interpreted as a choledochal cyst in the porta hepatis or a pancreatic neoplasm. This confusion is eliminated if flowing blood can be demonstrated by Doppler ultrasound analysis. Following intravenous contrast administration, CT scan shows dense enhancement of the residual lumen comparable to that seen in the adjacent aorta. The diagnosis of aneurysm is more difficult if the lumen is filled with thrombus. The possibility of aneurysm should be considered before biopsy of a presumed pancreatic mass. Although T1- and T2-weighted MR images show a signal void in the region of blood flow, slow or turbulent flow often results in heterogeneous increase in signal, which makes diagnosis of a vascular lesion more difficult. Subacute mural thrombus also increases T1 signal intensity. Gradient-echo sequences sensitive to flow show signal enhancement.

Aneurysms may be entirely free of clot or completely thrombosed. Figures 59–7 through 59–9 show images from the sonogram and arteriogram of a 70-year-old male who presented with an asymptomatic pulsatile mass. Sonography was performed without Doppler analysis and showed an anechoic mass lesion similar in appearance and location to a normal gallbladder. CT scan (not shown) was performed without intravenous contrast administration and showed a homogeneous soft tissue mass. Without mural calcification or IV contrast administration to suggest aneurysm, the appearance is nonspecific, and the etiology remains unknown. The diagnosis is difficult if blood flow has not been demonstrated. Potentially catastrophic hemorrhage may result from percutaneous needle biopsy of a lesion presumed to be solid. In this case, angiography finally proved the existence of aneurysmal dilatation of the hepatic artery.

Excision or embolization of hepatic artery aneurysms is performed to prevent catastrophic rupture. The goal of therapy is obliteration of the aneurysm with maintenance of arterial blood flow to the liver. Depending on the location of the aneurysm, its relationship to the gastroduodenal artery, and the presence of collateral arterial blood supply to the liver, simple surgical ligation or embolization may not be feasible. Reconstructive bypass grafting may be necessary to preserve adequate liver perfusion.

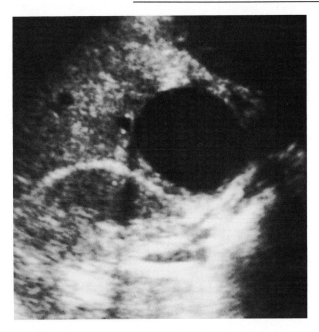

Figure 59-7. Sonography performed without Doppler shows an anechoic mass located posterior to the liver parenchyma and anterior to the right renal hilum.

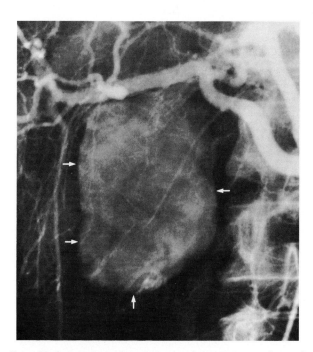

Figure 59-8. Selective celiac arteriogram demonstrates an abnormal contrast collection (arrows) in the early arterial phase.

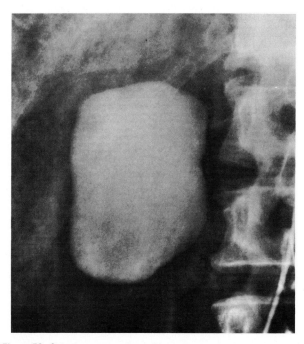

Figure 59-9. In the venous phase this contrast collection is dense and persistent.

REFERENCES

Gavin P, et al. Congenital hepatic artery aneurysm simulating pancreatic carcinoma. Radiology 1984; 152:607–608.

Guida P, Moore S. Aneurysm of the hepatic artery. Report of five cases with a brief review of the previously reported cases. Surgery 1966; 60(2): 299–310.

Kibbler C, et al. Use of CAT scanning in the diagnosis and management of hepatic artery aneurysm. Gut 1985; 26:752–756.

Petrin P, et al. Hepatic artery aneurysms. Am J Gastroenterol 1982; 77(12):934–935.

Shultz S, et al. Common hepatic artery aneurysm: pseudopseudocyst of the pancreas. AJR 1985; 144:1287–1288.

Case 60

HISTORY

A 3-year-old girl presented with intermittent fever and a left inguinal mass.

RADIOLOGY

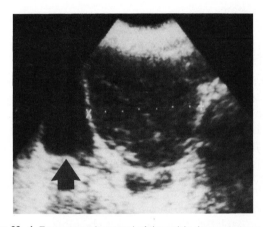

Figure 60-1. Transverse ultrasound of the pelvis demonstrates a solid, hypoechoic mass measuring 4.0 × 5.0 cm (measuring markers). The bladder (arrow) is deviated to the right and separated from the mass by an echogenic plane of fat.

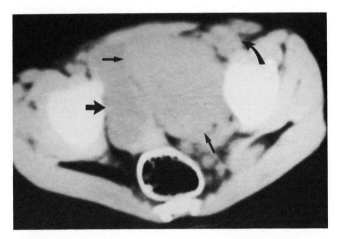

Figure 60-2. Noncontrast CT scan shows a left parailiac soft tissue mass (small arrows) that is homogeneous and isodense with the adjacent bladder (large arrow). There is left parailiac adenopathy (curved arrow).

DIFFERENTIAL DIAGNOSIS

The differential diagnosis includes lymphoma, rhabdomyosarcoma, abscess, primitive neural ectodermal tumor, neuroblastoma, and metastasis.

PATHOLOGY

A left inguinal lymph node resection was performed.

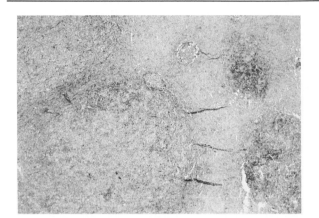

Figure 60-3. The specimen from the lymph node contains broad fibrous sclerotic septa that compartmentalize the node into nodules.

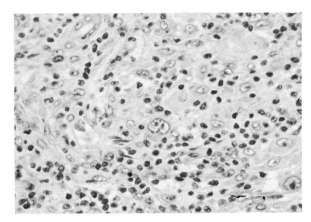

Figure 60-4. The nodules have a prominent inflammatory infiltrate and scattered large vesicular binucleated tumor cells that contain prominent eosinophilic nucleoli. These cells are Reed-Sternberg cells.

DIAGNOSIS

The final pathologic diagnosis was Hodgkin's disease.

DISCUSSION

Hodgkin's disease typically develops in patients older than 16 years with bimodal peaks during the third and sixth decades. Patients with Hodgkin's disease often present because of enlarged, palpable cervical or supraclavicular lymph nodes. Constitutional symptoms, including fever, night sweats, and weight loss, also occur.

Although no pathologic classification system is perfect, Hodgkin's disease is generally divided into four histologic subtypes: lymphocyte predominance, nodular sclerosis, mixed cellularity, and lymphocyte depletion. Although current therapy has nearly equalized the survival among these histologic subtypes, some prognostic significance is still attached to the different types. For example, the lymphocytic predominance subtype is relatively indolent in course, whereas the lymphocytic depletion subtype tends to be more aggressive. The most common variant is nodular sclerosis, which occurs more frequently in women and usually involves the mediastinum. The mixed cellularity variant occurs more frequently in men and involves the periphery more commonly than the mediastinum.

Hodgkin's disease is staged according to the Ann Arbor classification. In brief, stage I disease is limited to a single nodal group. Stage II disease is defined by involvement of two or more lymph node groups on the same side of the diaphragm. Stage III disease is defined by lymph node involvement on both sides of the diaphragm. The spleen may also be involved in stage III. In stage IV disease one or more extralymphatic organs may be involved with or without lymph node involvement. Physical examination is best for peripheral lymph node enlargement, and CT is best for evaluation of the thorax and abdomen. Exploratory laparotomy is performed when its outcome may change treatment from radiation to chemotherapy.

The Reed-Sternberg cell is the hallmark of Hodgkin's disease. This cell is large and bilobed with prominent nucleoli and abundant cytoplasm. Because the Reed-Sternberg cell may sparsely populate the lymphomatous mass, the diagnosis of Hodgkin's disease often requires a larger tissue sample than can be obtained by needle biopsy. Once the diagnosis has been established, fine-needle aspiration can be used to obtain specimens for cell markers and other special studies.

Hodgkin's disease is unusual in young children and, when it occurs, is rarely isolated below the diaphragm. Disease occurring both above and below the diaphragm is more common and typically involves the lymph nodes and spleen. The majority of patients with subdiaphragmatic Hodgkin's disease present with palpable, inguinal adenopathy or an abdominal mass due to enlarged retroperitoneal or mesenteric lymph nodes. Rarely, a patient presents with a fever of unknown origin. Subdiaphragmatic Hodgkin's disease rarely is isolated to the liver, pancreas, bladder, or gastrointestinal tract. These sites are more frequently involved in non-Hodgkin's lymphoma.

The primary imaging modalities include plain radiography, computed tomography, and lymphangiography. The chest film is abnormal in half of all patients with Hodgkin's disease. The lymph node mass shows peripheral lobulations on the posteroanterior radiograph and opacification of the retrosternal clear space on the lateral radiograph. Associated findings include hilar adenopathy, pleural effusion, and pulmonary parenchymal nodules. Thoracic CT should be performed in patients with a normal chest radiograph and often shows extensive adenopathy or thymic involvement. Contrast-enhanced CT helps to differentiate vessels from hilar adenopathy. If thoracic CT is performed without contrast enhancement, MR images can distinguish between vessels and enlarged lymph nodes.

Although abdominal CT shows para-aortic as well as mesenteric lymph node masses, lymphangiography can detect early architectural changes due to lymphoma in normal-sized retroperitoneal and pelvic lymph nodes. Because of the paucity of intra-abdominal fat in children, CT delineation of retroperitoneal mass lesions and adenopathy can be difficult without careful administration of oral and intravenous contrast material. Sonography of lymphoma typically shows homogeneous hypoechogenicity and enhanced through-transmission. Central necrosis of a lymphomatous mass causes a nonspecific complex cystic appearance.

Figures 60–5 through 60–7 show the plain film, CT, and MR image of a 14-year-old girl who presented because of a palpable supraclavicular lymph node. The studies show a soft tissue mass in the expected location of the thymus. The diagnosis in this case is also Hodgkin's disease. In children Hodgkin's disease is the most common cause of an anterior mediastinal mass. Teratoma is the second most common cause.

The treatment of patients with Hodgkin's disease varies according to the pathologic staging of the disease. Various protocols for radiation and chemotherapy exist but, in general, stages I and II are treated with radiation alone. Stage III is treated with a combination of radiotherapy and chemotherapy, and stage IV is often treated with chemotherapy alone. The prognosis for patients with Hodgkin's disease is excellent, particularly for those with the nodular sclerosing and lymphocyte predominant subtypes.

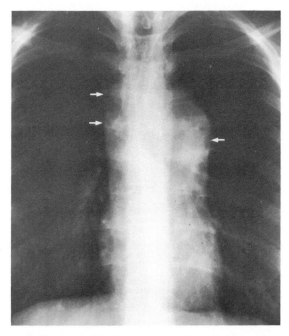

Figure 60–5. AP chest film shows abnormal left and right mediastinal contours (arrows).

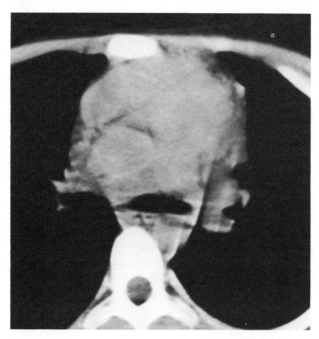

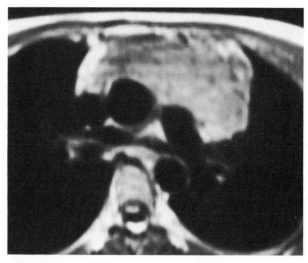

Figure 60–7. Axial T1-weighted (TR = 650, TE = 20) MR image shows that the mass is solid and contiguous with the ascending aorta and the main pulmonary trunk.

Figure 60–6. Noncontrast CT scan confirms an anterior mediastinal mass that is identical in attenuation with the great vessels.

REFERENCES

Cabanillas F, Fuller LM. The radiologic assessment of the lymphoma patient from the standpoint of the clinician. Radiol Clin North Am 1990; 28(4):683–695.

Cohen M, et al. Hodgkin disease and non-Hodgkin lymphoma in children: utilization of radiologic modalities. Radiology 1986; 158:499–505.

Jenkin R, et al. Hodgkin's disease in children: a retrospective analysis. Cancer 1975; 35:979–990.

Krikorian J, et al. Hodgkin's disease presenting below the diaphragm: a review. J Clin Oncol 1986; 4(10):1551–1562.

Osborne BM. Contextual diagnosis of Hodgkin's disease and non-Hodgkin's lymphoma. Radiol Clin North Am 1990; 28(4):669–682.

Case 61

HISTORY

A 59-year-old male presented with slowly increasing left lower thigh pain of several years' duration. At another institution he had been told that he had Paget's disease of the femur.

RADIOLOGY

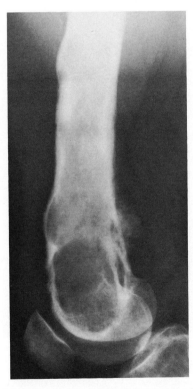

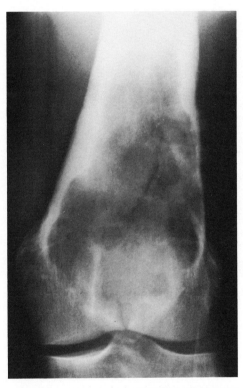

Figure 61-1. A lateral view of the femur demonstrates a large intramedullary lytic lesion. Multiple nodular outgrowths have eroded the endosteal surface of the cortex over the entire distal half of the femoral shaft. Multiple tiny nodular and flocculent calcifications are centrally located within the medullary canal. In addition, there is cloudlike ossification in the posterior soft tissues.

Figure 61-2. AP radiograph demonstrates a pathologic fracture extending into the intercondylar notch at the location of the soft tissue calcifications.

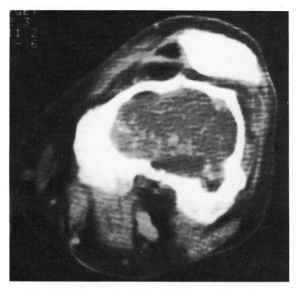

Figure 61-3. CT image obtained through the distal metaphysis of the femur demonstrates dense central medullary flocculent calcification corresponding to the findings on the lateral radiograph.

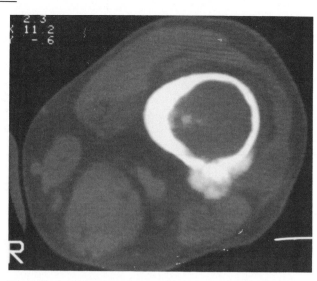

Figure 61-4. A CT image obtained slightly more caudally demonstrates ill-defined cloudlike ossifications extending posteriorly from the femur into the soft tissue.

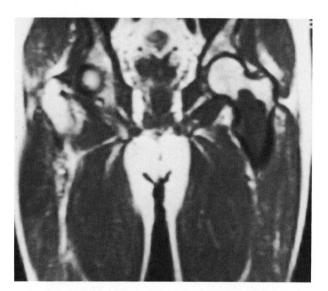

Figure 61-5. Coronal MR image obtained with relative T1 weighting (TR = 400, TE = 20) demonstrates the proximal end of the lesion within the femoral neck.

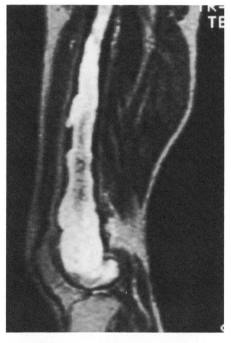

Figure 61-6. A sagittal MR image obtained with T2 weighting (TR = 2000, TE = 120) demonstrates complete replacement of the medullary canal of the femur by abnormal tissue. The periphery of the lesion is extremely bright.

DIFFERENTIAL DIAGNOSIS

The differential diagnosis includes enchondroma, chondrosarcoma, bone infarction, and Paget's disease.

PATHOLOGY

The femur was resected and limb-sparing reconstruction was performed.

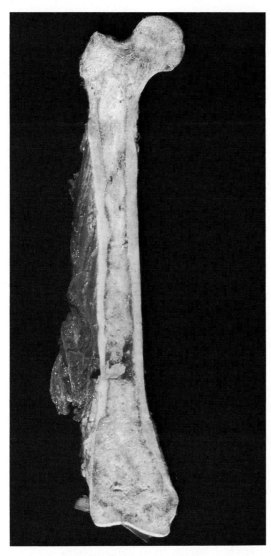

Figure 61-7. The resected femur shows a glistening opalescent mass that extends along almost its entire length.

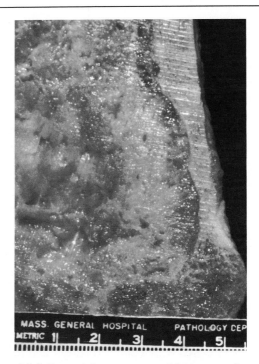

Figure 61-8. The medullary component of the tumor scallops the endosteal surface of the cortex and permeates the ends of the medullary cavity.

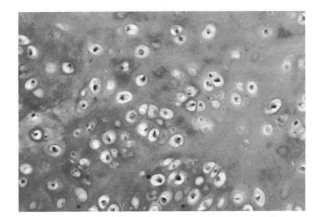

Figure 61-9. Histologically, most of the neoplastic matrix is hyaline cartilage, which shows a mild increase in cellularity and cytologic atypia.

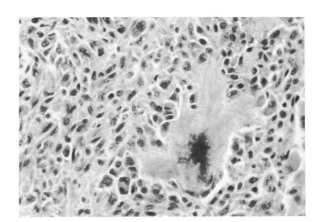

Figure 61-10. In one area the hyaline cartilage is surrounded by a much more cellular and pleomorphic component of the tumor that produces a coarse eosinophilic trabecular matrix typical of neoplastic bone.

DIAGNOSIS

The final pathologic diagnosis was dedifferentiated chondrosarcoma.

DISCUSSION

Chondrosarcoma, the third most common primary bone tumor (after myeloma and osteogenic sarcoma), accounts for 20% of all primary malignant bone tumors and arises from chondroblasts or collagenoblasts. This tumor may be primary, arising de novo in a previously normal bone, or secondary (in about 15% of cases), arising from a preexisting osteochondroma or enchondroma. Males are affected in 60% of cases. In 80% of cases, the hips, shoulder, proximal femur, or proximal humerus is involved. Chondrosarcoma is the most common primary malignancy of the scapula, ribs, sternum, and hand.

Chondrosarcomas are generally slow growing tumors that may reach huge proportions, especially when they involve the pelvis. Patients often complain of dull pain that has been present for years, with a mean duration of 1 to 2 years in one report.

A chondrosarcoma is central if it arises in the interior of a bone and peripheral if it arises on its surface (as from a degenerated osteochondroma). Chondrosarcoma may also arise in juxtacortical and extraosseous sites. Histologic variants include rare mesenchymal chondrosarcomas, which occur in bones or soft tissues of young patients and are associated with a poor prognosis, and the clear cell variant, a tumor featuring cells with clear cytoplasm that occur near the epiphysis or secondary ossification centers, typically of low grade.

Central chondrosarcomas occur most frequently in the metaphysis of the proximal humerus and in the proximal and distal femur. Extension into the diaphysis and occasionally into the epiphysis may occur. The joint is rarely involved. These larger lesions may contain calcific foci and may result in endosteal scalloping, cortical breakthrough, soft tissue mass, periosteal reaction, and pathologic fracture. Otherwise, tumor margins are highly variable. CT is helpful in detecting a calcified matrix not seen on plain films and in assessing the integrity of the cortex. MR is superior in assessing intramedullary involvement and in defining the relationship of an associated soft tissue mass to adjacent neurovascular structures.

Microscopically, the tumors are graded from 1 to 3 (or, in some institutions, 1 to 4). Grade 1 lesions are low grade, and differentiation of grade 1 lesions from benign chondromas may be very difficult. Grade 2 and 3 lesions demonstrate increasing disarray of the matrix, increased cellularity with anaplasia, and more frequent mitoses. Most lesions are grade 1 or 2 at presentation.

Plain film findings are variable and reflect the histologic grade. A lytic, often expansile lesion is seen. Matrix calcification is present in two thirds of cases, characteristically in the form of rings and broken arcs. Endosteal scalloping is frequently observed. A cortical break and soft tissue mass may be present. Radionuclide scanning demonstrates a solitary focus of increased activity. CT is useful for detection of calcification, evaluation of marrow, and assessment of soft tissue masses. Recent literature suggests that MR imaging is more sensitive for detecting marrow involvement and may provide better detail of soft tissue masses; however, CT remains superior for the evaluation of cortical changes and calcifications.

Definitive treatment requires prompt and complete surgical resection. Prognosis is worse for large lesions, lesions of high grade, and central lesions, with a 10-year survival of 70% to 80% for grade 1 lesions, 35% to 60% for grade 2, and 0 to 35% for grade 3. For the typical lesion of low or moderate grade, local recurrence occurs in approximately one third of cases, whereas hematogenous metastases (usually lung) and lymphatic metastases are less common. High-grade tumors are often treated by chemotherapy, but dosage is limited by the advanced age of many of these patients, the response is limited, and prognosis is poor. Dedifferentiation of primary lesions (usually to fibrosarcomas or osteosarcomas) has been reported and is associated with a less than 10% survival at 5 years. Finally, there have been reports of soft tissue seeding by tumor cells after biopsy, emphasizing the importance of careful consideration of any possible biopsy procedure.

Malignant transformation of a solitary benign enchondroma is said to occur in 1% to 2% of patients. It is more likely to occur in enchondromas of the long tubular or flat bones than in the small bones of the hands or feet. Malignant degeneration to chondrosarcoma is most frequent. Malignant transformation to another cell type, or dedifferentiation, may also occur, usually resulting in high-grade lesions. In order of descending frequency, fibrosarcoma, osteosarcoma, malignant fibrous histiocytoma, angiosarcoma, or rhabdomyosarcoma may be seen.

More than 100 dedifferentiated chondrosarcomas have been reported. Pain is the most common complaint. Characteristic sites of involvement include the diaphysis of the femur and proximal portions of the humerus and tibia. Pathologic fractures are seen in 10% to 40%. The radiologic diagnosis of a dedifferentiated chondrosarcoma depends on identification of adjacent features of a low-grade cartilage lesion along with an aggressive osteolytic component.

REFERENCES

Frassica FJ, et al. Dedifferentiation of chondrosarcomas: a report of 78 cases. Radiology 1987; 163:590.

Resnick D, Kyriakos M, Greenway GD. Tumors and tumor-like conditions of bone: imaging and pathology of specific lesions. *In*: Resnick D, Niwayama G (eds). Diagnosis of Bone and Joint Disorders (2nd ed). Philadelphia: Saunders, 1988:3720–3735.

Zimmer WD, et al. Bone tumors: MRI vs CT. Radiology 1985; 155:709–718.

Case 62

HISTORY

A 54-year-old female with history of resected esophageal squamous cell carcinoma presented with new onset of weakness and ataxia.

RADIOLOGY

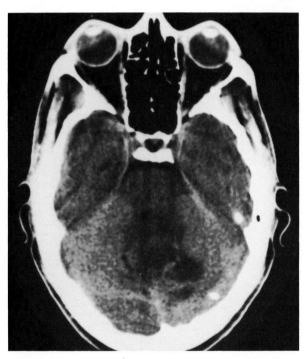

Figure 62–1. Noncontrast CT scan through the posterior fossa shows an irregular low attenuation mass in the left cerebellar hemisphere and vermis. The fourth ventricle is compressed, but the temporal horns are not enlarged.

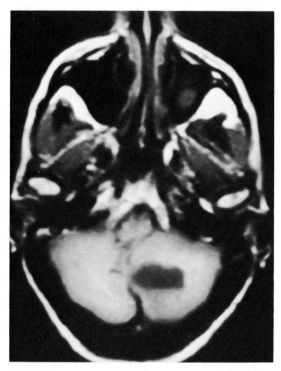

Figure 62–2. On the T1-weighted axial MR image, a fluid-fluid level becomes visible. The dependent fluid is isointense with brain, whereas the superior component is hypointense.

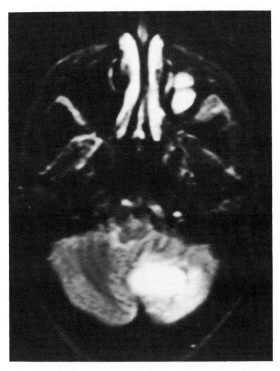

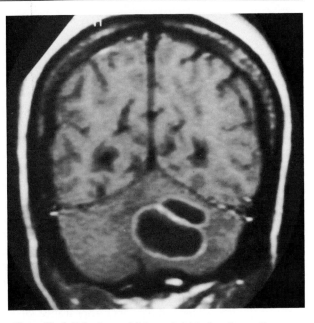

Figure 62-4. Following gadolinium administration, the cystic mass enhances peripherally and demonstrates a septation.

Figure 62-3. On the late echo T2-weighted image the dependent fluid layer is relatively hypointense compared with the markedly hyperintense superior component. This appearance is consistent with hemorrhage and a hematocrit effect.

DIFFERENTIAL DIAGNOSIS

The differential diagnosis includes metastasis, cystic astrocytoma, abscess, ependymoma, and hemangioblastoma.

PATHOLOGY

A stereotactic needle biopsy was obtained.

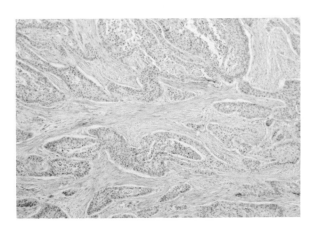

Figure 62-5. Histologically the solid component of the lesion consists of irregular nests of tumor cells surrounded by septa of fibrous tissue.

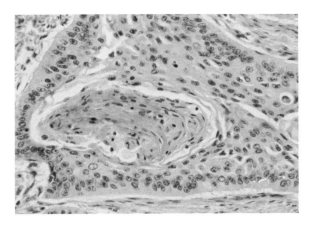

Figure 62-6. The tumor cells are keratinized and form squamous pearls.

DIAGNOSIS

The final pathologic diagnosis was esophageal carcinoma metastatic to the posterior fossa.

DISCUSSION

Metastasis is the most common intra-axial posterior fossa tumor in the adult. The most common primary tumors that metastasize to the brain are lung, breast, melanoma, colorectal cancer, and renal neoplasms. Metastases from other sites are unusual but do occur. In this case, the histology of the intracranial mass was similar to that of the patient's esophageal mass.

In 1978 a review by Irie found only four cases of brain metastasis from esophageal carcinoma. Since then, several case reports of this occurrence have been published. Metastases from esophageal carcinoma most frequently affect the lungs, liver, and adrenal glands. Autopsy series of patients with esophageal carcinoma found a 3.3% incidence of brain metastases. CNS metastasis is probably a late event in the course of the disease, but the incidence may rise as treatments improve.

The radiographic appearance of brain metastasis is generally nonspecific. Thirty percent of these lesions are solitary. Metastases are typically located at the junction of the gray and white matter and are commonly surrounded by moderate to severe edema. Metastases from choriocarcinoma, melanoma, and lung and renal carcinomas are more likely to be hemorrhagic. Central necrosis is not uncommon. With intravenous contrast, 90% of metastases enhance, either in a homogeneous fashion or at the rim, depending on the amount of central necrosis present.

On MR images metastases generally demonstrate decreased T1 and increased T2 signal intensity relative to gray matter, with prominent surrounding bright edema on T2-weighted images. The presence of hemorrhage and necrosis complicates this appearance. The enhancement pattern is similar to that of CT. MR imaging with gadolinium is now the most sensitive method for detecting metastatic disease.

REFERENCES

Irie K, Austin E, Morgansten L. Solitary meningocerebral metastasis from squamous cell carcinoma of the esophagus: a case report. Cancer 1978; 42: 2461–2465.

Latchaw RE, Johnson DW, Kanal E. Metastases. *In*: Latchaw RE (ed). MR and CT Imaging of the Head, Neck and Spine (2nd ed). St. Louis: Mosby Year-Book, 1991.

Odaimi M, Ajani JA. Brain metastases with elevated alpha-fetoprotein level in a patient with esophageal carcinoma. South Med J 1986; 79:1304–1306.

Case 63

HISTORY

A 26-year-old woman who was 1 month post partum presented following recent episodes of right upper quadrant pain.

RADIOLOGY

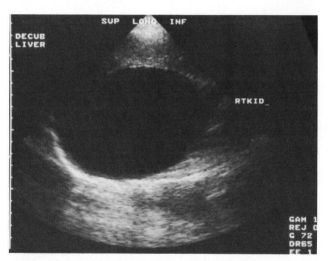

Figure 63-1. Ultrasound reveals a 10- × 12-cm anechoic cyst superior to the right kidney. The cyst is contiguous with the kidney but does not obviously arise from the renal parenchyma.

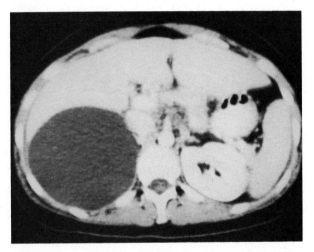

Figure 63-2. A contrast CT demonstrates a large low attenuation cyst in the right suprarenal space displacing the right kidney inferiorly.

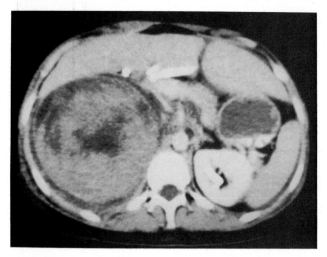

Figure 63-3. A second CT was done 10 days later following cholecystectomy. The cyst is now complex in appearance with high attenuation areas consistent with hemorrhage. The cyst appears to have increased slightly in size.

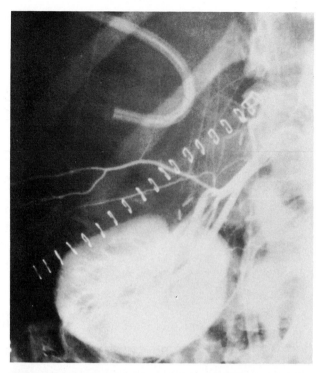

Figure 63-4. The angiogram shows that the right kidney is inferiorly displaced. The mass does not involve the renal parenchyma. Right adrenal vessels are stretched and draped around an avascular mass. No neovascularity is demonstrated.

DIFFERENTIAL DIAGNOSIS

The differential diagnosis includes renal cyst, hepatic cyst, pancreatic pseudocyst, and cystic degeneration of an adrenal neoplasm.

PATHOLOGY

The patient underwent a right retroperitoneal exploration. Submitted to pathology was a membranous tissue specimen, which was reconstructed to a cyst measuring 13 cm in diameter.

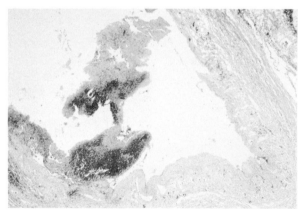

Figure 63-5. Adrenal cyst with intraluminal hemorrhage. The cyst wall is composed of a layer of fibrous tissue with entrapped small groups of adrenal cortical cells.

DIAGNOSIS

The final pathologic diagnosis was adrenal pseudocyst.

DISCUSSION

Adrenal cysts are rare. On postmortem studies the incidence is 0.06%, with a male to female ratio of 1:2. The lesions occur with equal frequency on both sides. Bilateral adrenal cysts are found in 15% of cases, typically in children. A modified classification system divides adrenal cysts into four major categories: (1) parasitic cysts (7%), (2) epithelial cysts (9%), (3) endothelial cysts (45%), and (4) pseudocysts (39%). The quoted frequencies are based on both surgical and autopsy studies. Pseudocysts are the most common symptomatic cysts. Pseudocysts are further categorized into hemorrhagic cysts and cysts associated with tumor necrosis (either benign or malignant).

Most adrenal cysts are small and asymptomatic and are discovered incidentally or at autopsy. Cysts may be detected radiologically owing to calcification within their walls. Large cysts may produce symptoms owing to their mass. Patients may present with dull lower back pain and vague abdominal complaints such as nausea or vomiting, eructation, or epigastric distress.

Pseudocysts are thought to originate from hemorrhage within a pathologic or normal adrenal gland. Liquefaction, reabsorption, and encapsulation occur with time. The wall of a pseudocyst is composed of fibrous connective tissue and lacks an epithelial or endothelial lining. Cystic degeneration also occurs within adrenal tumors such as pheochromocytoma, functioning and nonfunctioning adenomas, and carcinoma. Consequently, surgical removal of all adrenal cysts has been recommended.

The clinical management of adrenal cysts has become more controversial with the introduction of percutaneous aspiration and cystography. Large cysts can be easily punctured for cytologic and chemical analysis. The internal structure of the cyst can be examined by contrast instillation, and drainage can be done to relieve symptoms. Only 19 cases of adrenal cyst aspiration have been reported in the literature, and further studies are needed to determine the recurrence rate.

Radiographically, 15% of adrenal cysts demonstrate peripheral curvilinear calcification. An intravenous pyelogram demonstrates the extrarenal location of the cyst; the involved kidney may be inferiorly or medially displaced. On ultrasound the cystic nature of the lesion is obvious. Classically, the cysts are anechoic and their walls thin. However, atypical features such as scattered echoes within the cyst, irregularities of the wall, and central calcification are sometimes present. On angiography the mass is avascular, and the adrenal vessels are splayed and stretched over the cyst. CT demonstrates a well-defined, low attenuation mass in the suprarenal region. Large cysts are often difficult to differentiate from the liver, adrenal gland, or kidney. Multiplanar imaging modalities such as MR imaging and ultrasound are extremely useful in this situation.

REFERENCES

Abeshouse G, et al. Adrenal cysts: review of the literature and report of three cases. J Urol 1959; 81(6):711–717.

Cheema P, et al. Adrenal cysts: diagnosis and treatment. J Urol 1981; 126:396–399.

Davenport M, et al. Adrenal cysts—report, review and classification. Postgrad Med J 1988; 64:71–73.

Incze J, et al. Morphology and pathogenesis of adrenal cysts. Am J Pathol 1979; 95(2):423–432.

Kearney G, et al. Functioning and nonfunctioning cysts of the adrenal cortex and medulla. Am J Surg 1977; 134:363–368.

Tung G, et al. Adrenal cysts: imaging and percutaneous aspiration. Radiology 1989; 173:107–110.

Case 64

HISTORY

A 41-year-old Guatemalan with a 3-month history of malaise, anorexia, sore throat, and cough presented following 2 days of fever and chills.

RADIOLOGY

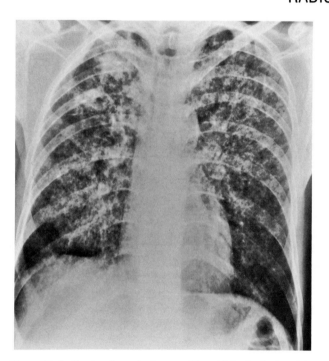

Figure 64–1. Chest radiograph shows a diffuse bilateral reticulonodular pattern with some areas of confluence in the right upper lobe.

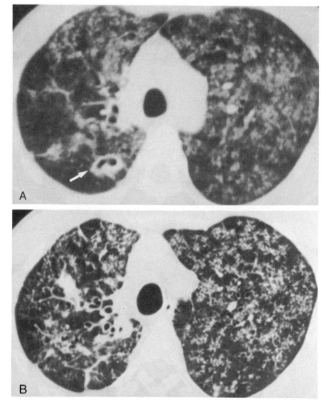

Figure 64–2. *A–B.* CT scan demonstrates right upper lobe volume loss, bronchiectasis, cavitation (arrow), and diffuse bilateral peribronchial irregular densities with areas of confluence.

DIFFERENTIAL DIAGNOSIS

The differential diagnosis includes granulomatous disease, viral infection, interstitial pneumonitis, drug-related pneumonitis, and pulmonary edema with atypical distribution. Sarcoidosis, lymphoma, Wegener's granulomatosis, bronchiolo-alveolar cell carcinoma, and eosinophilic granulomatosis are less likely.

PATHOLOGY

An endoscopic bronchial biopsy was performed.

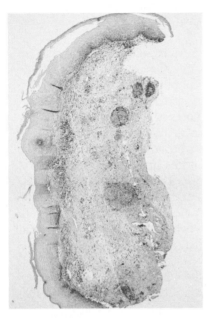

Figure 64-3. The bronchial biopsy shows squamous metaplasia of the bronchial mucosa with granulomas within the submucosa.

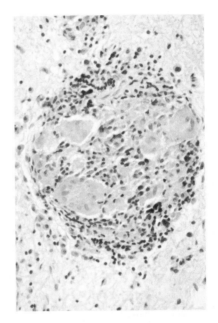

Figure 64-4. The granulomas contain epithelioid histiocytes as well as multinucleated giant cells and lymphocytes.

DIAGNOSIS

The final diagnosis was pulmonary tuberculosis with endobronchial spread.

DISCUSSION

Tuberculous infection has primary and postprimary (secondary) forms. The former usually occurs in childhood and is generally self-limited. It is evident as a focal parenchymal density in any lobe, associated with hilar adenopathy and sometimes pleural effusion. Postprimary tuberculosis most often occurs between the ages of 50 and 60 years; men are affected in 60% of cases, and there is a significantly higher incidence among blacks. Involvement of the upper lobes occurs in more than 80% of patients, and adenopathy or effusions may be present. Cavitation was reported to occur in 56% of cases in one series, the cavity wall being characteristically thick.

Endobronchial spread of tuberculosis begins when a walled-off caseous focus ruptures into an adjacent bronchus, discharging its contents into the airways. Spread of the contents through the bronchial tree results in widespread pulmonary lesions. Radiographically, multiple small shadows 4 to 10 mm in size (typical acinar air shadows) are seen. Direct extension through the canals of Lambert and the pores of Kohn can lead to areas of confluent disease that are indistinguishable from lobar or diffuse pneumonia.

Postprimary tuberculosis results from reactivation of a primary focus or from exogenous reinfection. A hypersensitivity immune response results in intense inflammatory reaction fibrosis and cicatrization. Typically, reactivation occurs in the apical and posterior segments of the upper lobes and the superior segment of the lower lobe; although it is unclear why this distribution is seen, it is thought to reflect sites of either increased oxygen tension (which increases virulence) or reduced lymph flow (which decreases clearance of a primary focus of disease). CT studies in secondary tuberculosis have demonstrated that cavitation is always present.

Tuberculosis is especially common in places where there are crowding and poverty. It is also common among the institutionalized, the chronically ill or disabled, and the immunosuppressed.

Tuberculosis is treated with multidrug regimens to decrease the incidence of resistance, but resistance is still seen in about 2% of patients, probably due to inadequate follow-up. In successfully treated patients the number of bacilli in the sputum is reduced by 99.75% within 4 weeks.

REFERENCES

Murata K, Itoh H, Todo G, et al. Centrilobular lesions of the lung: demonstration by high resolution CT and pathologic correlation. Radiology 1986; 161:641–645.

Nadich DP, Zerhouni EA, Siegelman SS, et al. Computed Tomography of the Thorax. New York: Raven Press, 1984.

Pare JAP, Fraser RG. Synopsis of Diseases of the Chest. Philadelphia: Saunders, 1983.

Woodring JH, Vandiviere HM, Fried AM, et al. Update: the radiographic features of pulmonary tuberculosis. AJR 1986; 146:497–506.

Case 65

HISTORY

A 59-year-old male presented after 1 year of weight loss and 4 months of crampy abdominal pain.

RADIOLOGY

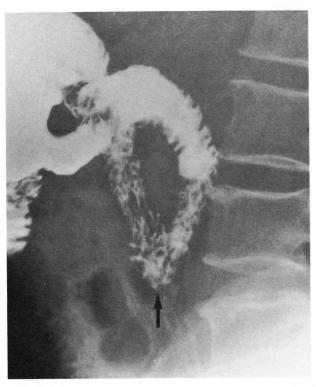

Figure 65-1. A lateral view from an upper GI series demonstrates focal inferior displacement and tethering of the third part of the duodenum (arrow). The bowel mucosa is normal.

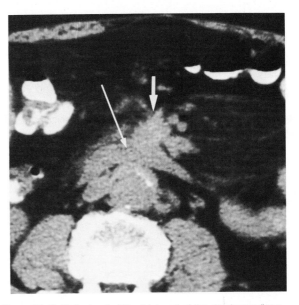

Figure 65-2. At the level of the third part of the duodenum (long arrow), CT scan shows a spiculated soft tissue mass (short arrow) at the mesenteric pedicle.

DIFFERENTIAL DIAGNOSIS

The differential diagnosis includes metastatic disease, inflammatory mass, pancreatic neoplasm, lymphoma, pancreatic pseudocyst, and carcinoid tumor.

PATHOLOGY

Surgical biopsy specimens were obtained from a hard mass and a matted collection of mesenteric nodes in the peripancreatic region.

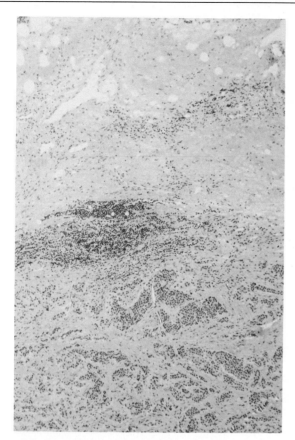

Figure 65-3. Specimen from the mesentery shows mesenteric fat with adjacent tumor.

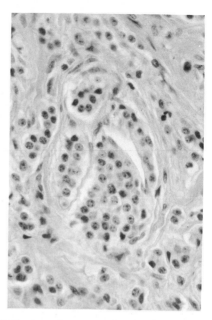

Figure 65-4. The tumor is composed of round nests of polyhedral cells that have centrally placed nuclei and a moderate amount of cytoplasm. There is minimal pleomorphism and little mitotic activity.

DIAGNOSIS

The final pathologic diagnosis was mesenteric carcinoid tumor.

DISCUSSION

Carcinoid tumors are derived from the enterochromaffin (Kulchitsky) cells of neural crest ectodermal origin, which are located within the mucosal basement membrane of the small bowel. Because these cells stain with silver salts, carcinoid tumor is also termed argentaffinoma.

Carcinoid tumor of the bowel occurs most frequently in the appendix, followed by the rectum and distal ileum. Less than 10% of tumors are located in the proximal small bowel. Carcinoid tumor represents the most common primary neoplasm of the small bowel. It typically presents in the sixth and seventh decades with no gender or racial predominance. The tumor is slow growing, and patients typically survive 5 to 10 years after diagnosis.

Presenting symptoms result either from local mass effect, including pain and bowel obstruction, or from the carcinoid syndrome. This syndrome, which is present in approximately 30% of patients, includes diarrhea, skin flushing, bronchoconstriction, cardiac valve lesions (especially of the tricuspid and pulmonic valves), and hypotension. Symptoms result from the systemic release of hormonally active substances by the tumor, in particular serotonin. Serotonin is metabolized by the liver to 5-hydroxyindoleacetic acid (5-HIAA), which is metabolically inactive. Therefore, in patients with abdominal carcinoid, the presence of the carcinoid syndrome usually indicates hepatic metastases with secretion of serotonin directly into the hepatic veins. Serotonin produced within the bowel lesions is not expected to cause systemic manifestations owing to portal blood flow to the liver and metabolism by hepatocytes.

Histologically, carcinoid of the small bowel arises at the mucosal basement membrane. Because the mucosal surface remains intact, barium studies show a smooth contour abnormality and obtuse margins typical of a submucosal lesion. Abdominal CT demonstrates the primary tumor in less than 50% of patients. Secondary signs are more easily visualized, especially stranding of adjacent mesenteric fat, which results from a desmoplastic response evoked by the tumor. A small or microscopic tumor may be detected if a significant fibrotic reaction occurs. This desmoplastic reaction can distort the mesentery, thicken the adjacent fat with soft tissue density, and cause tethering of adjacent bowel loops. Lymphadenopathy is common at the time of presentation. Metastases are rare in primary tumors measuring less than 1 cm, but tumors greater than 2 cm metastasize in most cases. The angiographic features of carcinoid tumor may be distinctive. The tumor is recognized by its marked vascularity and often demonstrates a stellate configuration in the arterial phase followed by a dense capillary blush. Metastases to the liver and regional lymph nodes show the same tumor blush.

Discrete carcinoid tumors are surgically resected. In patients with carcinoid syndrome, the primary tumor may be resected or debulked for palliation, and hepatic metastases may be treated by selective arterial embolization. Nonsurgical treatment of the carcinoid syndrome includes use of cytotoxic agents, adrenergic and anticholinergic agents, glucagon, and somatostatin.

REFERENCES

Cockery B, et al. CT manifestations of abdominal carcinoid. J Comput Assist Tomogr 1985; 9: 38–42.

Picus D, Glazer HS, et al. CT of abdominal carcinoid. AJR Am J Roentgenol 1984; 143:581–585.

Case 66

HISTORY

An 11-year-old boy presented with abdominal pain after a sledding accident.

RADIOLOGY

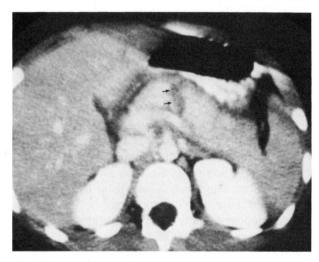

Figure 66-1. Contrast-enhanced CT scan demonstrates a linear low attenuation region (arrows) traversing the body of the pancreas.

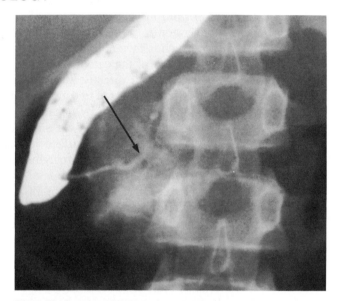

Figure 66-2. A spot image obtained during endoscopic retrograde cholangiopancreatography (ERCP) shows abrupt termination of the proximal pancreatic duct (arrow). This abrupt termination is associated with surrounding leakage of contrast material.

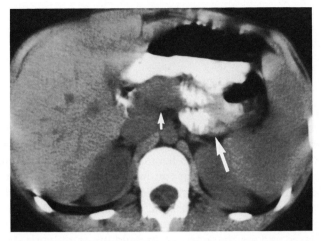

Figure 66-3. Eight months following distal pancreatectomy, noncontrast CT scan shows the remaining proximal pancreas (small arrow) and small bowel filling the surgical bed (large arrow).

DIFFERENTIAL DIAGNOSIS

The differential diagnosis includes pancreatic fracture or laceration, cystic neoplasm, and pancreatic pseudocyst.

PATHOLOGY

Distal pancreatectomy was performed. There was peripancreatic soft tissue hemorrhage.

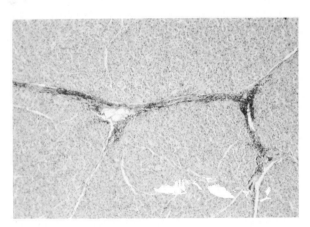

Figure 66-4. Lobules of pancreatic parenchyma show extravasated red blood cells within the connective tissue septa.

DIAGNOSIS

The final diagnosis was pancreatic fracture.

DISCUSSION

Pancreatic trauma accounts for 3% to 12% of abdominal injuries. Penetrating and blunt trauma account for 70% and 30% of pancreatic injuries, respectively. The high mortality in patients with pancreatic trauma usually is due to coincidental injury to the vascular system resulting in catastrophic hemorrhage or to late complications such as sepsis. One third of patients with pancreatic injury develop complications. The most common complications include hemorrhagic (sac) necrosis, phlegmonous collection, abscess, pseudocyst, pancreatico-enteric fistula, and pancreatic insufficiency.

Pancreatic injury due to blunt trauma may be difficult to diagnose clinically. Symptoms are often delayed and are characterized by mild upper abdominal pain. The serum amylase level may or may not be elevated; a complete pancreatic transection may be associated with normal amylase level. Because patients with penetrating trauma undergo exploratory laparotomy, pancreatic injury may be visualized directly. The presence of retroperitoneal or peripancreatic hematoma requires meticulous exploration of the pancreas and, if injury is detected, determination of ductal integrity.

CT accurately depicts pancreatic morphology and screens the entire abdomen for associated injury, retroperitoneal hemorrhage, and intraperitoneal fluid. Pancreatic laceration or transection results in focal edema and hemorrhage that is relatively low in attenuation compared with adjacent pancreatic parenchyma. Focal hematoma may be similar to or increased in attenuation compared with adjacent pancreatic parenchyma. Fluid often collects in the lesser sac. Endoscopic retrograde cholangiopancreatography (ERCP) is used both pre- and intraoperatively to evaluate pancreatic duct integrity.

Evaluation of the pancreas by CT is more difficult in children because of their decreased retroperitoneal fat. Intravenous contrast administration enhances pancreatic tissue and increases visualization of the nonenhancing, intrapancreatic hematoma. The advantage of contrast administration is shown in Figures 66–5 and 66–6. This 7-year-old girl was an unrestrained passenger in a motor vehicle accident and suffered blunt abdominal trauma. Before contrast administration an ill-defined, low attenuation region is of unclear significance. After contrast administration the transverse fracture plane remains unenhanced and is sharply distinguished from the enhanced pancreas.

Pancreatic fracture can be complicated by pancreatitis, retroperitoneal hemorrhage, phlegmonous collection, sac necrosis, infection with abscess, or pseudocyst formation. CT scan accurately diagnoses and stages the severity of pancreatic injury and its subsequent complications. During the acute illness CT examination is performed without and with intravenous contrast administration. Noncontrast CT scan shows acute hemorrhage, which is hyperdense. Contrast-enhanced CT scans can be used to identify focal regions of intrapancreatic hematoma or necrosis and, in cases of extensive necrosis, areas of residual viable pancreatic tissue. Ultrasound, although less sensitive than CT in the diagnosis of pancreatic injury, is useful in following pancreatic fracture and its complications, including pseudocyst formation.

CT scan guides interventional procedures when complications develop. Needle aspi-

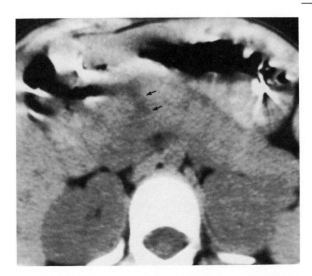

Figure 66-5. At the level of the pancreatic body noncontrast CT scan shows an ill-defined transverse region of low attenuation (arrows) that is of unclear significance and possibly represents volume averaging or a beam-hardening artifact.

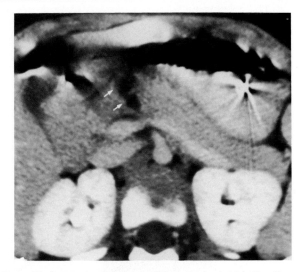

Figure 66-6. Following intravenous (IV) contrast administration, the transverse fracture plane (arrows) becomes conspicuous adjacent to opacified pancreatic tissue.

ration of pancreatic fluid can be used to diagnose an infected phlegmon, pseudocyst, or frank abscess and may lead to aggressive radiologic intervention or surgery. Percutaneous CT-guided catheter drainage of pancreatic fluid collections is effective in most patients.

Figures 66-7 through 66-9 show sequential images of a 32-year-old female who presented with multiple trauma following a motor vehicle accident. In this patient pancreatic fracture resulted in transection of the duct and subsequent complications that were followed by CT scan. Two weeks following trauma the pancreatic fracture plane was widened by fluid. This collection became infected and, 4 weeks following trauma, was drained by percutaneous catheter placement. One year following trauma a well-defined pseudocyst was located at the site of the original fracture. Pancreatic tissue distal to the fracture became atrophic.

At the time of presentation the presence or absence of pancreatic duct injury determines surgical therapy. Simple pancreatic contusions without ductal injury are managed by sump drainage. Because transection of the duct results in leakage of enzymes and necrosis of surrounding tissues, patient management often requires distal pancreatectomy. Associated duodenal injury may require pancreaticoduodenectomy.

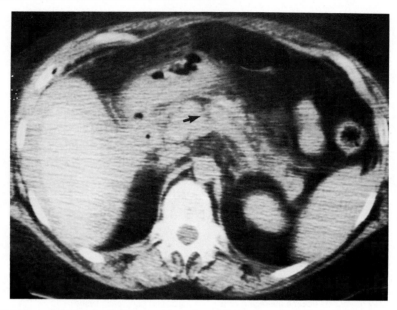

Figure 66–7. Following blunt abdominal trauma, intraperitoneal fluid surrounds the liver. A linear region of low attenuation (arrow) traverses the pancreatic body at the same level and represents a fracture plane.

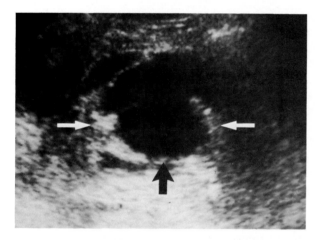

Figure 66–8. Two weeks later, transverse sonography of the pancreas shows a fluid collection (black arrow) that separates the margins of the distracted pancreatic fragments (white arrows).

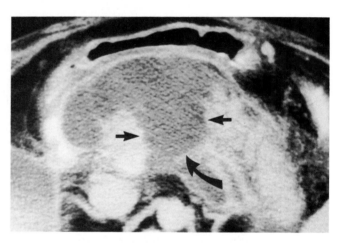

Figure 66–9. Contrast-enhanced CT scan shows fluid (curved arrow) widening the pancreatic fracture plane (straight arrows).

REFERENCES

Gorenstein A, et al. Blunt injury to the pancreas in children: Selective management based on ultrasound. J Pediatr Surg 1987; 22:1110–1116.

Jeffrey RB, et al. Computed tomography of pancreatic trauma. Radiology 1983; 147:491–494.

Jeffrey RB, et al. Ultrasound in acute pancreatic trauma. Gastrointest Radiol 1986; 11:44–46.

Case 67

HISTORY

A 7-year-old girl was referred for cervical spine films after a seizure.

RADIOLOGY

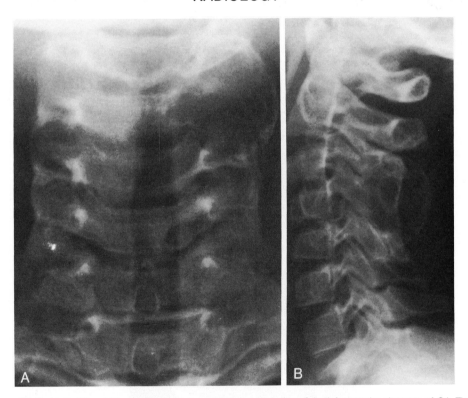

Figure 67-1. *A-B.* AP and lateral plain films demonstrate a lytic lesion of the left posterior elements of C4. The lesion has produced an expanded periosteal shell.

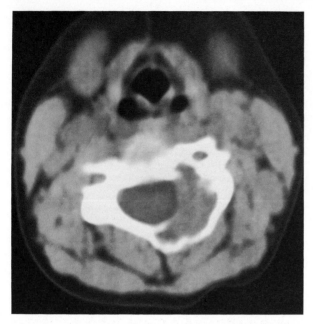

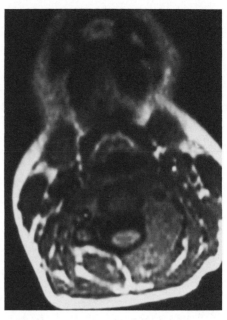

Figure 67-2. On CT scan there is a lytic destructive lesion involving all of the left lamina, articular mass, and spinous process of C4. Most of the lesion is of soft tissue density (compare with cerebrospinal fluid [CSF]). Small, subtle low attenuation areas represent tiny cystic components.

Figure 67-3. T1-weighted MR image shows that the lesion has much brighter signal characteristics than adjacent CSF.

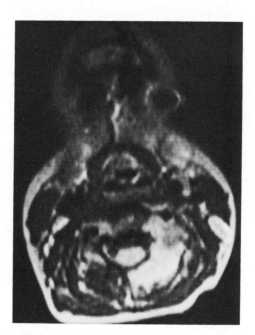

Figure 67-4. On T2-weighted MR images the lesion brightens considerably.

DIFFERENTIAL DIAGNOSIS

The differential diagnosis includes aneurysmal bone cyst, osteoblastoma, fibrous dysplasia, metastasis, giant cell tumor, and brown tumor.

PATHOLOGY

The lesion was resected.

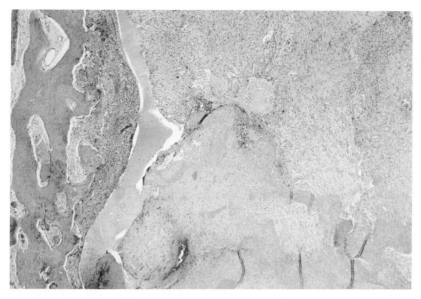

Figure 67–5. Microscopically the lesion is surrounded peripherally by a layer of relatively well-formed reactive woven bone.

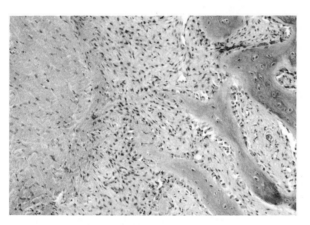

Figure 67–6. Most of the lesion is solid, but there are small cystic spaces filled with red blood cells.

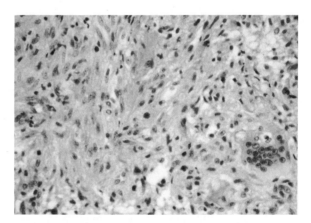

Figure 67–7. The solid areas contain many fibroblasts and multinucleated osteoclast-type giant cells.

DIAGNOSIS

The final pathologic diagnosis was aneurysmal bone cyst, solid variant.

DISCUSSION

Aneurysmal bone cyst (ABC) is a benign, solitary non-neoplastic lesion that typically contains thin-walled, blood-filled cystic cavities. Aneurysmal bone cysts are usually primary lesions. Up to 30% of lesions, however, may result from cyst formation within another bone lesion. Chondroblastoma, chondromyxoid fibroma, osteoblastoma, giant cell tumor, fibrous dysplasia, and osteosarcoma have all been reported to give rise to aneurysmal bone cysts. The genesis of the cyst is unclear. Some authors suggest venous obstruction or arteriovenous fistula formation as a possible cause. A history of previous trauma is frequently present.

ABC usually occurs during the first three decades of life. Eighty percent of patients are less than 20 years old, but the age range extends from 3 to 70 years. There is a slight female predominance. Symptoms may progress slowly over years or may progress with alarming rapidity, raising questions about malignancy. Pain and swelling are typical, including radicular pain related to nerve compression in spinal lesions. An ABC may affect practically any bone; half of the lesions involve the long tubular bones, and about one third involve the spine. In the long tubular bones an eccentric and metaphyseal location is most common. Epiphyseal extension, usually following closure of the growth plate, is rare. In the spine an ABC usually arises from the posterior elements. The vertebral body may be affected but rarely in isolation.

Radiographic findings vary with the location and maturity of the lesion. Although osteolysis and expansion are dominant findings, four general stages of development are identified. The initial lytic phase appears as a circumscribed area of rarefaction, which, when located eccentrically, thins and expands the cortex. The active growth phase results in aggressive expansile bone destruction, a paper-thin outer cortical margin, and a prominent periosteal reaction. In the stabilization phase a well-defined sclerotic margin surrounds distinct internal septa and trabeculations (the characteristic "soap bubble" appearance). Finally, in the healing phase the cystic lesion progressively calcifies and ossifies into a mass of irregular bone. The lesion may resemble a giant cell tumor (usually more epiphyseal), enchondroma (usually less expanded), osteoblastoma, or brown tumor.

In the spine, ABC involves the posterior elements alone or in combination with the vertebral body. In a child, a specific diagnosis may be made if the lesion expands the transverse or spinous process. Less specific changes occur in the lamina and pedicle, and differentiation from osteoblastoma may be impossible. When the lesion involves the vertebral body, extends from one vertebra to another (or to a rib), results in pathologic fracture, and encroaches upon the spinal canal or adjacent soft tissues, malignant tumors and infection should be considered.

Bone scan usually demonstrates tracer uptake at the periphery of the lesion with relative central photopenia; however, this finding is nonspecific and may be seen in a number of benign and malignant conditions.

CT scan defines the size, location, and matrix of both intraosseous and extraosseous components. Both CT and MR can sometimes detect fluid-fluid levels. Fluid-fluid levels are thought to be the result of hemorrhage into the cyst. Similar findings of fluid-fluid levels have been reported in osteosarcoma. Demonstration of fluid-fluid levels requires that the patient remain stationary for approximately 10 minutes prior to scanning. MR can clearly define the margin of the lesion and its relationship to neural structures, which is especially important for lesions in the spine.

Although they are composed of dilated vascular channels, aneurysmal bone cysts are angiographically hypovascular. There may be small regions of hypervascularity but not marked vascularity or tumor vessels.

The usual ABC measures less than 10 cm but can grow to a much larger size, especially if it is located in the ilium or scapula. Grossly, there may be a single cyst cavity or multiple communicating spaces separated by fibrous septa that are not lined by endothelium. These spaces contain blood and a variable amount of solid material. Microscopically, this solid material consists of fibroblasts and multinucleated osteoclast-type giant cells.

Rarely, as in this case, a lesion may be entirely solid. The solid variant of ABC is most commonly seen in patients in the first two decades of life. It has a greater predilection than the classic lesion for the axial skeleton. Radiographically, the solid variant has a greater variety of appearances, looking identical to the classic lesion or demonstrating highly aggressive moth-eaten bone destruction. Calcification is more common. Histologically, the lesion is richer in fibroblasts, osteoblasts with osteoid production, and osteoclast-type giant cells.

Although the ABC is benign and does not metastasize, surgical resection, curettage with bone grafting, or cryosurgery is usually recommended because of its potential for aggressive growth, bone destruction, and soft tissue extension. When a lesion is incompletely excised, recurrence occurs in 10% to 20% of patients. Because the ABC is a histologically benign lesion, radiation therapy may incur an unacceptable risk of malignant transformation.

REFERENCES

Dahlin D, et al. Aneurysmal bone cyst and other nonneoplastic conditions. Skel Radiol 1982; 8: 243–250.

Hudson T. Fluid levels in aneurysmal bone cysts: a CT feature. AJR 1984; 141:1001–1004.

Hudson T, et al. Magnetic resonance imaging of fluid levels in an aneurysmal bone cyst and in anticoagulated human blood. Skel Radiol 1985; 13:267–270.

Resnick D, Kyriakos M, Greenway GD. Tumors and tumor-like lesions of bone: imaging and pathology of specific lesions. *In*: Resnick D, Niwayama G (eds). Diagnosis of Bone and Joint Disorders (2nd ed). Philadelphia: Saunders, 1988:3831–3842.

Sanerkin NG, et al. An unusual intraosseous lesion with fibroblastic, osteoclastic, osteblastic, aneurysmal and fibromyxoid elements. Cancer 1983; 51:2278–2286.

Case 68

HISTORY

A 49-year-old male presented with episodic dizziness and easy fatigability. Personality changes had been noted during the several months prior to admission.

RADIOLOGY

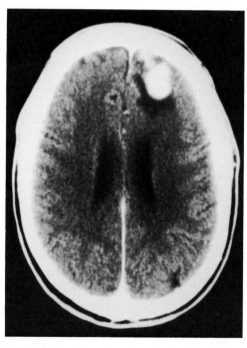

Figure 68-1. Contrast-enhanced cranial CT scan shows an enhancing mass in the left frontal lobe. There is moderate surrounding white matter edema.

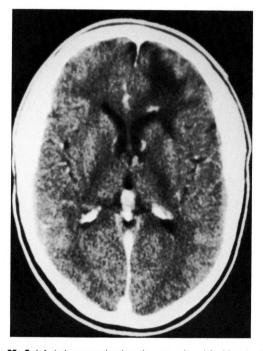

Figure 68-2. Inferiorly, several enhancing ependymal foci involve the anterior portion of the left frontal horn and the left lateral ventricle near the head of the caudate nucleus. A dense focus of enhancement is located in the pineal region.

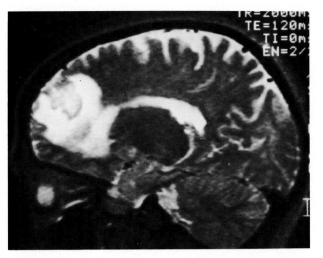

Figure 68-3. On the sagittal late echo T2-weighted MR image, the left frontal lobe mass shows mild and heterogeneous hyperintensity with surrounding edema.

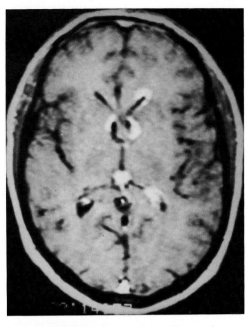

Figure 68-4. Postgadolinium T1-weighted axial image shows multiple enhancing intraventricular and subependymal foci.

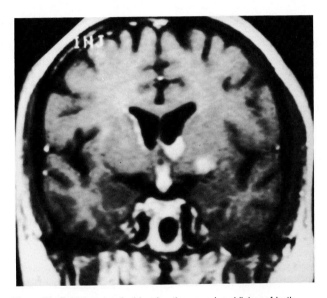

Figure 68-5. Enhancing foci involve the ependymal lining of both lateral ventricles, the suprachiasmatic recess of the third ventricle, and the left thalamus.

DIFFERENTIAL DIAGNOSIS

The differential diagnosis includes high-grade glioma with subarachnoid seeding, metastatic disease, lymphoma, sarcoidosis, toxoplasmosis, and fungal disease.

PATHOLOGY

A stereotactic needle biopsy under CT guidance was performed.

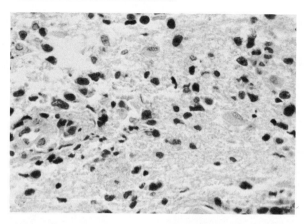

Figure 68-6. A small biopsy specimen shows that the neoplasm consists of small to moderately sized cells that have irregular hyperchromatic nuclei and scant cytoplasm.

DIAGNOSIS

The final diagnosis was primary CNS lymphoma.

DISCUSSION

Lymphoma accounts for 1% of all intracranial neoplasms, but it has tripled in incidence over the last 10 years. The tumor occurs both sporadically and with increased frequency in organ transplant recipients and in patients with acquired immune deficiency syndrome (AIDS) or congenital immunodeficiency. Nearly all CNS lymphomas are of the non-Hodgkin's type. Histologically, neoplastic lymphoid tissue is seen within the walls of blood vessels and along perivascular spaces. Immunohistochemical study generally demonstrates a monotypic B-cell population.

Primary CNS lymphoma affects males more commonly than females in a 2 : 1 ratio. The disease is most common in patients in the fifth and sixth decades of life. The most common initial presentation is an intraparenchymal cerebral mass, which involves the supratentorial compartment in about 80% of patients. Multiple lesions are seen in about 50% of cases. In contrast, subarachnoid space involvement is more common in metastatic lymphoma to the CNS and virtually always precedes the development of intracerebral metastatic disease. Typical symptoms are nonfocal, such as headache, nausea, vomiting, and memory loss.

The CT appearance of primary CNS lymphoma is that of an isodense to hyperdense mass, commonly involving the basal ganglia, corpus callosum, or thalamus. Peritumoral edema tends to be minimal or moderate. Calcification and hemorrhage are unusual. Enhancement of the masses is generally uniform. Although the MR appearance is variable, there is a tendency for tumors to be isointense or only mildly hyperintense to gray matter on T2-weighted images. This characteristic is nonspecific, however, and is also seen in metastatic melanoma or adenocarcinoma, sarcoid, and meningiomas.

Radiotherapy is the most common mode of therapy for CNS lymphoma. Steroid administration can result in dramatic reductions in tumor mass. Late recurrences, however, are common. The role of chemotherapy is under study but remains uncertain. The average survival time is 45 months for patients presenting with single parenchymal tumors.

REFERENCES

Atlas S. Intraaxial brain tumors. *In*: Atlas S (ed). Magnetic Resonance Imaging of the Brain and Spine. New York: Raven Press, 1991:302–307.

Burger PC, Scheithauer BW, Vogel FS. Surgical Pa-

thology of the Nervous System and Its Coverings (3rd ed). New York: Churchill Livingstone, 1991:359–365.

Hochberg FH, Miller DC. Primary central nervous

system lymphoma. J Neurosurg 1988; 68: 835–853.

Pittman KB, Olveny CL, North JB, et al. Primary central nervous system lymphoma. A report of 9 cases and review of the literature. Oncology 1991; 48:184–187.

Schwaighofer BW, Hesselink JR, Press GA, et al. Primary intracranial CNS lymphoma: MR manifestations. AJNR 1989; 10:725–729.

Case 69

HISTORY

A 45-year-old woman presented with acute left flank pain.

RADIOLOGY

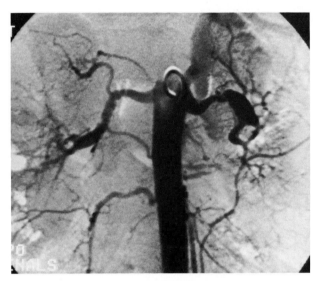

Figure 69-1. An abdominal aortic angiogram demonstrates a stenotic right main renal artery, which shows changes consistent with ectasia or aneurysm and has a beaded appearance. The left renal artery also appears stenotic and exhibits a small extraluminal collection.

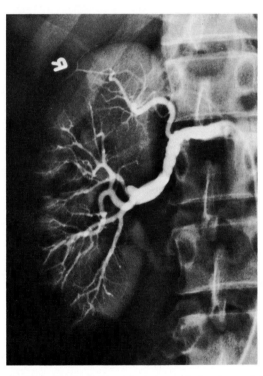

Figure 69-2. A selective right renal arteriogram better demonstrates the beaded stenotic appearance.

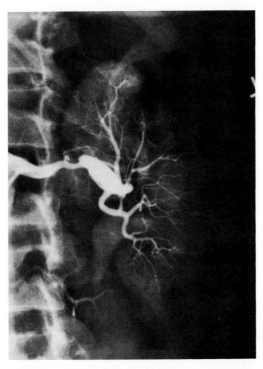

Figure 69-3. A 1.5-cm lobulated aneurysm is seen in the proximal left renal artery together with an associated persistent contrast collection containing an intimal flap. A peripheral wedge-shaped defect is present in the lower pole of the left kidney, consistent with a dissection. Two weeks later the previously noted right renal artery stenosis was not seen. This occurrence is consistent with vasospasm, and angioplasty was not performed.

DIFFERENTIAL DIAGNOSIS

The differential diagnosis includes fibromuscular dysplasia with spontaneous dissection and cortical infarcts. The proximal renal artery distribution, dissection, and beaded appearance exclude other vasculitides such as polyarteritis nodosa.

PATHOLOGY

Specimen from a similar case in another patient is submitted. Biopsy of such lesions is rarely performed.

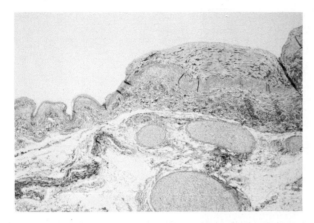

Figure 69-4. Trichrome stain, which stains collagen blue and smooth muscle red, demonstrates marked irregularity in the thickness of the arterial wall.

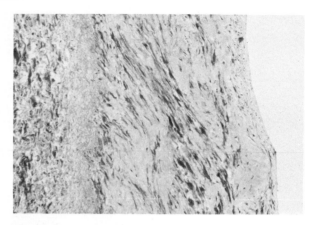

Figure 69-5. Thickened portion of arterial wall with disorganized media and increased fibrous tissue.

DIAGNOSIS

The final diagnosis was fibromuscular dysplasia of the renal artery with dissection.

DISCUSSION

Fibromuscular dysplasia is the cause of renal artery stenosis in approximately one third of patients with renovascular hypertension. It is observed in all age groups, and the majority of patients are women (ratio 3:1). The patients are younger than those affected by atherosclerosis. Fibromuscular dysplasia is the most common cause of renovascular hypertension in children.

Dysplastic lesions of the renal artery result from collagen deposition, hyperplasia of smooth muscle and fibroblasts, and disruption or thinning of the elastica interna. Typically the lesions involve the mid and distal renal artery and occasionally the entire renal artery. The lesions involve the main renal artery in the great majority of adults; in children branch vessel disease predominates either alone or in association with main renal artery disease. Renal artery dysplasia is bilateral in two thirds of patients. Unilateral disease occurs more frequently in the right renal artery. No venous abnormalities have been described.

Lesions are classified according to the predominant site of involvement within the vessel wall—intimal, medial, or adventitial. Medial fibroplasia accounts for 60% to 70% of all cases of renal artery dysplasia. Fibromuscular dysplasia and atherosclerosis may coexist in older patients.

Treatment of renovascular disease may be indicated to normalize blood pressure or to preserve renal function. In contrast to atherosclerotic renovascular disease, preservation of renal function is rarely a primary reason for treatment. Nephrectomy was the first curative intervention in renovascular hypertension. Surgical vascular reconstruction has been done, with cure rates ranging from 38% to 85%. Most recently, percutaneous transluminal angioplasty has become the treatment of choice, with cure rates ranging from 25% to 85% at 5 years.

REFERENCES

Davidson A. Radiology of the Kidney. Philadelphia: Saunders, 1985.

Kadir S. Diagnostic Angiography. Philadelphia: Saunders, 1986.

Luscher T, Lie J, Stanson A, et al. Subject review— arterial fibromuscular dysplasia. Mayo Clin Proc 1987; 62:931.

Scully R, Mark E, McNeely W, et al. Case report 9-1990. N Engl J Med 1990; 322:612.

Case 70

HISTORY

A 77-year-old asymptomatic woman presented following the incidental discovery of a mass on routine chest radiograph.

RADIOLOGY

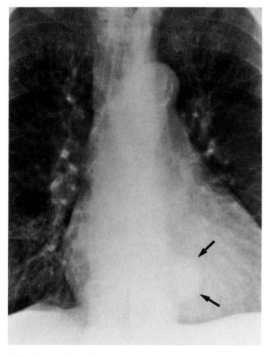

Figure 70-1. Initial chest film reveals a smooth, rounded, soft tissue mass localized to the left lower posterior mediastinum or lung (arrows).

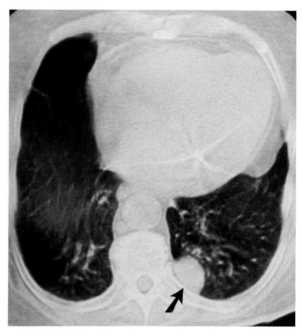

Figure 70-2. CT shows the lesion (arrow) to be smooth and contiguous with the pleura.

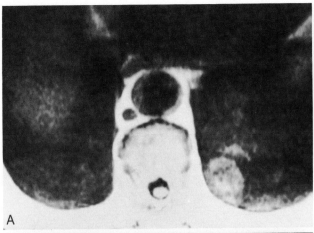

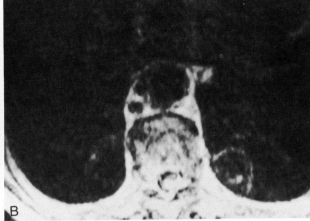

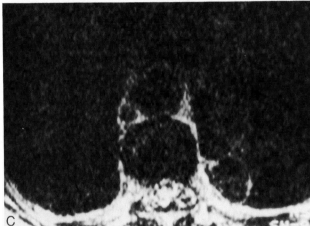

Figure 70-3. *A*. MR image shows that the 3- × 2-cm left paraspinal mass has a homogeneous signal that is isointense to muscle on a T1-weighted sequence. Decreased signal is evident on the T2-weighted images at TE 60 (*B*) and TE 120 (*C*). There is no extension of the mass into the neural foramina. On fluoroscopically guided biopsy (not shown) the lesion moved with the lung but was freely mobile within the pleural space in a fashion consistent with a lesion on a pedicle arising from the visceral pleura.

DIFFERENTIAL DIAGNOSIS

The differential diagnosis includes mesothelioma, metastatic disease, loculated pleural effusion, neurogenic tumor, and paravertebral mass.

PATHOLOGY

The lesion was resected.

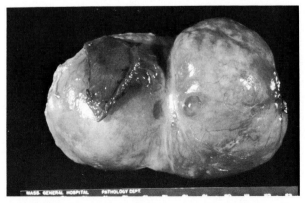

Figure 70-4. The surgical specimen shows a triangular segment of lung attached to a large, well-encapsulated, shiny mass.

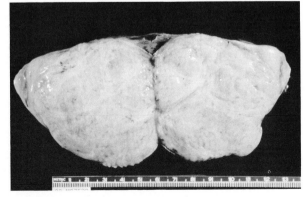

Figure 70-5. On bisection the mass was found to be solid, leathery, and tan-white.

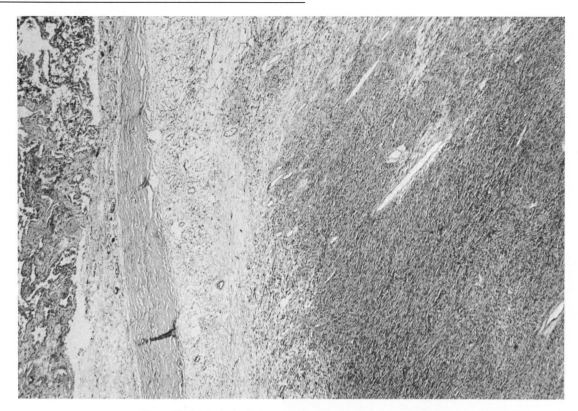

Figure 70-6. Histologically the tumor arises from the adjacent pleura.

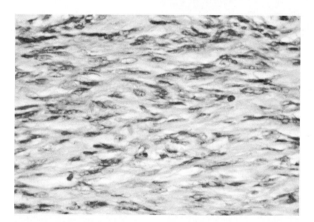

Figure 70-7. The tumor is composed of uniform, cytologically benign spindle cells with intervening bundles of collagen.

DIAGNOSIS

The final pathologic diagnosis was benign fibrous mesothelioma.

DISCUSSION

Mesotheliomas are rare tumors of mesodermal origin that arise from the visceral or parietal pleura and represent fewer than 5% of all neoplasms that involve the pleura. The great majority of neoplasms that involve the pleura do so secondarily.

The benign fibrous mesothelioma (pleural fibroma) is a localized growth. Seventy percent arise from the visceral pleura, 30% from the parietal pleura. They vary in size, from small lesions 1 to 2 cm in diameter to masses that can fill the entire hemithorax. They are often attached to the pleural surface by a pedicle. They remain confined to the lung surface and usually do not produce a pleural effusion. However, invasion of chest wall structures or the lung can occur following incisional biopsy.

Benign fibrous mesothelioma is uncommon and is distinctly different from the malignant mesothelioma that is associated with exposure to asbestos. Malignant mesothelioma is a diffuse lesion that spreads widely in the pleural space, usually is associated with extensive pleural effusion, and invades contiguous structures by direct extension.

Grossly, benign fibrous mesotheliomas consist of dense fibrous tissue with occasional cysts of viscid fluid. Microscopically, spindle cells resembling fibroblasts are distributed among whorls of reticulin and collagen fibers.

About half of affected individuals are asymptomatic, and the lesion is first detected on a routine chest radiograph. Symptoms can include dyspnea, fever, hypertrophic pulmonary osteoarthropathy (15%), and hypoglycemia (10%).

Radiologically, fibrous mesotheliomas present as pleural-based masses that can simulate intrapulmonary masses if they are located in a fissure. They may also simulate mediastinal masses. Up to 10% have pleural effusion. CT may demonstrate a well-defined, smoothly contoured, noncalcified mass with a smoothly tapering margin, compressive atelectasis of adjacent lung, and crural thickening. The MR signal characteristics are consistent with fibrous lesions: dark on both T1- and T2-weighted images.

Surgery is the treatment of choice. Recurrences may result in about 10% of patients, but repeat surgical intervention may be successful in eradicating the tumor, and long-term survival can be expected.

REFERENCES

Cotran RS, Kumar V, Robbins SL. Robbins' Pathologic Basis of Disease (4th ed). Philadelphia: Saunders, 1989.

Dedrick CG, McLoud TC, Shepard JA, et al. Computed tomography of localized pleural mesothelioma. AJR 1985; 144:275–280.

Case 71

HISTORY

A 33-year-old HIV-positive Haitian male presented with a history of 1 week of upper abdominal pain.

RADIOLOGY

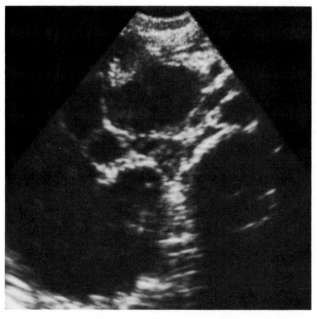

Figure 71-1. Transverse sonogram of the central abdomen shows a complex cystic mass that encompasses the entire field of view.

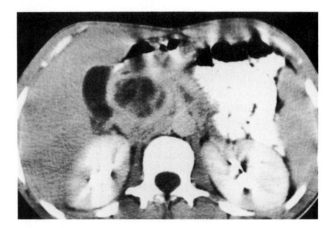

Figure 71-2. Contrast-enhanced CT scan shows a mesenteric mass with heterogeneous peripheral enhancement and central necrosis. The mass is adjacent to the pancreas and extends caudally into the mesenteric pedicle.

DIFFERENTIAL DIAGNOSIS

The differential diagnosis includes lymphoma, Kaposi's sarcoma, tuberculous lymphadenitis, and lymphadenopathy syndrome.

PATHOLOGY

Exploratory laparotomy was performed. A biopsy of the mass was obtained.

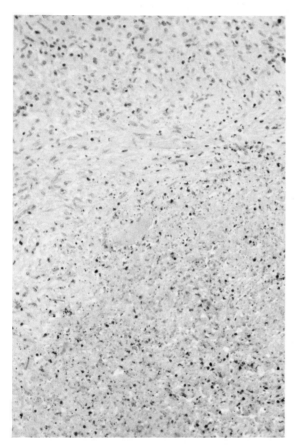

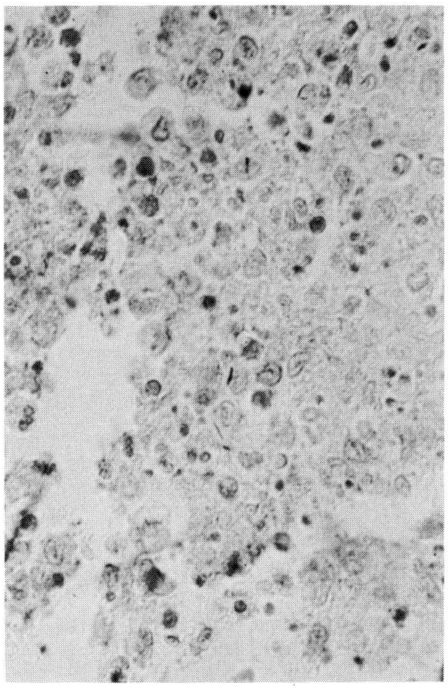

Figure 71-4. Acid-fast stain shows scattered intracytoplasmic acid-fast–positive beaded organisms.

Figure 71-3. Histologically, focally necrotic granulomas surrounded by a cuff of histiocytes and lymphocytes were found.

DIAGNOSIS

The final diagnosis was mesenteric lymphadenitis due to *Mycobacterium avium-intracellulare.*

DISCUSSION

The abdominal manifestations of the acquired immune deficiency syndrome (AIDS) are numerous. All components of the gastrointestinal system are involved including the bowel, visceral organs, and lymphatic system. *M. avium-intracellulare* (MAI) is a ubiquitous organism but an uncommon pathogen in immunocompetent persons. As a pathogen, this mycobacterium is usually confined to the lungs in patients with underlying pulmonary disease. MAI has been detected clinically in 10% to 20% of AIDS patients, and autopsy studies suggest a prevalence as high as 50%. The organism disseminates from a pulmonary source and can be cultured from blood, bone marrow, lymph nodes, and visceral abdominal organs.

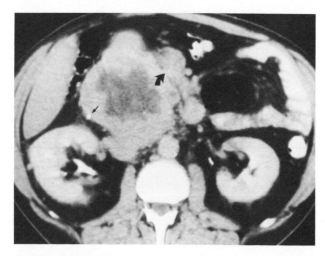

Figure 71-5. Contrast-enhanced CT scan shows a retroperitoneal mass with irregular margins and central necrosis. The mass is paracaval, displaces the pancreas (curved arrow) anteriorly, contains a punctate calcification (small arrow), and appears to extend into the mesenteric pedicle.

Abdominal adenopathy in patients with AIDS is commonly detected by sonography or CT. The lymphadenopathy syndrome, which occurs in patients with AIDS or AIDS-related-complex (ARC), results in "shotty" retroperitoneal and mesenteric lymph node enlargement. The lymph nodes in ARC typically measure up to 1.5 cm, do not undergo necrosis or cavitation, and show follicular hyperplasia on microscopic examination. Lymph nodes measuring more than 1.5 cm in diameter suggest another diagnosis including Kaposi's sarcoma, lymphoma, or MAI lymphadenitis. Retroperitoneal and mesenteric lymph node masses may require percutaneous needle biopsy or exploratory laparotomy for a definitive diagnosis.

It may be extremely difficult to differentiate a lymph node mass from a primary retroperitoneal tumor, especially if it incites a surrounding inflammatory response. Figure 71-5 shows the CT scan from a patient with malignant paraganglioneuroma. Although the abnormality closely resembles necrotic, matted lymph nodes, this retroperitoneal neoplasm represented a discrete lesion and was resected entirely.

MAI infection can involve the GI tract or retroperitoneal and mesenteric lymph nodes. Mucosal involvement of the bowel wall simulates Whipple's disease and results in dilated small bowel loops, thickened mucosal folds with nodularity, and associated peripancreatic lymph node enlargement. More commonly, MAI infection is isolated to the retroperitoneal and mesenteric lymph chains. Enlarged lymph nodes frequently develop low attenuation centers owing to caseation necrosis. Lymph nodes may become matted into necrotic mass lesions, which are detected by sonography or CT.

A presumptive diagnosis of MAI infection is made by histologic examination and the presence of caseation necrosis. Detection of acid-fast organisms indicates mycobacterial infection. MAI is differentiated from other mycobacteria by culture, which often takes weeks to complete. MAI is resistant to standard antituberculous treatment regimens. There is no effective antibiotic therapy.

REFERENCES

Frager D, et al. Gastrointestinal complications of AIDS: radiologic features. Radiology 1986; 158: 597–603.

Jeffery R, et al. Abdominal CT in acquired immunodeficiency syndrome. AJR 1986; 146:7–13.

Marinelli D, et al. Nontuberculous mycobacterial infection in AIDS: clinical, pathologic and radiographic features. Radiology 1986; 160:77–82.

Megibow A, et al. Radiology of nonneoplastic gastrointestinal disorders in acquired immunodeficiency syndrome. Semin Roentgenol 1987; 22:31–41.

Nyberg D, et al. Abdominal CT findings of disseminated mycobacterium avium-intracellulare in AIDS. AJR 1985; 145:297–299.

Case 72

HISTORY

A 4-year-old boy with a 9-month history of anterior right leg mass presented following the recent onset of pain. There was no history of trauma.

RADIOLOGY

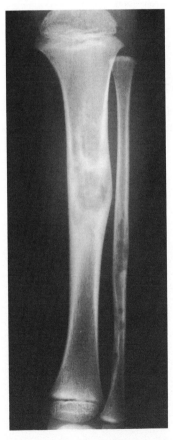

Figure 72-1. An AP radiograph of the right tibia and fibula demonstrates lesions of both bones. Each lesion consists of multiple lytic areas surrounded by well-formed sclerotic walls. The bony contours have been enlarged by periosteal apposition.

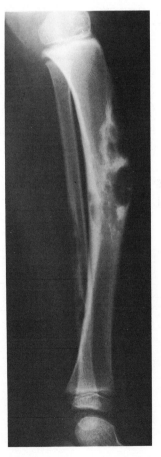

Figure 72-2. A lateral radiograph demonstrates a moderate amount of bowing of the mid tibia.

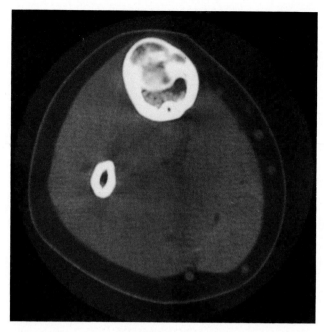

Figure 72-3. A CT scan through the lesion demonstrates its multilocular nature. A large anterior lesion is seen with a small daughter lesion medially and a second focus occupying the posterior cortex. The lesion contains amorphous, cloud-like mineralization and is bounded by moderately well-formed periosteal and endosteal bone.

DIFFERENTIAL DIAGNOSIS

The differential diagnosis includes osteofibrous dysplasia (ossifying fibroma), adamantinoma, fibrous dysplasia, neurofibromatosis, cystic angiomatosis, and hemangioendothelioma (angiosarcoma).

PATHOLOGY

The lesion was resected.

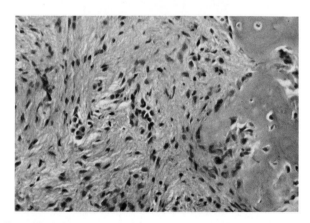

Figure 72-4. The lesion contains various components including reactive woven bone, a spindle cell proliferation, and small nests of epithelial-like cells.

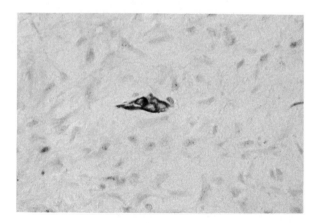

Figure 72-5. Using immunohistochemistry, the nests of epithelial cells stain positively with antibody to the cytoskeletal intermediate-filament keratin.

DIAGNOSIS

The final pathologic diagnosis was osteofibrous dysplasia (ossifying fibroma of the tibia, differentiated adamantinoma).

DISCUSSION

This case is an example of a lesion that has been the subject of much controversy. Osteofibrous dysplasia was first described in 1921 as a slow-growing, painless enlargement of the cortex of the tibia and fibula occurring in children less than 15 years old. At puberty the lesion stops growing and may regress. Bowing and pathologic fracture are frequent. Histologically, it closely resembles monostotic fibrous dysplasia except for its strong predilection for the tibia, its histologic finding of osteoblastic rimming of trabeculated bone, and its zonal architecture (sparse woven bone centrally and frequent lamellar bone peripherally).

Malignant adamantinoma may coexist with the histologic features of osteofibrous dysplasia. Adamantinoma in which the osteofibrous-like features predominate may be clinically and pathologically indistinguishable from osteofibrous dysplasia except for the additional histologic feature of scarce, scattered nests of epithelial-like cells. Pain is also typical of adamantinoma but is atypical for osteofibrous dysplasia. Cases have been reported of recurrent osteofibrous dysplasia demonstrating epithelial elements, osteofibrous dysplasia that progressed to adamantinoma in adulthood, and adult cases of adamantinoma with osteofibrous stroma. These reports have led investigators to postulate that the two entities are really one process, with the osteofibrous stroma representing a reactive response. This postulate is of great concern because it was once thought that osteofibrous dysplasia had features so typical that biopsy was unnecessary. The benign course and histologic absence of epithelial elements in childhood osteofibrous dysplasia may in fact represent tumor regression, a process known to occur in other tumors like neuroblastoma.

REFERENCES

Alguacil-Garcia A, et al. Osteofibrous dysplasia of the tibia and adamantinoma. Am J Clin Pathol 1984; 82:470–474.

Czerniak A, et al. Morphologic diversity of long bone adamantinoma. Cancer 1989; 64:2319–2334.

Dahlin DC, Unni KK. Bone Tumors: General Aspects and Data on 8,542 Cases (4th ed). Springfield, IL: Thomas, 1986:346–356.

Gebhardt M, et al. The treatment of adamantinoma of the tibia by wide resection and allograft bone transplantation. J Bone Joint Surg 1987; 69A: 1177–1188.

Hudson T. Radiologic-Pathologic Correlation of Musculoskeletal Lesions. Baltimore: Williams & Wilkins, 1987:399–405.

Keeney GL, et al. Adamantinoma of the long bones: a clinicopathologic study of 85 cases. Cancer 1989; 64:730–737.

Mirra J. Bone Tumors. Philadelphia: Lea & Febiger, 1989.

Moon NF, Mori H. Adamantinoma of the appendicular skeleton—updated. Clin Orthop 1986; 204: 215–237.

Perez-Atayde AR, et al. Adamantinoma of the tibia: an ultrastructural and immunohistochemical study. Cancer 1985; 55:1015–1023.

Schajowicz F, et al. Adamantinoma of the tibia masked by fibrous dysplasia. Clin Orthop 1989; 238:294–301.

Case 73

HISTORY

A 68-year-old male with a 55-year history of "chronic osteomyelitis" involving the proximal right tibia presented with pain in the left shoulder.

RADIOLOGY

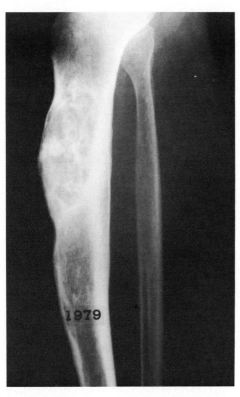

Figure 73-1. A lateral plain film made in 1979 reveals a 4- × 8-cm lytic lesion involving the metadiaphysis of the tibia. The lesion is well defined and multicystic in appearance and has reactive sclerosis surrounding its margins. The anterior cortex is thinned and expanded.

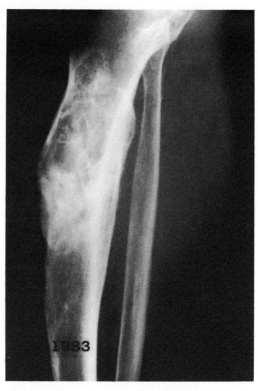

Figure 73-2. A lateral film made 4 years later shows further enlargement of the bone and thinning of both anterior and posterior cortices.

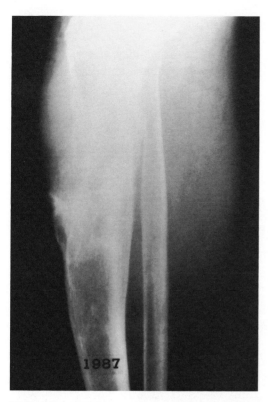

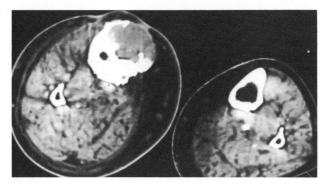

Figure 73-4. A CT scan confirms these findings. No tumor matrix is visible.

Figure 73-3. Lateral radiograph obtained in 1987 demonstrates a large area of destruction of the anterior cortex of the tibia and a soft tissue mass.

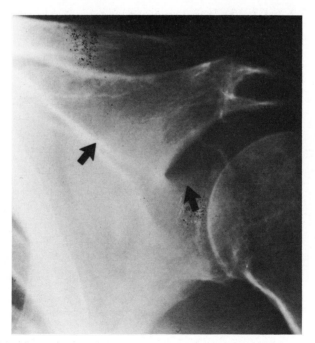

Figure 73-5. An AP radiograph of the left shoulder demonstrates a lytic process involving the scapula near the base of the scapular spine.

DIFFERENTIAL DIAGNOSIS

The differential diagnosis includes chronic osteomyelitis, squamous cell carcinoma, fibrous dysplasia, chondromyxoid fibroma, metastasis, lymphoma, and ossifying fibroma.

PATHOLOGY

The lesion was resected.

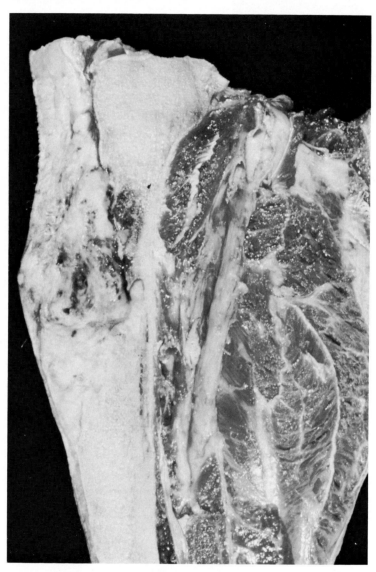

Figure 73-6. The resected specimen shows a large tumor that has destroyed much of the medullary cavity and overlying cortical bone. Tumor invades the subcutaneous fat and causes the overlying skin to bulge.

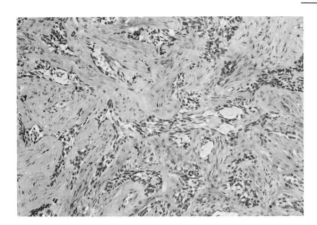

Figure 73-7. Microscopically the tumor consists of irregular nests of tumor cells surrounded by reactive fibroblasts.

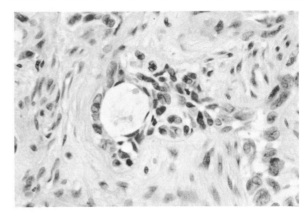

Figure 73-8. The nests of tumor cells are composed of spindle and epithelioid cells, some of which form tubular structures.

DIAGNOSIS

The final pathologic diagnosis was adamantinoma with skeletal metastases.

DISCUSSION

Maier first noted a case of this primary bone neoplasm with epithelial characteristics in 1900. Fischer is credited with the first complete description of this tumor (1913), noting its similar histologic appearance to the more common adamantinoma of the jaw. The dental profession now uses the term ameloblastoma when referring to an adamantinoma of the mandible, whereas adamantinoma of the appendicular skeleton is the preferred name for the less common and unrelated tumor noted peripherally. For the sake of brevity, adamantinoma will be used in this outline to refer to an adamantinoma of the appendicular skeleton.

Adamantinomas are exceedingly rare bone tumors. In Dahlin's description of 4774 malignant bone tumors in 1978, only 17 were adamantinomas, a prevalence of 0.36%. Approximately 200 cases have been described in the literature. More than 80% of adamantinomas occur in the tibia, usually the diaphysis or metaphysis. Although malignant, the tumors are indolent in nature, and patients may describe long-term swelling or pain at the site of the lesion. The peak incidence occurs between the ages of 10 and 30, although the youngest reported patient was a 4-year-old child and the oldest patient was a 74-year-old woman. Interestingly, more than 60% of patients report a history of significant trauma to the area prior to the onset of symptoms and diagnosis of the tumor. The association between adamantinoma and osteofibrous dysplasia has received a great deal of attention. Numerous cases have been reported in which these two lesions have been found in close proximity or even intermingled (see discussion for Case 72).

The etiology of the tumor is the subject of much debate because of its varied histologic patterns. The basic features include epithelioid nests of cells within a dense fibrous stroma. The fibrous stroma has two possible causes. Although these cells may represent tumor cells (ie, the tumor is bimodal), most investigators believe that the stroma is reactive. Five patterns of the epithelioid nests have been described: (1) basaloid, with nests of epithelioid cells surrounded by palisading layers of larger cells; (2) spindle-like, with packed palisades of spindle mesenchyme-like cells; (3) tubular, with small flattened or cuboidal cells lining spaces of varying size, giving the impression of vascular or glandular structures; (4) squamoid; and (5) osteofibrous dysplasia–like, with small nests of epithelioid cells in a stroma that contains trabeculated bone rimmed by osteoblasts resembling osteofibrous dysplasia.

Despite the varied histologic patterns, immunohistochemical and electron microscopic investigations have confirmed the epithelial derivation of adamantinoma. The nests of cells stain strongly for cytokeratin and vimentin, both markers of epithelial cells.

They do not stain for factor VIII antigen and *Ulex europaeous*, which are specific endothelial markers, and are negative for S100, excluding a neural origin. On electron microscopy one sees further evidence of the tumor's epithelial origin with basement membranes, microvilli, tonofilaments, well-developed desmosomes, and gap junctions. There are no Weibel-Palade granules, nor is there evidence of pinocytosis, which would indicate endothelium-derived tissue. Given the tumor's epithelial origin and its characteristic location in bones that are close to the skin surface, many have postulated that the tumor is derived from nests of epithelial cells displaced either after trauma or during embryogenesis.

Adamantinomas most often present as large lesions located in the diaphysis or metaphysis of the tibia. The typical appearance is that of a multicystic osteolytic lesion with surrounding sclerosis. The "soap bubble" appearance of a classic adamantinoma is attributed to the multiple cysts found within the lesion. The cortex may be thinned or inapparent but is most often intact. No significant periosteal reaction is identified. Multicentric lesions are frequently found, and this finding may help explain the high local recurrence rate after excision or curettage. The definitive diagnosis depends on open biopsy.

Adamantinomas are malignant tumors despite their indolent presentation and appearance. Local excision and curettage results in an unacceptably high rate of local recurrence. These tumors are refractory to chemotherapy or radiotherapy. Amputation has been the accepted surgical therapy. Wide resections with bone grafting have become more popular as a limb-saving procedure. The tumor can metastasize to lymph nodes, lung, or other bones. Late metastasis (after several years) is not unusual. The 10-year tumor-free survival is only 9%.

REFERENCES

Gebhardt M, et al. The treatment of adamantinoma of the tibia by wide resection and allograft bone transplantation. J Bone Joint Surg 1987; 69A(8):1177–1188.

Hudson T. Radiologic-Pathologic Correlation of Musculoskeletal Lesions. Baltimore: Williams & Wilkins, 1987:399–405.

Moon NF, Mori H. Adamantinoma of the appendicular skeleton—updated. Clin Orthop 1986; 204: 215–237.

Unni K, et al. Adamantinomas of long bones. Cancer 1974; 34:1796–1805.

Weiss S, Dorfman H. Adamantinoma of long bone. Hum Pathol 1977; 8:141–153.

Case 74

HISTORY

A 17-month-old girl was presented with lethargy, nausea, and irritability. Her head circumference was greater than the 95th percentile for her age.

RADIOLOGY

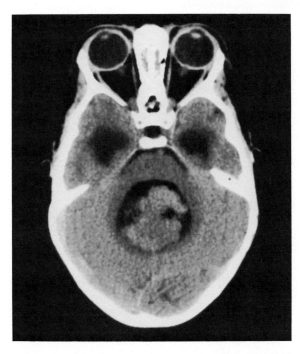

Figure 74-1. Noncontrast cranial CT scan demonstrates a polypoid mass in the fourth ventricle and obstructive hydrocephalus. There is no evidence of calcification or hemorrhage.

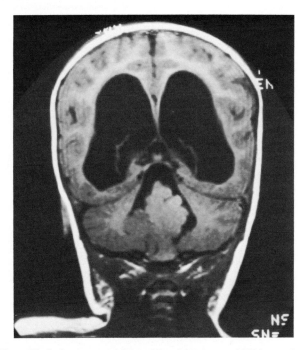

Figure 74-2. On a postgadolinium, T1-weighted coronal MR image the mass arises from the floor of the fourth ventricle and extends through the right foramen of Luschka. Some areas of tumor showed minimal enhancement (not shown).

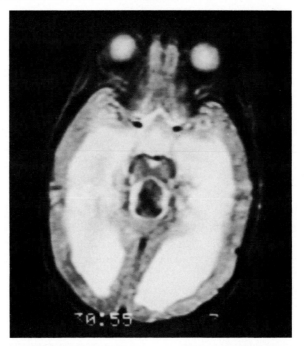

Figure 74-3. The mass extends superiorly into the aqueduct and is heterogeneously dark on T2-weighted images.

DIFFERENTIAL DIAGNOSIS

The differential diagnosis includes ependymoma, primitive neuroectodermal tumor (medulloblastoma), choroid plexus papilloma, and astrocytoma.

PATHOLOGY

The lesion was resected.

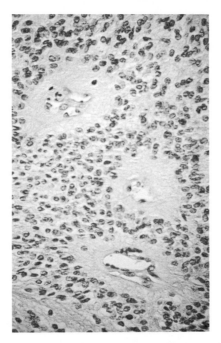

Figure 74-4. Photomicrograph of histologic specimen shows three blood vessels surrounded by eosinophilic cuffs of tumor cell cytoplasm separating nuclei of tumor cells from vessel walls (perivascular pseudorosettes). Nuclei are of uniform size and shape.

DIAGNOSIS

The final pathologic diagnosis was ependymoma.

DISCUSSION

Ependymomas arise from the layer of differentiated ependymal cells that line the ventricles of the brain and the central canal of the spinal cord. Grossly, it is not unusual for ependymomas to demonstrate areas of cyst formation, hemorrhage, and calcification. Microscopically, they are composed of cells containing granular chromatin and regular, round to oval nuclei. A characteristic feature is the formation of perivascular pseudorosettes, in which blood vessels are surrounded by tumor cytoplasmic processes, leaving nucleus-free halos around the vessels.

Ependymomas constitute 8% of intracranial gliomas in children and 1% to 6% of intracranial gliomas in adults. The majority of these tumors occur in children in the first decade of life. A second peak occurs in the fourth decade. In children they commonly arise in the fourth ventricular floor. Symptoms and signs are usually the result of space-occupying effects and secondary obstructive hydrocephalus: headache, vomiting, and ataxia. Most ependymomas grow slowly and are well circumscribed. Soft and often frondlike, they have a propensity for plastic growth and may protrude through the ventricular foramina into the subarachnoid space.

Approximately 50% of lesions are calcified on CT, and most show irregular, patchy enhancement. They are frequently markedly heterogeneous on T2-weighted MR images owing to hemorrhage, calcification, necrosis, and tumor vascularity; thus, differentiation of ependymoma from other lesions is based on their location and morphology rather than on appearance. Gadolinium-enhanced imaging is useful for evaluating possible seeding of the cerebrospinal fluid (CSF) pathways.

Treatment includes surgery and irradiation, but the prognosis is generally poor because of the tumor's location and the technical difficulty of performing a complete resection. Cytologic evidence of malignancy is usually absent, but histologic appearance does not correlate well with prognosis.

REFERENCES

Prince MR, Chew FS. Ependymoma of the fourth ventricle. AJR 1991; 157:1278.

Ross GW, Rubenstein LJ. Lack of histopathological correlation of malignant ependymomas with postoperative survival. J Neurosurg 1989; 70:31–36.

Rubenstein LJ. Tumors of the Central Nervous System. Washington DC: Armed Forces Institute of Pathology, 1972:104–114.

Shuman RM, Alvord EC, Leech RW. The biology of childhood ependymomas. Arch Neurol 1975; 32:731–739.

Spoto GP, Press GA, Hesselink JR, et al. Intracranial ependymoma and subependymoma: MR manifestations. AJNR 1990; 11:83–91.

Case 75

HISTORY

A 63-year-old female with a history of partial colectomy for adenocarcinoma presented with pelvic pain and fullness.

RADIOLOGY

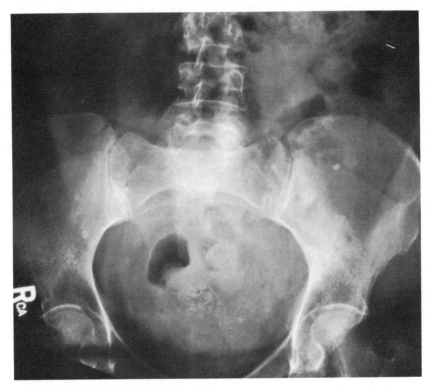

Figure 75-1. Plain film demonstrates a large, noncalcified, pelvic soft tissue mass.

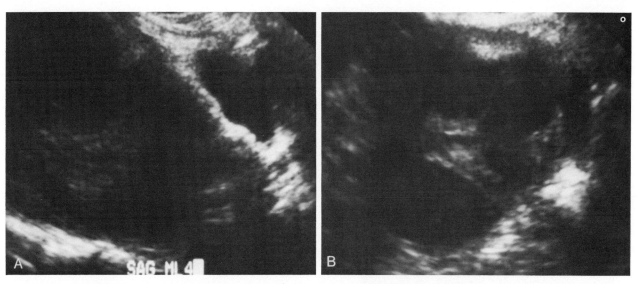

Figure 75-2. Sagittal (*A*) and transverse (*B*) ultrasound examination of the pelvis reveals a 14- X 18- X 10-cm heterogeneous pelvic mass. The uterus, bladder, and ovaries were not identifiable.

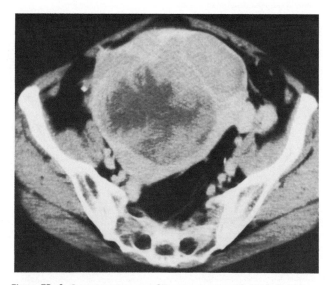

Figure 75-3. Contrast-enhanced CT scan shows a 13- X 13- X 13-cm heterogeneous pelvic mass with areas of contrast enhancement that probably arise from the uterus. The ovaries are not visible, and the mass displaces bowel loops. The ureters are mildly dilated.

DIFFERENTIAL DIAGNOSIS

The differential diagnosis includes ovarian or uterine neoplasms, retroperitoneal sarcomas, and metastases.

PATHOLOGY

A total hysterectomy was performed.

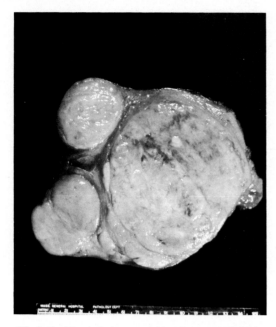

Figure 75-4. The bisected uterus contains a large, round pink-tan mass.

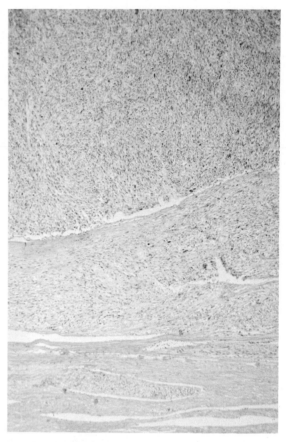

Figure 75-5. The tumor margins push into the adjacent myometrium. A smaller portion of the tumor (bottom) is within a vascular space.

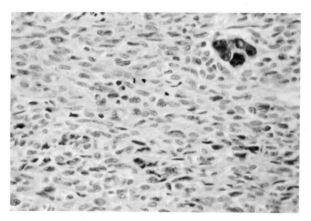

Figure 75-6. The tumor is composed of malignant spindle cells with scattered large pleomorphic cells.

DIAGNOSIS

The final pathologic diagnosis was leiomyosarcoma of the uterus.

DISCUSSION

Uterine sarcomas are rare, comprising only 3% to 6% of all uterine neoplasms. Carcinomas and leiomyomas are much more common neoplasms. It is unclear whether uterine leiomyosarcomas originate de novo or arise from preexisting leiomyomas. In one series comprising 13,000 fibroids (leiomyomas) a 0.3% incidence of sarcomatous degeneration was found.

Uterine leiomyosarcomas produce pelvic pain, mass, weight loss, and irregular bleeding. They are seen in postmenopausal women, who have a mean age of 58. Risk factors are said to include previous radiation therapy, hypertension, diabetes, and obesity. Once the diagnosis has been made, total hysterectomy and oophorectomy are usually performed. The value of oophorectomy is unknown because, unlike with carcinoma, the influence of hormones is uncertain. Radiation and chemotherapy are sometimes recommended, depending upon the stage of the disease. Overall 5-year survival is 40%.

REFERENCES

Callen, PW. Ultrasound in Obstetrics and Gynecology. Philadelphia: Saunders, 1988.

Jones HW, Wentz AC, Burnett LS. Novak's Textbook of Gynecology. Baltimore: Williams & Wilkins, 1988.

Trelo SO, Fishman EK, Kuhlman J. Computed tomography of uterine sarcomas. Clin Imaging 1989; 13:208.

Worthington JL, Balfe DM, Lee JKT, et al. Uterine neoplasms: magnetic resonance imaging. Radiology 1986; 159:725–730.

HISTORY

An otherwise healthy 23-year-old man presented with a dry cough of 6 months duration.

RADIOLOGY

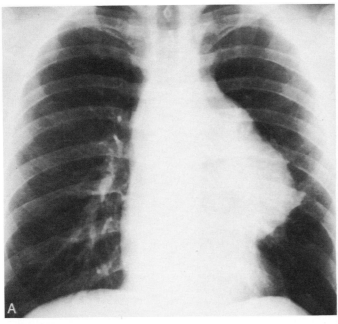

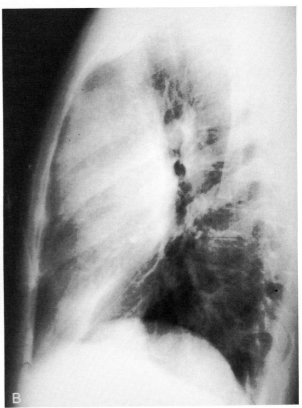

Figure 76-1. *A–B.* Chest films demonstrate a large, predominantly left-sided anterior mediastinal mass with clear lungs and no chest wall abnormalities.

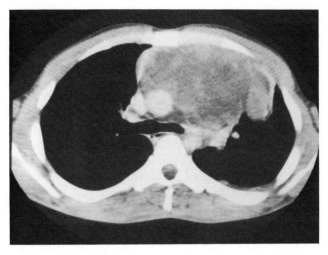

Figure 76–2. Contrast-enhanced CT demonstrates a heterogeneous mass that narrows the left main stem bronchus and displaces posteriorly the left main pulmonary artery. No internal calcifications are identified. There is a large, low attenuation, round region along the right lateral border of the mass.

DIFFERENTIAL DIAGNOSIS

The differential diagnosis includes lymphoma, undifferentiated carcinoma, mediastinal germ cell tumor, thymoma, thymic carcinoid, thyroid lesion, and metastatic disease.

PATHOLOGY

Biopsy was performed.

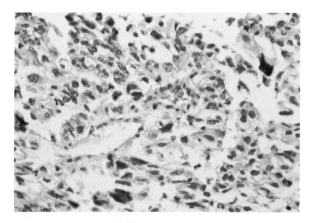

Figure 76–3. Microscopically the tumor is found to contain scattered blood vessels around which palisade stellate and elongated tumor cells. The tumor cells have atypical hyperchromatic nuclei and a moderate amount of eosinophilic cytoplasm.

DIAGNOSIS

The final pathologic diagnosis was yolk sac tumor (endodermal sinus tumor).

DISCUSSION

Primary mediastinal germ cell tumors are unusual malignant lesions that are thought to arise from germ cells that migrate into the mediastinum during development. A thymic origin has been postulated to account for their occurrence in the anterior mediastinum. Primary germ cell tumors of the mediastinum are histologically identical to germ cell tumors of the testes. These tumors can be classified into seminiferous germ cell tumors and embryonal carcinomas. The seminiferous germ cell tumors include seminoma, dysgerminoma, and germinoma. The embryonal carcinomas may be undifferentiated or differentiated. The differentiated forms include embryonic forms, teratoma and teratocarcinoma, and extraembryonic forms, choriocarcinoma and yolk sac (endodermal sinus) tumor.

Yolk sac tumor is among the most unusual of the primary mediastinal germ cell tumors. These were originally called mesonephromas because of the presence of structures resembling primitive glomeruli. The term endodermal sinus tumor derives from a histologic resemblance to intraplacental perivascular structures in the rat called endodermal sinuses. The term yolk sac tumor applies because the tumor originates from the endoderm of the yolk sac. Although the majority of yolk sac tumors occur in the gonads, 20% are extragonadal. Reported sites include the sacrum and coccyx, vagina, retroperitoneum, liver, central nervous system, and mediastinum, nearly all in males under the age of 50 years. As with most of the primary germ cell tumors of the mediastinum, endodermal sinus tumors are generally large at the time of discovery. Most patients present with symptoms of short duration referable to mass effect, but 42% may also have systemic complaints.

The appearance on plain films of yolk sac tumors is nonspecific: that of a large anterior mediastinal mass. On CT they usually exhibit low density regions that correspond to necrosis or hemorrhage; calcification is absent if they are untreated. CT is useful in staging the tumors. Monitoring the response to therapy can be done with CT or with alphafetoprotein levels.

Yolk sac tumors of the anterior mediastinum have the poorest prognosis among the primary germ cell tumors and are more aggressive than their testicular counterparts. Therapy consists of chemotherapy and surgery and sometimes radiotherapy as well. A dramatic response to chemotherapy is common but transient. The single most important prognostic factor is the resectability of the mass. Widespread metastatic disease is common.

REFERENCES

Fox MA, Vix VA. Endodermal sinus (yolk sac) tumors of the anterior mediastinum. AJR 1980; 135:291–294.

Levitt RG, Husband JE, Glazer HS. CT of primary germ cell tumors of the mediastinum. AJR 1984; 142:73–78.

Mori K, Eguchi K, Moriyama H, et al. Computed tomography of anterior mediastinal masses: differentiation between thymoma and germ cell tumor. Acta Radiol 1987; 28:395–398.

Truong LD, Harris L, Mattioli C, et al. Endodermal sinus tumor of the mediastinum: a report of 7 cases and review of the literature. Cancer 1986; 58: 730–739.

Case 77

HISTORY

A 58-year-old female presented with a 4-day complaint of lower abdominal pain. She had a history of aortoiliac vascular grafting.

RADIOLOGY

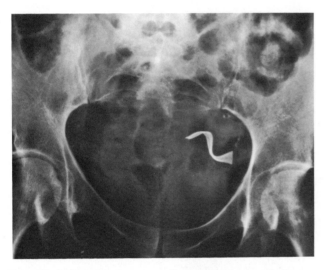

Figure 77-1. Pelvic film shows a curvilinear foreign body projecting over the left hemipelvis.

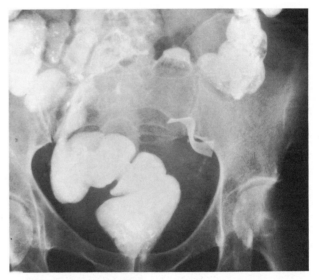

Figure 77-2. The sigmoid colon, which is partially opacified by residual barium and Gastrografin, is displaced by an extrinsic soft tissue mass that surrounds the foreign body.

295

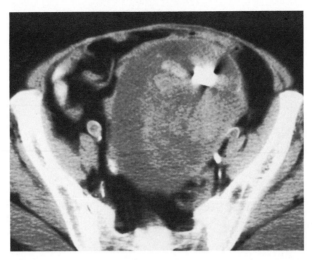

Figure 77-3. Noncontrast CT scan demonstrates bi-iliac vascular grafts. The foreign body is surrounded by a sharply circumscribed 10- × 15-cm heterogeneous collection, which is located in the surgical bed between the iliac bypass grafts.

DIFFERENTIAL DIAGNOSIS

The differential diagnosis includes retained foreign body, diverticular abscess, hematoma, false aneurysm, and cystic neoplasm.

PATHOLOGY

Laparotomy was performed.

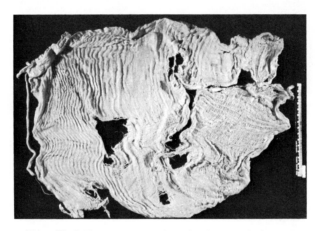

Figure 77-4. The removed specimen is a long surgical sponge.

DIAGNOSIS

The final pathologic diagnosis was gossypiboma.

DISCUSSION

Gossypiboma should be included in the differential diagnosis of a complex mass detected in the postoperative patient. Gossypiboma results from a foreign body composed of cotton material. The most common example of gossypiboma is a retained surgical sponge. Although cotton sponges do not rapidly decompose and are not resorbed by the body, they may elicit an inflammatory response. Two inflammatory reactions occur, fibrinous and exudative. The fibrinous reaction results in encapsulation and local adhesions with eventual foreign body granuloma formation. The exudative reaction results in sterile abscess formation and usually presents sooner than the fibrinous reaction owing to local mass effect. Although one or the other predominates, fibrinous and exudative reactions occur simultaneously.

Like other foreign bodies, a retained surgical sponge may remain quiescent, but usually it causes complications including secondary infection with abscess, fistula formation, and migration with perforation of adjacent structures and viscera. The reported mortality from infected sponges approaches 75%. When symptoms occur, the foreign body must be resected. When the sponge is detected incidentally during radiographic examination, the risk of surgical excision must be weighed against the potential for future complications.

Surgical sponges used in the western hemisphere are manufactured with radiopaque markers incorporated. Owing to overlying osseous or other radiodense structures, however, these markers may not always be visible on plain film examination. If a radiograph is obtained shortly after surgery, gas that has become trapped in the interstices of the sponge may be visible. In chronically retained sponges, CT usually shows a surrounding sharply marginated soft tissue mass in the surgical bed. The peripheral rim or pseudocapsule may be partially calcified or may be enhanced following intravenous contrast administration. The central component may show alternating layers of low and high attenuation due to fluid, hemorrhage, and fibrosis. The foreign body may not be recognizable as a sponge if significant distortion has occurred.

Ultrasound detection of a mass lesion suggests the presence of a gossypiboma in the postoperative patient. The sponge is echogenic with an intense and sharply defined distal acoustic shadow. The surrounding soft tissue component is reniform in morphology and complex or nonspecific in echogenicity. Although CT is more sensitive and specific in detecting gas or calcification in the soft tissue mass, ultrasound may be more sensitive in detecting a centrally located sponge.

REFERENCES

Choi B, et al. Retained surgical sponge: diagnosis with CT and sonography. AJR 1988; 150: 1047–1050.

Kokubo T, et al. Retained surgical sponges: CT and US appearance. Radiology 1987; 165:415–418.

Sheward S, et al. CT appearance of a surgically re-tained towel (gossypiboma). J Comput Assist Tomogr 1986; 10(2):343–345.

Yamato M, et al. CT and ultrasound findings of surgically retained sponges and towels. J Comput Assist Tomogr 1987; 11(6):1103–1106.

Case 78

HISTORY

A 53-year-old man presented with hematuria and complained of occasional flank pain.

RADIOLOGY

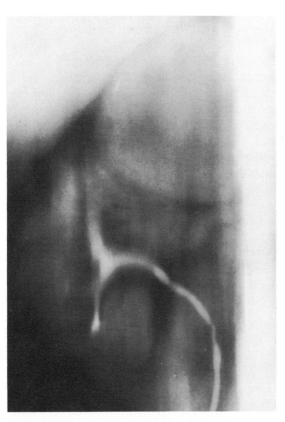

Figure 78-1. Nephrotomogram shows a mass superior to the right kidney with peripheral curvilinear calcifications. The mass is slightly inhomogeneous.

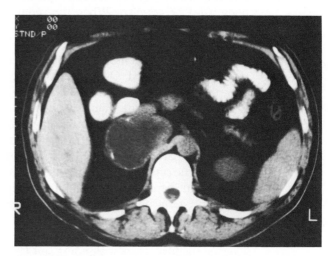

Figure 78-2. On CT scan a 9-cm right adrenal mass with a low attenuation center and a marginated rim of calcification is seen. No retroperitoneal lymphadenopathy is visible.

DIFFERENTIAL DIAGNOSIS

The differential diagnosis includes adrenal carcinoma, nonfunctioning pheochromocytoma, calcified hematoma, tuberculosis, and calcified adrenal hemorrhage

PATHOLOGY

The lesion was resected.

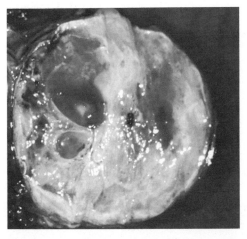

Figure 78-3. The solid pale yellow and hemorrhagic tumor is
encapsulated by a thin layer of white fibrous tissue.

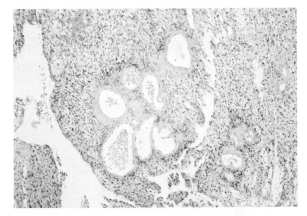

Figure 78-4. The lesion contains prominent dilated capillaries and is
surrounded by a proliferation of benign spindle cells.

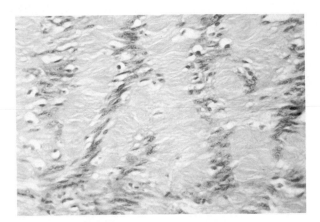

Figure 78-5. In some areas the spindle cells are arranged in parallel
array and separated by fibrillar eosinophilic tissue, forming Verocay
bodies.

DIAGNOSIS

The final pathologic diagnosis was periadrenal schwannoma.

DISCUSSION

For a general discussion of schwannomas, please refer to Case 22.

Case 79

HISTORY

A 31-year-old human immune deficiency virus (HIV)-positive female intravenous drug abuser presented with dysarthria of 1 day and headaches of 1 week.

RADIOLOGY

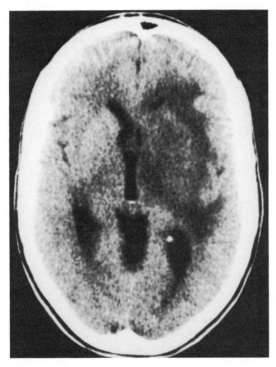

Figure 79-1. Noncontrast CT scan shows a low attenuation area centered in the left lenticular nucleus and caudate head, with edema involving the left internal capsule and external capsule. The frontal horn of the left lateral ventricle is compressed.

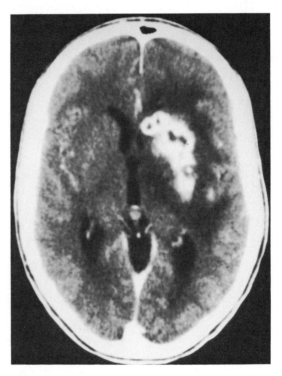

Figure 79-2. The enhanced CT scan demonstrates areas of patchy and ring enhancement.

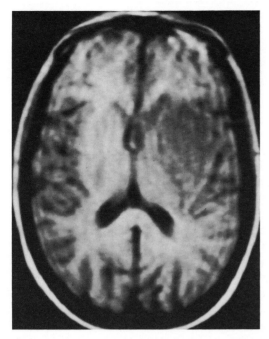

Figure 79-3. The lesion is hypointense on T1-weighted MR images.

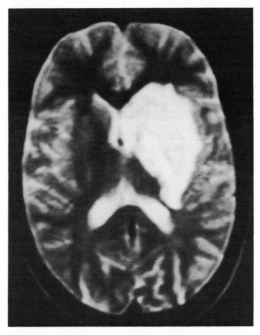

Figure 79-4. T2-weighted images demonstrate hyperintense signal, representing both the lesion and the surrounding edema in the internal and external capsules.

DIFFERENTIAL DIAGNOSIS

The differential diagnosis includes lymphoma, Kaposi's sarcoma, toxoplasmosis, bacterial, fungal, or tuberculous abscess, and viral infection (such as cytomegalovirus).

PATHOLOGY

A stereotactic needle biopsy of the lesion was obtained.

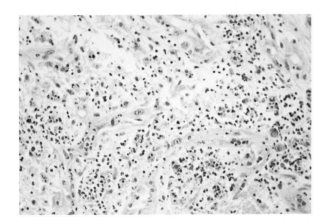

Figure 79-5. The specimen consists of granulation tissue with acute and chronic inflammatory cells.

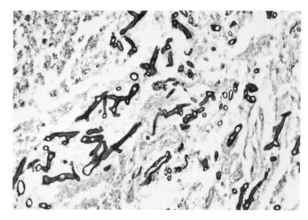

Figure 79-6. Silver stain shows numerous large branching hyphae growing in the inflammatory tissue.

DIAGNOSIS

The final pathologic diagnosis was mucormycosis.

DISCUSSION

Mucormycosis is an uncommon opportunistic infection caused by fungal species of the family Mucoracea. The principal pathogenic genera are *Rhizopus*, *Rhizomucor*, and *Absidia*. These molds are ubiquitous and grow on decaying vegetation and foods with a high sugar content. Infections occur in immunocompromised patients, most frequently diabetics with a history of ketoacidosis. In this population, the infection typically first involves the nose or paranasal sinuses (rhinocerebral mucormycosis). Several other groups of patients are at increased risk and present with characteristic syndromes. These include patients with leukemia, who may present with rhinocerebral, pulmonary, or disseminated mucormycosis; patients with kwashiorkor, who generally exhibit gastrointestinal mucormycosis; patients on deferoxamine therapy for iron or aluminum overload, who have an increased risk of disseminated infection; and intravenous drug abusers, who also more often present with disseminated disease.

Histologically, a mucormycotic abscess is composed of a neutrophilic infiltrate surrounding broad, irregularly shaped hyphae that branch at right angles. As in aspergillosis, hyphal invasion of blood vessels is not unusual.

About 50% of patients with isolated intracerebral mucormycosis have a history of intravenous drug abuse. In these patients, the fungus is thought to reach the CNS through either direct intravenous injection of organisms or through spread from the injection site. The symptoms include fever, headache, nuchal rigidity, nausea, vomiting, and confusion. The abscesses have a predilection for the basal ganglia, particularly in intravenous drug abusers with intracerebral involvement. Cavernous sinus thrombosis is a frequent complication.

On CT imaging, a large irregular area of intracerebral low attenuation with associated mass effect may be seen. On MR imaging, the appearance of the lesion is nonspecific; it is usually hypointense on T1-weighted images and hyperintense on T2-weighted images. Both CT and MR demonstrate patchy, irregular enhancement, unlike the thin ring-enhancing pattern seen with many bacterial abscesses. Abscess can be difficult to differentiate from bland infarcts, which may result from hyphal invasion and obstruction of blood vessels.

Treatment of intracerebral mucormycosis generally includes radical surgical debridement and intravenous amphotericin B. The value of adjunctive therapies such as rifampin, tetracycline, and hyperbaric oxygen is unclear. Close serial follow-up with MR imaging has been suggested to monitor the results of therapy. Close surveillance of patients with rhinocerebral infection may also be warranted; in one study, two of four patients showed intracranial extension on imaging studies before clinical signs developed.

REFERENCES

Anand VK, Alemar G, Griswold JA. Intracranial complications of mucormycosis: an experimental model and clinical review. Laryngoscope 1992; 102(6):656–663.

Case 52-1990. A 31-year-old HIV-seropositive woman with a cerebral lesion seven years after treatment of carcinoma of the cervix. N Engl J Med 1990; 323(26):1823–1833.

Gaing AA, Corbalan F, Weinberger J. Phycomycosis

(mucormycosis) in differential diagnosis of cerebral mass lesions in intravenous drug users. Mt Sinai J Med 1992; 59:69–71.

Sugar AM. Mucormycosis. Clin Infect Dis 1992; 14 Suppl. 1:S126–129.

Terk MR, Underwood DJ, Zee CS, et al. MR imaging in rhinocerebral and intracranial mucormycosis with CT and pathologic correlation. Magn Reson Imaging 1992; 10(1):81–87.

Case 80

HISTORY

A 68-year-old man with chronic renal insufficiency presented with microhematuria.

RADIOLOGY

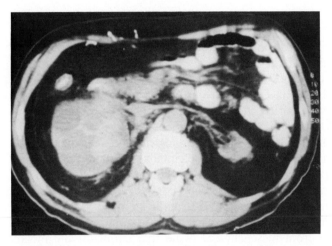

Figure 80-1. A noncontrast abdominal CT demonstrates a 9- × 8- × 12-cm complex mass that totally replaces the right kidney. The kidney has a lobulated contour. No pyelocaliectasis is present. The renal mass is associated with multiple peripheral cystic areas. The left kidney is atrophic. Shotty lymph nodes are present in the para-aortic and retrocaval regions, but there is no obvious involvement of the right renal vein or inferior vena cava.

DIFFERENTIAL DIAGNOSIS

The differential diagnosis includes renal cell carcinoma, multilocular cystic nephroma, lymphoma, and metastatic neoplasm.

PATHOLOGY

The patient underwent a right radical nephrectomy.

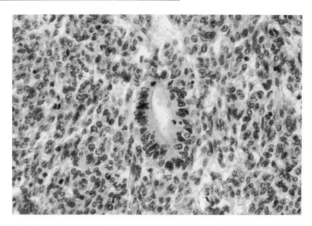

Figure 80–2. The malignant spindle cell element of the blastema surrounds the tubular components of the neoplasm.

DIAGNOSIS

The final diagnosis was Wilms' tumor in an adult.

DISCUSSION

Wilms' tumor (or nephroblastoma) is a very common childhood neoplasm, accounting for 20% of all pediatric malignancies. Eighty-five percent of patients are 6 years old or less, and peak incidence occurs in the third or fourth year of life. Wilms' tumors are extremely rare in adults. Only 1% occur in patients over 15 years old, and less than 200 cases have been reported in the literature. The oldest patient with a documented nephroblastoma was 80.

It is often difficult to distinguish pathologically between an adult Wilms' tumor and a renal cell carcinoma with sarcomatous elements (carcinosarcoma). The following criteria have been adopted for the diagnosis of an adult Wilms' tumor: (1) primary renal neoplasm, (2) presence of primitive blastema (fetal-type renal cells), (3) formation of abortive or embryonal tubular or glomeruloid structures, (4) no areas consistent with renal cell carcinoma, and (5) age over 15 years. Wilms' tumor in both children and adults is thought to arise from mesenchymal tissue that simulates the metanephrogenic renal blastema, which is the precursor for both the nephrons and the interstitial elements of the kidney. Microscopically, there is no difference between a nephroblastoma in adults and children. It is thought that many of the previously reported cases of adult Wilms' tumor were in fact renal cell carcinomas with sarcomatous elements. A renal cell carcinoma lacks fetal renal tissue.

Adult nephroblastomas typically occur in young adults, who present with a slowly enlarging abdominal mass with or without associated flank pain. Hematuria is a frequent associated symptom. Constitutional symptoms such as weight loss, fatigue, and fever are often not present at the time of diagnosis.

Preoperative diagnosis of an adult Wilms' tumor is understandably difficult. Most patients enter surgery with the diagnosis of a renal cell carcinoma, although this neoplasm tends to occur in an older patient population. Wilms' tumors are typically very large at presentation. They are believed to arise in the cortex of the kidney where the highest concentration of blastemal tissue is found.

A mass effect is demonstrated on intravenous urography. Calcification is present in 10% to 30% and is always subtle in appearance. CT shows a large, well-circumscribed, exophytic, inhomogeneous mass, possibly arising from the cortex. Cystic areas are usually described. A pseudocapsule is present in 75% of cases. In addition, a crescent-shaped area of increased attenuation has been described at the periphery of the lesion, which is thought to represent compressed normal kidney. Renal cell carcinoma generally is a smaller and more infiltrating tumor than a nephroblastoma. On angiography Wilms' tumors are most often hypovascular with a "creeping-vine" neovascularity, although avascular and hypervascular tumors have been described. No significant arteriovenous shunting is seen.

The staging of adult Wilms' tumors is the same as that used for children: stage 1, tumor limited to the kidney; stage 2, tumor extends beyond the kidney but is entirely resected; stage 3, residual tumor confined to the abdomen; stage 4, hematogenous metastases; and stage 5, bilateral nephroblastomas. Only one case of bilateral adult nephroblastoma has been recorded. The most common site for metastasis is the lungs; other reported sites include the liver, bone, skin, orbit, brain, and spinal cord.

Fortunately, the preoperative metastatic workups for both adult Wilms' tumor and renal cell carcinoma are identical, given their propensity to metastasize to similar areas. In addition, both are treated initially by radical nephrectomy. Only one case of bilateral adult Wilms' tumor has been recorded. As with children, an aggressive multimodal approach is recommended for the treatment of adult Wilms' tumor. This includes surgery, postoperative radiation (to both the renal bed and metastatic sites), and adjunctive chemotherapy. The prognosis for adult Wilms' tumor is poor compared to that in children with the same clinical stage but has improved with more aggressive therapy. Overall 18-month disease-free survival has recently been reported at 44%.

REFERENCES

Babain R, et al. Wilms' tumor in the adult patient. Cancer 1980; 45:1713–1719.

Fishman E, et al. The CT appearance of Wilms' tumor. J Comput Assist Tomogr 1983; 7(4): 659–665.

Kilton L, et al. Adult Wilms' tumor: a report of pro-

longed survival and review of literature. J Urol 1980; 124:1–5.

Kioumehr F, et al. Wilms' tumor (nephroblastoma) in the adult patient. AJR 1989; 152:299–302.

Roth D, et al. Nephroblastoma in adults. Urology 1984; 24(3):275–277.

Case 81

HISTORY

A 17-year-old male presented with acute shortness of breath resulting from a pulmonary embolus.

RADIOLOGY

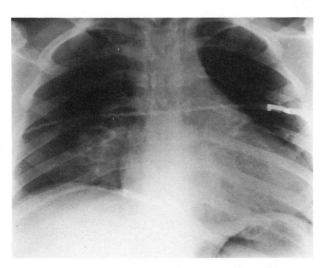

Figure 81-1. Initial chest radiographs demonstrate diffuse bibasilar patchy densities.

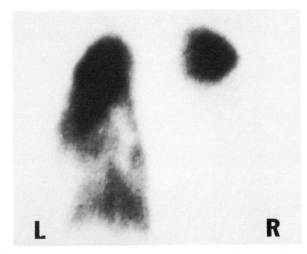

Figure 81-2. There are perfusion defects in the left lower lobe with nonperfusion of the right lower lobe on the posterior nuclear ventilation-perfusion (V/Q) scan.

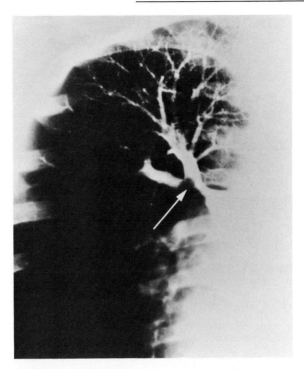

Figure 81-3. A pulmonary arteriogram shows a saddle embolus (arrow) completely occluding the right interlobar artery.

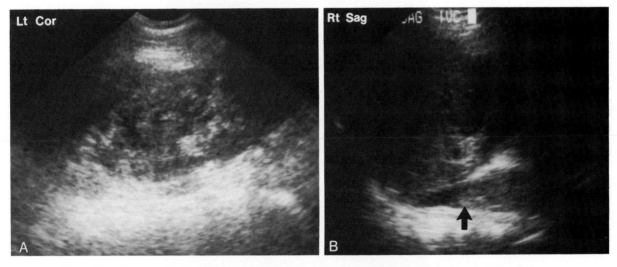

Figure 81-4. Following streptokinase administration, the patient was transferred to Massachusetts General Hospital. Sonography demonstrates a large left renal mass involving the lower and midpoles. Cystic components are present (*A*, left coronal projection), and tumor extension into the inferior vena cava is seen (*B*, right sagittal projection, arrow).

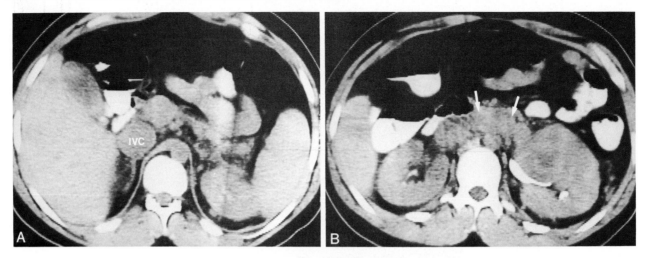

Figure 81-5. *A-B.* Abdominal CT scan demonstrates a large heterogeneous, nonenhancing left renal mass, along with expansion of the left renal vein (arrows) and inferior vena cava. Small left renal lymph nodes are present.

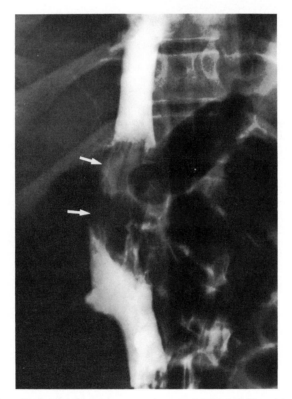

Figure 81-6. Inferior vena cavagram shows an intraluminal filling defect.

DIFFERENTIAL DIAGNOSIS

The differential diagnosis includes Wilms' tumor and renal cell carcinoma.

PATHOLOGY

Embolectomy was performed.

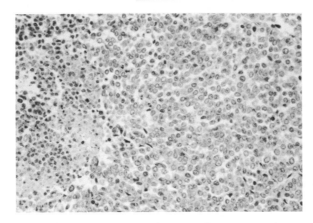

Figure 81-7. The tissue removed from the pulmonary artery shows sheets of small round cells that contain a scant amount of eosinophilic cytoplasm. In some areas there are foci of necrosis.

DIAGNOSIS

The final diagnosis was Wilms' tumor presenting as pulmonary embolus.

DISCUSSION

The kidney is the most common site of origin of abdominal neoplasms in children. Wilms' tumor, also called nephroblastoma, is the most common primary malignant renal tumor of childhood and accounts for about 10% of all childhood malignant tumors. Wilms' tumor is slightly more common in males. More than 90% of these tumors occur at 8 years of age or less, and the average age of presentation is 2 to 3 years. The most frequent (90%) clinical presentation of Wilms' tumor is an abdominal mass. Other clinical findings include hypertension (0% to 60%), abdominal pain (20% to 30%), anorexia with nausea and vomiting (15%), fever (10% to 20%), and gross hematuria (5% to 10%). Venous obstruction can result in leg edema, the formation of a varicocele, or the Budd-Chiari syndrome.

Pathologically, Wilms' tumors are fleshy, predominantly solid tumors, often well circumscribed with a pseudocapsule. Bilateral disease is reported in 4% to 10% of cases. Typically, the tumors are large; the average Wilms' tumor measures 12 cm at presentation. Renal nonfunction from tumor mass effect occurs in 10% of cases. Most of the tumors arise within the cortex, and many grow in an exophytic fashion. Focal hemorrhage and necrosis are common. On microscopic examination, the typical Wilms' tumor consists of a poorly differentiated (blastemal) element, a spindle cell element, and an epithelial element. Wilms' tumors metastasize by direct invasion of adjacent tissues, lymphatic spread to retroperitoneal nodes, hematogenous seeding, or, rarely, urothelial spread to the distal urinary tract. Renal vein invasion has been reported in up to 39% of cases (average 12% to 20%), accounting for the frequent incidence of hematogenous lung metastases. Inferior vena cava invasion is relatively infrequent but is associated with a higher incidence of pulmonary emboli. One study has documented two cases of Wilms' tumor presenting as sudden death due to a pulmonary embolus.

Sonography is the primary method of diagnosis. Tumors are predominantly solid, bulge beyond the kidney margin, and are slightly hyperechoic to adjacent liver. A clear margin is seen in 50% of cases. Calcification, hemorrhage, and focal necrosis are common. Occasionally, the cystic changes may be marked, appearing similar to multilocular cystic disease. Distorted or obstructed calyces may be present. Noncontrast CT typically demonstrates a large inhomogeneous, intrarenal mass, less dense than the surrounding kidney. Following contrast administration, the tumor enhances only slightly and may be seen only in the periphery. MR has not yet found a major role in the imaging of Wilms' tumors.

With chemotherapy and radiation therapy, long-term survival rates may exceed 80%. For further discussion, see case 80.

REFERENCES

Bisset GS, Strife JL, Kirks DR. Genitourinary tract. *In*: Kirks DR (ed). Practical Pediatric Imaging: Diagnostic Radiology of Infants and Children (2nd ed). Boston: Little, Brown, 1991:994–1010.

Cremin BJ. Wilms' tumor: ultrasound and changing concepts. Clin Radiol 1987; 38:465–474.

Case 82

HISTORY

A 56-year-old male receiving chemotherapy for acute myelogenous leukemia presented with persistent fevers.

RADIOLOGY

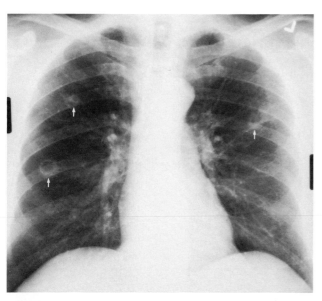

Figure 82-1. Plain chest radiograph shows bilateral cavitating nodules (arrows).

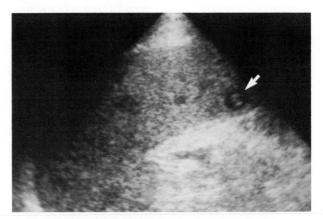

Figure 82-2. Transverse sonogram of the spleen demonstrates multiple round hypoechoic lesions. One of these lesions shows a "wheel within a wheel" or "target" morphology (arrow).

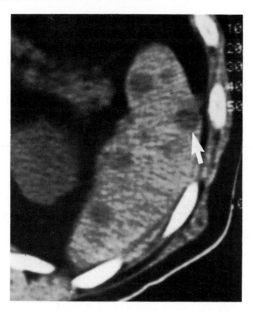

Figure 82-3. Noncontrast CT scan shows multiple, low density, round splenic lesions. One of these lesions has high central attenuation, giving it a target appearance (arrow).

DIFFERENTIAL DIAGNOSIS

The differential diagnosis includes pyogenic or fungal abscesses, leukemic infiltrates, and metastatic tumor.

PATHOLOGY

The patient underwent exploratory laparotomy and splenectomy. The spleen was enlarged.

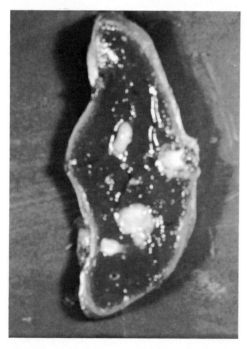

Figure 82-5. Microscopy shows that the centers of the nodules are rich in neutrophils. They are surrounded by layers of macrophages, chronic inflammatory cells, and fibrosis.

Figure 82-4. The bisected spleen contains numerous soft tan nodules.

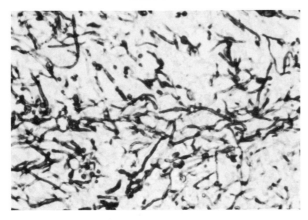

Figure 82-6. A silver stain of the inflammatory exudate shows that the areas with abundant neutrophils contain numerous black unicellular yeast organisms and branching pseudohyphae.

DIAGNOSIS

The final diagnosis was splenic candidal abscesses.

DISCUSSION

Candidal and other fungal splenic abscesses consist of pus, necrotic tissue, and fungus surrounded by layers of histiocytes, chronic inflammatory cells, and fibrosis. On sonography, one may see a "wheel within a wheel" appearance with a peripheral hypoechoic zone (fibrosis), an enclosed echogenic zone (inflammatory cells), and a hypoechoic center (pus, necrotic debris, and fungal elements). One may also see hypoechoic lesions with an echogenic center (fibrosis surrounding inflammatory cells without central necrosis). With healing, lesions become uniformly hypoechoic (fibrosis without central inflammatory mass), and eventually small and echogenic (scar, often calcified). On CT, the abscesses are well-defined, nonenhancing lesions of relatively low attenuation, occasionally with a central focus of higher attenuation.

Fungal abscesses in neutropenic patients may not be detectable in spite of widely disseminated infection. Typical lesions are smaller than 2 cm. Splenomegaly is usual. The liver may also be involved. The lesions become apparent with the return of neutrophil function and their capacity for mounting an inflammatory reaction.

Fungal splenic abscesses occur almost exclusively in immunosuppressed patients receiving multidrug chemotherapy. The diagnosis has become much more common in recent years as the population at risk has increased in size and as more sensitive imaging techniques have been applied. The presentation is nonspecific: persistent fevers, malaise, and weight loss. The most frequent pathogens are *Candida*, *Aspergillus*, and *Cryptococcus*. A histologic diagnosis is often necessary because blood and tissue cultures may be falsely negative. The treatment is usually splenectomy. Antifungal therapy with close radiologic follow-up may be sufficient in some cases. Without prompt treatment, the infection is often fatal.

REFERENCES

Chew FS, Smith PL, Barboriak D. Candidal splenic abscesses. AJR 1991; 156:474.

Nelken N, Ignatius J, Skinner M, et al. Changing clinical spectrum of splenic abscess. A multicenter study and review of the literature. Am J Surg 1987; 154:27–34.

Pastakia B, Shawker TH, Thaler M, et al. Hepato-splenic candidiasis: wheels within wheels. Radiology 1988; 166:417–421.

von Eiff M, Essink M, Roos N, et al. Hepatosplenic candidiasis, a late manifestation of *Candida* septicaemia in neutropenic patients with haematologic malignancies. Blut 1990; 60:242–248.

Case 83

HISTORY

A 40-year-old male presented with hemophilia and a history of pelvic fracture.

RADIOLOGY

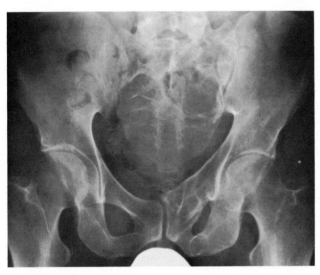

Figure 83-1. AP radiograph of the pelvis demonstrates deformity of the left superior pubis from a previous fracture. There is a large multilocular lytic lesion involving the S1 and S2 segments, primarily on the left side. A poorly defined soft tissue density is seen overlying the lytic area of bone.

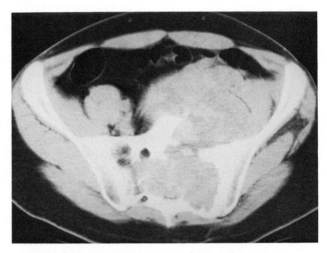

Figure 83-2. An unenhanced CT scan of the pelvis confirms the presence of a large destructive lesion of the sacrum. There is a soft tissue mass that measures 13 × 13 × 9 cm. The mass is of heterogeneous density and contains multiple areas of calcifications. No adenopathy is present.

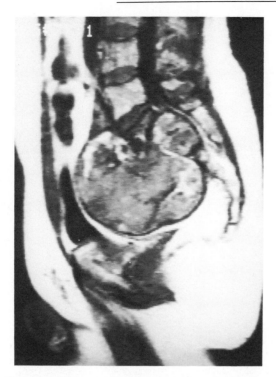

Figure 83–3. A T1-weighted (TR = 550, TE = 20) axial MR image of the pelvis reveals that the sacral and soft tissue mass is bounded by a low intensity rim, suggesting encapsulation. Within the lesion there are areas of bright signal intensity suggesting either fat or recent hemorrhage.

DIFFERENTIAL DIAGNOSIS

The differential diagnosis includes chordoma, giant cell tumor, neurofibroma or schwannoma, and osteomyelitis (including hydatid disease).

PATHOLOGY

A biopsy of the lesion was performed.

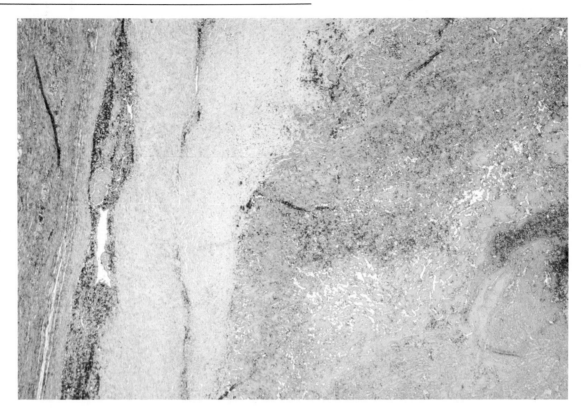

Figure 83-4. The specimen contains large areas of organizing hemorrhage separated from the surrounding tissues by a pseudocapsule.

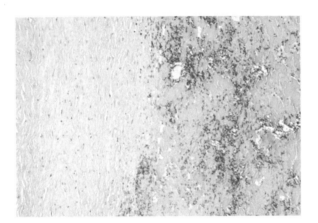

Figure 83-5. The pseudocapsule consists of hypocellular fibrous tissue. Fibroblasts and blood vessels grow into the blood from the pseudocapsule.

DIAGNOSIS

The final pathologic diagnosis was hemophilic pseudotumor.

DISCUSSION

Hemophilia is a bleeding disorder with frequent osseous manifestations and complications. The most common skeletal complication of hemophilia is hemarthrosis, which occurs in up to 90% of hemophiliacs. Hemophilic pseudotumors arise in only 1% to 2% of patients. Pseudotumors were first described in 1918. Since that time over 1000 cases have been reported. These lesions may occur in patients with either factor VIII or factor IX deficiency. Because hemophilia is an X-linked disease, pseudotumors occur only in males; female carriers are unaffected. The most common sites for development of pseudotumors are the long bones of the lower extremity and the osseous pelvis, with more than 75% of lesions occurring in these locations. The small bones of the hand are the next most frequent site of involvement.

Pathologically, hemophilic pseudotumors are composed of a thick fibrous capsule filled with coagulum. Three different theories have been proposed as possible causes of these lesions. Some believe that pseudotumors are secondary to soft tissue or subperiosteal bleeding with subsequent cyst formation. A competing theory is that these lesions are secondary to intraosseous bleeding with pressure necrosis of the bone. Alternatively, some authors think that pseudotumors may be the result of extension of hemarthroses under pressure.

The soft tissue component is variable. When present, the soft tissue mass can become quite large and can produce pressure necrosis of the skin. This is perhaps the most important complication of hemophilic pseudotumors because it exposes the patient to the possibility of severe infection and rupture of the pseudocyst, which may lead to rapid exsanguination.

Radiographically, pseudotumors frequently demonstrate periosteal elevation and destruction of bone. This appearance may make differentiation from Ewing's sarcoma or other malignancy difficult. Calcification or ossification is often evident on plain radiographs or CT. Periosteal new bone formation may be present in the form of arcuate ossific densities known as "struts" extending from the bone into the soft tissues. The pseudotumor is usually encapsulated by periosteum or fibrous tissue, leading to the appearance of a thin rim of decreased signal on both the T1- and T2-weighted MR images. The internal signal characteristics of pseudotumors vary depending on how recently bleeding has taken place.

When pseudotumors are slow growing, they can be managed medically by paying attention to the patient's coagulation status. In enlarging lesions, surgical intervention is necessary. The success of surgery depends on removal of the entire pseudocapsule of the lesion. Radiotherapy has been of some benefit in the treatment of small pseudotumors.

REFERENCES

Bonner G, et al. CT of hemophilic pseudotumors of the pelvis. AJR 1980; 135:167–169.

Brant E. Radiologic aspects of hemophilic pseudotumors in bone. AJR 1972; 115:525–539.

Hermann G, et al. Computed tomography and ultrasonography of the hemophilic pseudotumor and their use in surgical planning. Skel Radiol 1986; 15:123–128.

Resnick D. Bleeding disorders. *In*: Resnick D, Niwayama G (eds). Diagnosis of Bone and Joint Disorders (2nd ed). Philadelphia: Saunders, 1988:2497–2520.

Wilson D, Prince J. MR imaging of hemophilic pseudotumors. AJR 1988; 150:349–350.

Case 84

HISTORY

A 43-year-old male presented with left-sided ataxia and dysphagia.

RADIOLOGY

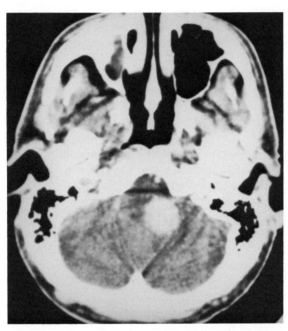

Figure 84-1. Contrast-enhanced cranial CT scan shows a sharply circumscribed homogeneously enhancing round mass. Intra- versus extra-axial location is difficult to determine.

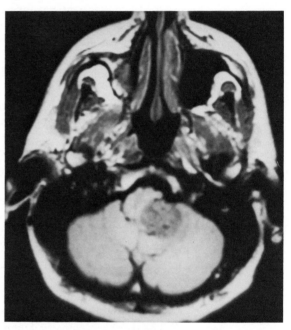

Figure 84-2. T1-weighted axial MR image shows an extra-axial mass in the left cerebellopontine angle with associated compression and displacement of the pons and left cerebral hemisphere.

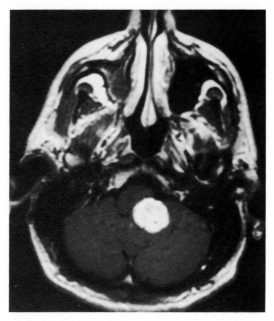

Figure 84–3. Following gadolinium administration, the mass enhances densely.

DIFFERENTIAL DIAGNOSIS

The differential diagnosis includes neurofibroma, schwannoma, meningioma, paraganglioma, metastasis, epidermoid, and glioma.

PATHOLOGY

The lesion was resected.

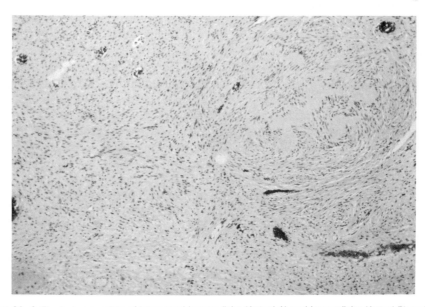

Figure 84–4. The lesion consists of interposed hypercellular (Antoni A) and hypocellular (Antoni B) regions.

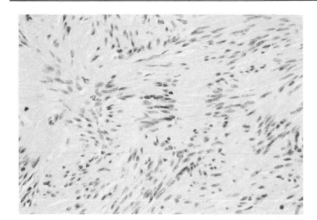

Figure 84-5. The hypercellular (Antoni A) regions contain Verocay bodies in which the spindle-shaped nuclei are arranged in columns and separated by eosinophilic fibrillar cytoplasmic processes.

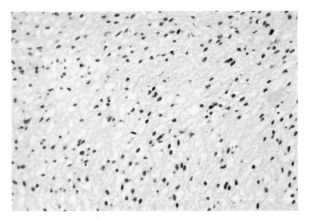

Figure 84-6. In the Antoni B regions the round to elongated neoplastic cells are haphazardly arranged in a loose myxoid background.

DIAGNOSIS

The final pathologic diagnosis was schwannoma originating from the vagus nerve sheath.

DISCUSSION

Schwannomas, benign tumors of nerve sheaths, were first described by Verocay in 1910. They are usually solitary and arise from Schwann cells enveloping nerve axons. All peripheral and all cranial nerves except the optic and olfactory nerves (which do not possess Schwann cell sheaths) can develop schwannomas. Frequently used synonyms for schwannoma include neurilemoma and neurinoma.

Histologic examination of schwannomas characteristically demonstrates proliferating Schwann cells and fibroblasts in areas of both high and low cell density (Antoni A and Antoni B tissue). This case also demonstrates foci of palisaded nuclei within Antoni A tissue, called Verocay bodies.

Schwannomas account for 8% of all primary intracranial tumors. The overwhelming majority involve the acoustic nerve. The trigeminal nerve is the second most commonly involved nerve. Tenth cranial nerve schwannomas are rare and are found in the thorax, parapharyngeal space, jugular foramen, or cerebellopontine angle. Symptoms of vagal nerve schwannoma depend on location; at the jugular foramen, symptoms are generally related to compression of the exiting vagus, spinal accessory, and glossopharyngeal nerves. In the posterior fossa, schwannomas may become large and present with cerebellar signs or deficits in the acoustic nerve, mimicking acoustic schwannoma.

On CT, a well-circumscribed, extra-axial, enhancing mass is noted. Bone remodeling rather than destruction is present when the neoplasm extends into the jugular foramen, implying a slow-growing tumor. In the posterior fossa the mass is centered more caudally than the typical acoustic schwannoma. Multiplanar MR imaging best characterizes the extra-axial location of the mass. The tumor is generally high in signal on T2-weighted images and enhances brightly with gadolinium, but it can be heterogeneous in signal owing to cystic change, particularly when large.

Surgical resection is the treatment of choice for symptomatic schwannomas. The tumors are not radiosensitive. Schwannomas rarely undergo malignant transformation.

REFERENCES

Chang SC, Schi YM. Neurilemmoma of the vagus nerve. A case report and brief literature review. Laryngoscope 1984; 94:946–949.

St. Pierre S, Theriault R, Leclerc JE. Schwannomas of the vagus nerve in the head and neck. J Otolaryngol 1985; 14:167–170.

Sigal R, d'Anthouard F, David P, et al. Cystic schwannoma mimicking a brain stem tumor: MR features. J Comput Assist Tomogr 1990; 14:662–664.

Case 85

HISTORY

A 44-year-old female presented with fever, chills, and myalgias. The patient reported a history of a "fractured right shoulder" as a young child.

RADIOLOGY

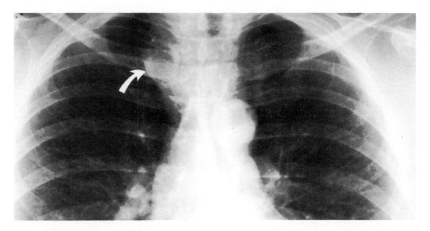

Figure 85-1. A chest radiograph reveals a soft tissue mass in the right paratracheal region (arrow) with extension to the thoracic inlet and deviation of the trachea to the left. Left upper lobe pneumonia is present.

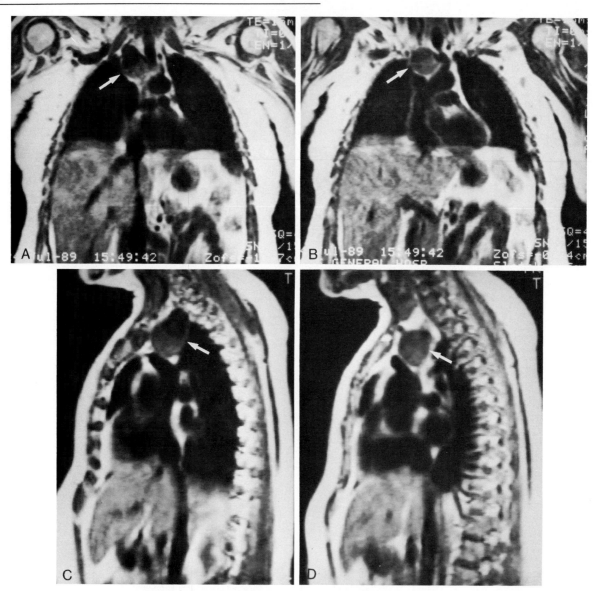

Figure 85-2. Coronal *(A–B)* and sagittal *(C–D)* T1-weighted MR images demonstrate a 4-cm rounded mass (arrow) adjacent to the right brachiocephalic and subclavian arteries. Heterogeneous signal is present within the mass and may be secondary to thrombus formation and/or slow flow.

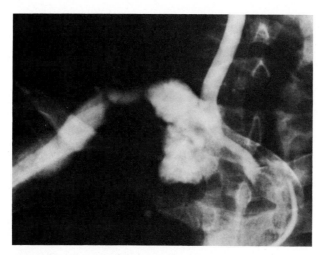

Figure 85-3. Angiogram shows a 4-cm aneurysm arising from the midsubclavian artery, with dilatation of the distal subclavian and axillary arteries. The right vertebral artery is not opacified and is presumably occluded.

DIFFERENTIAL DIAGNOSIS

The differential diagnosis includes thyroid goiter or neoplasm, lymphadenopathy, neurofibroma or schwannoma of the vagus or phrenic nerve, and abscess.

PATHOLOGY

The patient underwent resection of the right subclavian artery aneurysm.

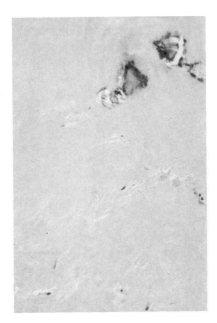

Figure 85-4. Portions of the subclavian artery show marked sclerosis with dystrophic calcification.

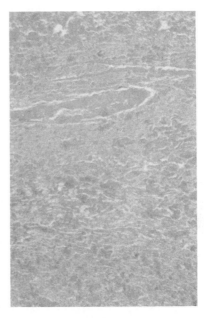

Figure 85-5. The contents of the vessel lumen are filled with layers of fibrin mixed with red blood cells and platelets.

DIAGNOSIS

The final diagnosis was subclavian artery aneurysm.

DISCUSSION

In general, the subclavian artery is one of the less common sites for aneurysm formation, but in the upper extremity it is one of the most common sites. The aneurysm results most often from trauma, as may have occurred in the case presented, or as a complication of cervical ribs and the thoracic compression syndrome. Other causes of aneurysm formation in the subclavian artery include infections such as tuberculosis and syphilis and congenital abnormalities of the arterial wall in conditions such as Ehlers-Danlos syndrome. Arteriosclerosis may also produce subclavian artery aneurysms.

Subclavian artery aneurysms may present with distal embolization to the digits, hemodynamic instability due to rupture, or ischemia of the extremity secondary to thrombosis. Aneurysms may also be discovered incidentally on chest radiographs obtained for unrelated reasons. It is relatively uncommon for subclavian aneurysms to present as pulsatile masses on physical examination.

On plain radiographs subclavian aneurysms may be evident as rounded soft tissue masses projecting over the lung apex at the thoracic inlet. The diagnosis may be confirmed by contrast-enhanced CT or angiography. MR can demonstrate the abnormality and the vascular anatomy in multiple planes.

Given the morbidity of the complications of subclavian artery aneurysm, surgical repair is usual. If the aneurysm is on the right, an approach through a median sternotomy is employed. If the abnormality is on the left, a left thoracotomy is used.

REFERENCES

Brown K, Poonam B. MR imaging of an aberrant right subclavian artery. J Comput Assist Tomogr 1987; 11:1071–1073.

Coselli J, Crawford E. Surgical treatment of aneurysms of the intrathoracic subclavian artery. Chest 1987; 91:704–708.

Kadir S. Diagnostic Angiography. Philadelphia: Saunders, 1986:172–206.

Case 86

HISTORY

A 31-year-old female presented with progressive right upper quadrant abdominal distention. She has been using birth control pills.

RADIOLOGY

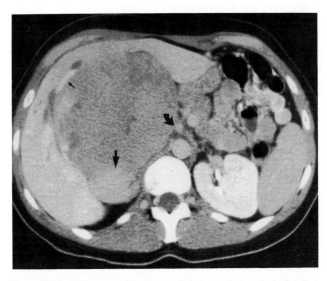

Figure 86-1. CT portography shows a heterogeneous mass lesion that displaces the portal vein (small arrow), kidney (large arrow), and superior mesenteric artery (curved arrow).

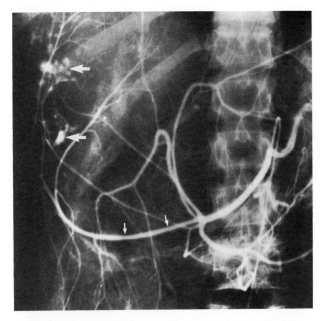

Figure 86-2. On angiography, the hepatic arteries are normal in size but displaced inferiorly (small arrows). Several peripheral contrast collections are visible (large arrows).

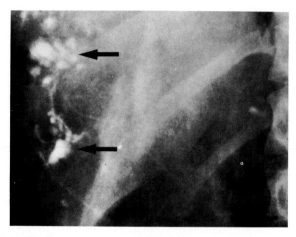

Figure 86-3. These contrast collections (arrows) persist into the venous phase.

DIFFERENTIAL DIAGNOSIS

The differential diagnosis includes hepatic adenoma, focal nodular hyperplasia, and hepatocellular carcinoma.

PATHOLOGY

The lesion was excised.

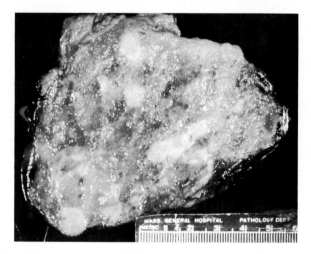

Figure 86-4. The resected lesion has a spongelike appearance with scattered pale tan, well-circumscribed round nodules.

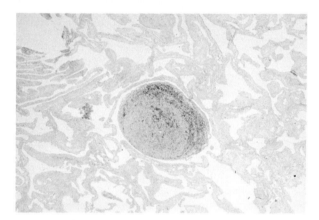

Figure 86-5. Microscopy shows that the lesion is composed of large, thin-walled vascular spaces with scattered intraluminal thrombi.

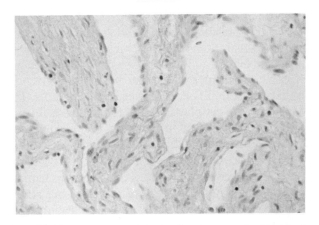

Figure 86-6. The interconnecting vascular spaces are lined by bland endothelial cells.

DIAGNOSIS

The final pathologic diagnosis was giant hepatic cavernous hemangioma.

DISCUSSION

Cavernous hemangioma is the most common benign tumor of the liver. It occurs in all age groups and has a female predominance. Many hepatic hemangiomas are located in the periphery of the posterior segment of the right liver lobe and are solitary, although multiple lesions occur in 10% of cases. The typical lesion measures less than 3 cm in diameter. The definitions of giant cavernous hemangiomas (GCH) vary in the literature and identify GCH as tumors measuring greater than 4 to 12 cm in at least one dimension. One article settled on a size criterion of 6 cm. Whereas hepatic hemangioma is usually asymptomatic and therefore is detected incidentally, GCH commonly causes symptoms owing to mass effect on adjacent structures, spontaneous hemorrhage, or thrombosis within the tumor. Although the size of the tumor and its imaging characteristics sometimes lend to a suspicion of malignancy, there is no malignant potential. Correct diagnosis of hemangioma can avoid angiography, biopsy, or exploratory laparotomy.

Histologically, cavernous hemangioma consists of large, thin-walled, blood-filled vascular spaces lined by endothelium and separated by fibrous septa. Blood flow is slow owing to dilatation of these venous channels. Small lesions are histologically uniform. Central fibrous scarring becomes more common as the hemangioma increases in size. The larger the GCH, the broader the spectrum of possible histopathologic changes, including hemorrhage, thrombosis, fibrosis, liquefaction, and hyalinization.

On sonography, the classic cavernous hemangioma is sharply marginated and homogeneously hyperechoic with posterior acoustic enhancement. Although GCH exhibits some of these findings, heterogeneous echogenicity is the rule and prohibits specific characterization of the lesion. GCH is often too large to be entirely visualized within the field of view of the sonographic probe.

On CT scanning, cavernous hemangioma can be diagnosed if several strict criteria are followed: on noncontrast scan, the lesion is relatively low in attenuation compared with normal liver; during contrast administration, the periphery of the hemangioma enhances first, and this is followed by progressive centripetal opacification; within 3 minutes delayed postcontrast images show homogeneous enhancement that is isodense with normal liver. GCH usually does not fulfill these criteria and therefore is more difficult to diagnose. On noncontrast scan, the central part of the lesion is lower in attenuation than the periphery. During intravenous contrast administration GCH shows heterogeneous peripheral enhancement. Although opacification tends to be centripetal, because of scarring, thrombosis, or hemorrhage, incomplete opacification may occur centrally even on delayed images. Incomplete opacification suggests the possibility of necrosis and therefore is difficult to differentiate from malignancy.

MR images of hepatic cavernous hemangioma show homogeneous signal that is isointense with spleen on T1-weighted images and markedly increased in intensity on T2-weighted images. The signal intensity on T2-weighted images is much greater than that expected for malignant lesions and usually permits a specific diagnosis. MR imaging of GHC shows peripheral signal intensity similar to that of conventional hemangioma and central heterogeneity on both T1- and T2-weighted sequences. The central region is typically lower in signal than the peripheral part of the tumor on T1-weighted images but may be relatively increased or decreased in signal on T2-weighted images depending on the proportion of cystic degeneration and liquefaction or fibrosis and hyalinization. The shape of the central region may be round, ovoid, linear, or irregular.

The angiographic appearance of small and giant cavernous hemangiomas is similar. The hepatic artery and its main branches may be displaced but remain normal in size. The smaller branches show no neovascularity. Contrast collections occur throughout the lesion and result from stasis in dilated vascular channels. Opacified venous lakes remain opacified late into the venous phase of the injection.

Because imaging findings are atypical for cavernous hemangioma, the appearance of GHC can be confused with malignancy including necrotic hepatoma or metastatic disease. Figures 86–7 through 86–9 are CT portogram and MR images from a 54-year-old patient with hepatocellular carcinoma. Like the GCH presented, this malignant lesion involves the left and right liver lobes and demonstrates central heterogeneity due to scarring or necrosis. The pathologic specimen (Figs. 86–10 and 86–11) confirmed the presence of central necrosis. Although the portal and hepatic veins are difficult to assess owing to displacement and distortion of the normal liver anatomy, there is no specific evidence of tumor thrombus to help differentiate between benign and malignant lesions. The presence of a focal high signal intensity on T2-weighted images suggests hemorrhagic necrosis and is not seen in hemangiomas. Other findings with hepatoma include pseudocapsule, central fatty degeneration, and daughter nodules.

Generally, cavernous hemangioma requires no treatment. Surgical excision of GCH may be necessary because of pain, mass effect, and the risk of spontaneous or traumatic hemorrhage. Depending on tumor size, segmental invasion, and vascular extension, hepatocellular carcinoma is resected.

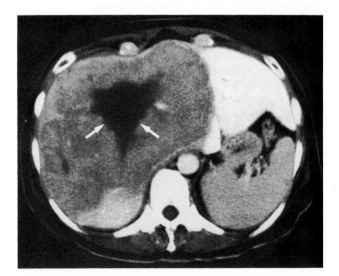

Figure 86–7. CT portography shows a large, heterogeneous mass with nonenhancing central necrosis or scar (arrows) located in the right hepatic and caudate lobes and the medial segment of the left hepatic lobe.

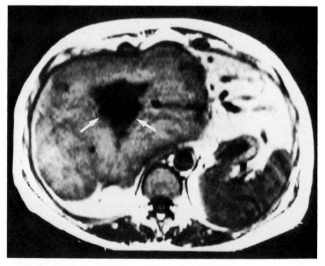

Figure 86–8. T1-weighted MR image (TR = 275, TE = 14) shows that the signal intensity of the mass is similar to that of the spleen. The central region (arrows) is low in signal intensity.

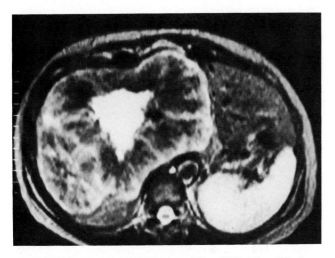

Figure 86-9. On T2-weighted MR image (TR = 2350, TE = 120), the mass is heterogeneous, and the central region shows markedly increased central signal intensity owing to necrosis and cavitation.

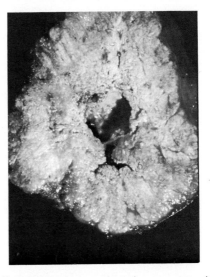

Figure 86-10. Partial hepatectomy showed a mass measuring 15 × 14 × 18 cm. The tumor eroded through the hepatic capsule and, on bisection, showed central cavitation and hemorrhage.

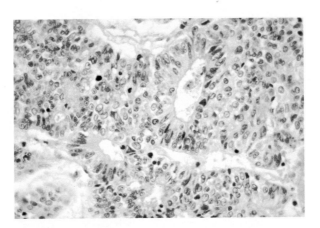

Figure 86-11. The histologic specimen contained dysplastic cells with a loose glandular organization and numerous mitoses. Special stains were positive for carcinoembryonic antigen and alphafetoprotein. The diagnosis was hepatocellular carcinoma.

REFERENCES

Brant WE, et al. The radiological evaluation of hepatic cavernous hemangioma. JAMA 1987; 257: 2471–2474.

Choi BI, Han MC, Park JH, et al. Giant cavernous hemangioma of the liver; CT and MR imaging in 10 cases. AJR 1989; 152:1221–1226.

Ferrucci JT: Liver tumor imaging: current concepts. AJR 1990; 155:473–484.

Itoh K, Nishimura K, Togashi K, et al. Hepatocellular carcinoma: MR imaging. Radiology 1987; 164:21–25.

Nelson RC, Chezmar JL: Diagnostic approach to hepatic hemangiomas. Radiology 1990; 176:11–13.

Case 87

HISTORY

A 60-year-old woman presented with shoulder pain.

RADIOLOGY

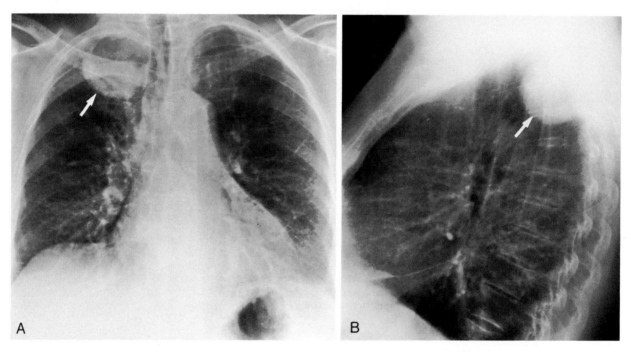

Figure 87-1. *A–B*. Plain radiographs of the chest and upper ribs reveal a 6-cm soft tissue mass (arrow) in the right apex with destruction of the 3rd rib.

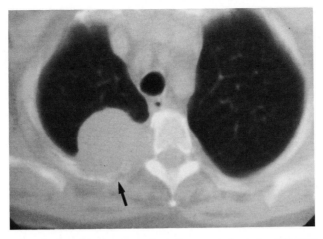

Figure 87-2. Chest CT scan confirms the mass lesion in the right apex abutting the posterior costovertebral region with rib destruction (arrow).

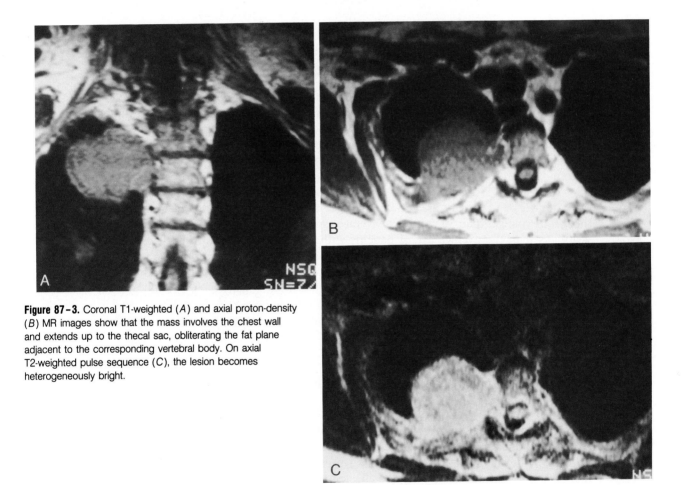

Figure 87-3. Coronal T1-weighted (*A*) and axial proton-density (*B*) MR images show that the mass involves the chest wall and extends up to the thecal sac, obliterating the fat plane adjacent to the corresponding vertebral body. On axial T2-weighted pulse sequence (*C*), the lesion becomes heterogeneously bright.

DIFFERENTIAL DIAGNOSIS

The differential diagnosis includes Pancoast tumor, metastases, and plasmacytoma.

PATHOLOGY

A bone biopsy was performed.

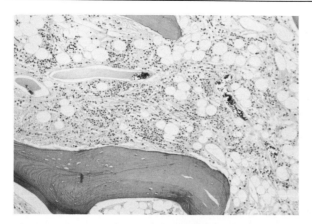

Figure 87-4. The biopsy specimen shows remodeled bony trabeculae surrounded by marrow that is infiltrated by tumor.

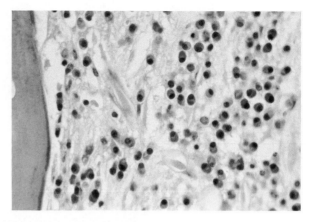

Figure 87-5. The tumor cells have eccentric nuclei, purple cytoplasm, and a perinuclear cuff.

DIAGNOSIS

The final pathologic diagnosis was solitary plasmacytoma.

DISCUSSION

Solitary plasmacytoma (plasma cell myeloma) is a hematologic malignancy composed of plasma cells and is a more uncommon form of the various plasma cell tumors, which include extramedullary plasmacytoma, osteosclerotic myeloma, and multiple myeloma. Solitary plasmacytoma of bone accounts for less than 10% of all plasma cell malignancies. Some authors feel that the disease entity represents an earlier stage of disseminated myeloma. By definition, anemia is absent and bone marrow remote from the solitary lesion is normal. Lesions may be intraosseous or be located in the soft tissues.

About 75% of patients are between the ages of 50 and 70 years, and the lesion is rare in persons younger than 30 years. The average age of patients with solitary myeloma is 10 years less than the average age of patients with multiple myeloma. Males are affected twice as often as females. Symptoms are insidious in onset, and complaints are often vague, varying from progressive bone pain (most commonly back pain), soft tissue masses, fever, and severe pain to paraplegia or other neurologic sequelae resulting from pathologic fractures or mass effect. In contrast to multiple myeloma, symptoms related to hyperviscosity, anemia, and renal failure are uncommon, as are complaints related to thyroid, gastrointestinal, or respiratory complications. A serum paraprotein level may or may not be present.

Pathologically, the tumors are grossly fleshy and red-brown. They are quite cellular with little or no supporting stroma, and the tumorous plasma cells vary in size from small to large.

Radiographically, these tumors have a wide range of appearances. Loss of bone density resulting from marrow involvement that reduces and thins the trabeculae and cortex can simulate osteoporosis. The central skeleton is most often affected owing to the primary involvement of the red marrow within the vertebrae, pelvis, ribs, skull, and mandible, though other bones may be affected as well. Rib involvement, as in this case, typically demonstrates expansile lesions of the outer ends. Alteration of bony texture is also seen, as are "punched out" lesions. Solitary plasmacytomas typically are bubbly, expansile lesions with endosteal scalloping. Occasionally, the lesions are osteosclerotic, with an appearance ranging from sclerotic rims around lucent lesions to ivory vertebrae. Tumors often invade the adjacent soft tissues, creating palpable, paraspinal, or extrapleural masses. Radionuclide bone scans can be misleading owing to failure of tracer uptake in lytic lesions. The high sensitivity of MR imaging in detecting marrow replacement makes it a quite valuable tool in the evaluation of tumor extent, particularly in the presence of a negative bone scan.

Progression to multiple myeloma becomes manifest in most patients with osseous plasmacytoma; however, extraosseous primaries, such as the lesions found in the lung, oropharynx, and sinuses, rarely disseminate and represent limited disease that usually can be cured by resection.

Standard therapy for solitary plasmacytoma includes localized radiotherapy. Surgical management includes fixation of pathologic fractures, prophylactic fixation to prevent fractures, and decompression and stabilization of spinal lesions. Disease progression warrants continued multimodal therapy with chemotherapy, radiotherapy, and orthopedic intervention because a substantial proportion of patients are still alive 5 years after treatment failure.

REFERENCES

Dahlin DC, Unni KK. Bone Tumors: General Aspects and Data on 8,542 Cases. Springfield, IL: Thomas, 1986:193–207.

Frassica DA, Frassica FJ, Schray MF, et al. Solitary plasmacytoma of bone: Mayo Clinic experience. Int J Radiat Oncol Biol Phys 1989; 16:43–48.

Hudson TM. Radiologic-Pathologic Correlation of Musculoskeletal Lesions. Baltimore: Williams & Wilkins, 1987:359–365.

Case 88

HISTORY

A 15-year-old girl presented with a 1-year history of pain in the distal left humerus.

RADIOLOGY

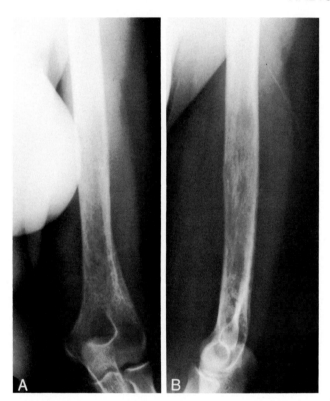

Figure 88-1. *A–B.* Plain films demonstrate subtle permeated bone destruction of the distal half of the humerus. No soft tissue mass is visible.

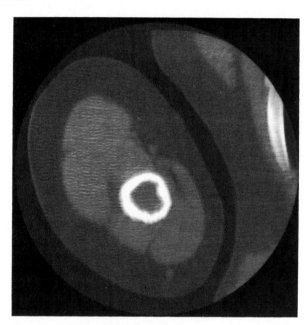

Figure 88-2. On CT scan tiny lucent areas within the cortex represent permeation by tumor. No soft tissue mass is present.

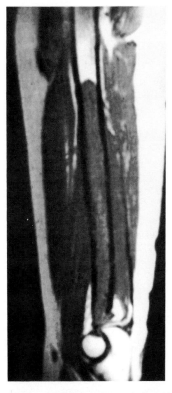

Figure 88-3. T1-weighted MR image demonstrates extensive replacement of the bone marrow by neoplasm.

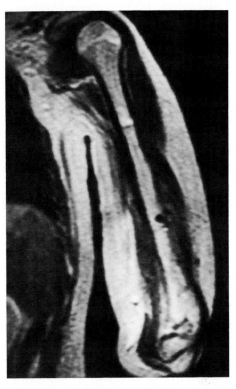

Figure 88-4. T2-weighted MR images are helpful in excluding a soft tissue mass; however, the transition zone between tumor and bone marrow is poorly delineated.

DIFFERENTIAL DIAGNOSIS

The differential diagnosis includes lymphoma, leukemia, histiocytosis, Ewing's sarcoma, and osteomyelitis. Osteosarcoma is less likely given the radiologic appearance.

PATHOLOGY

The lesion was resected.

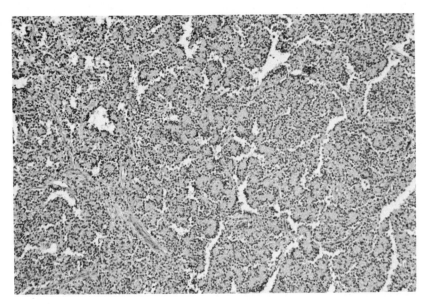

Figure 88-5. The tumor has a uniform appearance with neoplastic tumor cells surrounding ovoid eosinophilic structures.

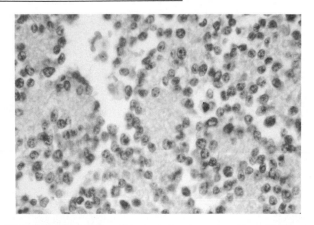

Figure 88-6. The tumor cells are small and round and have ill-defined cytoplasm. The central eosinophilic fibrillar tissue and the surrounding collar of tumor cells are rosettes.

DIAGNOSIS

The final pathologic diagnosis was primitive neuroectodermal tumor (PNET).

DISCUSSION

Primitive neuroectodermal tumors have recently been recognized as a type of "round cell" lesion distinct from Ewing's tumor. These tumors are identical to the malignant small cell tumor of the thoracopulmonary region described by Askin and colleagues in 1979. The lesions resemble the peripheral neuroepitheliomas seen in the soft tissue and are thought to be derived from the germinal neuroepithelial cell, which exhibits the potential to differentiate along a number of neural and mesenchymal lines. Others in this group include medulloblastoma, cerebral neuroblastoma, pineoblastoma, retinoblastoma, and ependymoblastoma. PNETs, however, form a distinct entity compared with other malignant small round cell tumors (neuroblastoma, Ewing's sarcoma, rhabdomyosarcoma, and lymphoma). Although first distinguished on the basis of light and electron microscopic analysis, their neuroectodermal origin has been confirmed by immunohistochemical methods.

On light microscopy one sees evidence of neural differentiation. There is an overall lobular pattern with reticular fibers surrounding large cell groups in a basketlike fashion. In particular, the cells are often arranged in rosettes with a central fibrillary core. On electron microscopy one sees dendritic processes interdigitating between cells, dense neurosecretory granules, and bands of neurotubulelike figures and intermediate filaments. On immunohistochemistry the cells are PAS positive (indicating the presence of glycogen) and stain positive for neuron-specific enolase (NSE), protein S100, and proteins specific for intermediate filaments (vimentin, neurofilaments, glial fibrillary acid protein [GFAP]).

In comparison, Ewing's sarcoma, which is also composed of sheets of small round cells and is PAS positive, is negative for those proteins specific for neurons—NSE, S100, vimentin, neurofilaments, and GFAP. On electron microscopy there is no evidence of dendritic processes or dense neurosecretory granules. In contrast, neuroblastoma is PAS negative, although it shares the other histochemical findings with peripheral PNET. Neuroblastoma, however, often elaborates norepinephrine and its byproducts, which can be reliably detected in the urine. PNET and Ewing's sarcoma do not elaborate catechols.

There have been two recent and exciting advances in the classification of Ewing's tumor, neuroblastoma, and PNET. Both Ewing's sarcoma and PNET demonstrate a reciprocal translocation on the long arms of chromosomes 11 and 22— rcp(11;22)(q24;q12). The proto-oncogene c-sis is located on the distal arm of chromosome 22. Using in situ hybridization techniques, it has been shown to be translocated onto chromosome 11 in Ewing's sarcoma and PNET. In contrast, neuroblastoma demonstrates a different chromosomal abnormality, namely amplification of the n-myc gene, which it shares with its close relative retinoblastoma.

Furthermore, a tumor-specific monoclonal antibody, HBA-71, has been found that recognizes an antigen on the glycocalyx of Ewing's and PNET cells but not on neuroblastoma cells. This observation suggests a close relationship between these two tumors. Some investigators speculate that Ewing's sarcoma is a more primitive form of the peripheral PNET. Peripheral PNET shares many clinical characteristics with Ewing's sarcoma. The peak age range is 9 to 23 (mean 15) years, and there is a male predominance of 2:1 (the Askin tumor shows a female predominance). Most PNETs are accompanied by a soft tissue component. Occasionally soft tissue masses without bone involvement can be seen in the lower extremity and the paravertebral area. Metastases to bone, lung, liver, bone marrow, spleen, and lymph nodes are noted at presentation in 50%, as in Ewing's sarcoma. Unlike Ewing's sarcoma (which is most common in the pelvis and the lower extremities), peripheral PNET is found most often in the thoracopulmonary region, followed by the extremities.

Radiographically, the two tumors are also very similar. One sees a permeated pattern of lysis with soft tissue extension, reflecting the tumor's aggressive behavior, in a diaphyseal or metadiaphyseal location. There may be extensive periosteal reaction, often with an onion-skin or hair-on-end appearance. CT and MR imaging can be helpful in clarifying the extent of disease, and bone scans are useful in looking for metastases.

Peripheral PNET has a poor prognosis. Despite aggressive surgical, chemical, and radiation therapy, mean survival is only 25 months. Although its prognosis is worse than that for Ewing's sarcoma, treatment regimens derived from Ewing's sarcoma therapy are more successful than those derived from neuroblastoma therapy. The high tendency of these tumors to recur locally emphasizes the role of extensive surgery in initial therapy.

REFERENCES

Askin FB, Rosai J, Sibley RK, et al. Malignant small cell tumor of the thoracopulmonary region in childhood: a distinctive clinicopathologic entity of uncertain histogenesis. Cancer 1979; 43: 2438–2451.

Dehner, L. Peripheral and central primitive neuroectodermal tumors. A nosologic concept seeking a consensus. Arch Pathol Lab Med 1986; 110: 997–1005.

Hamilton, G et al. Ewing's sarcoma associated HBA-71 tumor antigen represents a new differentiation marker of human thymocytes. J Cancer Res Clin Oncol 1989; 115:592–596.

Hamilton, G et al. Expression of a new human Thy-1–related antigen in Ewing's sarcoma and primitive neuroectodermal tumors. Immunol Lett 1989; 22:205–209.

Hudson TM. Radiologic-Pathologic Correlation of Musculoskeletal Lesions. Baltimore: Williams & Wilkins, 1987:359–397.

Jurgens H et al. Malignant peripheral neuroectodermal tumors: a retrospective analysis of 42 patients. Cancer 1988; 61:349–357.

Llambart-Bosch A, et al. Malignant peripheral neuroectodermal tumours of bone other than Askin's neoplasm. Virchows Arch [A]; Pathol Anat Histopathol 1988; 412:421–430.

Case 89

HISTORY

A 48-year-old female with symptoms of nasal obstruction for 1½ years presented for imaging after a large right nasal cavity mass was found on physical examination.

RADIOLOGY

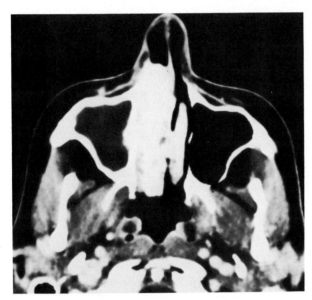

Figure 89-1. Contrast-enhanced CT scan demonstrates a heterogeneously enhancing mass in the inferior nasal cavity that extends posteriorly to the level of the choana. The right maxillary sinus is opacified. The nasal septum is deviated to the left.

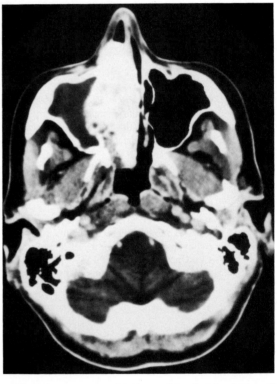

Figure 89-2. The mass remodels the medial wall of the right maxillary sinus and displaces it to the right. There are foci of low density necrosis.

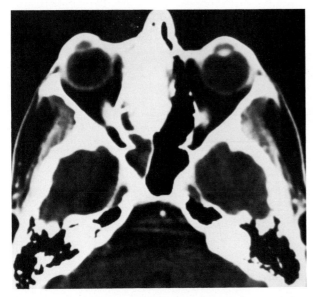

Figure 89-3. The mass extends superiorly into the right ethmoid air cells causing associated opacification of the right ethmoid air cells and the right sphenoid sinus.

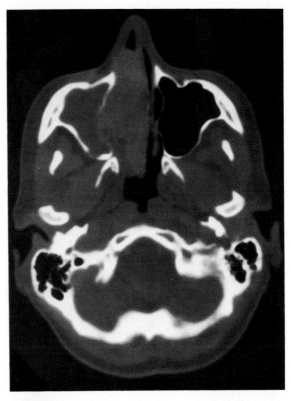

Figure 89-4. Bone windows show that the bowed medial wall of the right maxillary sinus may be eroded.

DIFFERENTIAL DIAGNOSIS

The differential diagnosis includes vascular lesions of the nasal cavity, including hemangiopericytoma, angiofibroma, benign or malignant fibrous histiocytoma, hemangioma, hemangioendothelioma, glomus tumor, angiomatous polyp, and granulation tissue.

PATHOLOGY

The lesion was embolized by catheter and resected through a right lateral rhinotomy and maxillectomy.

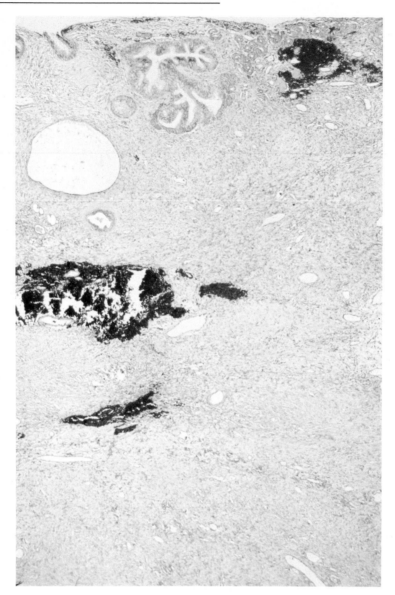

Figure 89-5. The nasal mucosa overlies the focally hemorrhagic and cellular tumor.

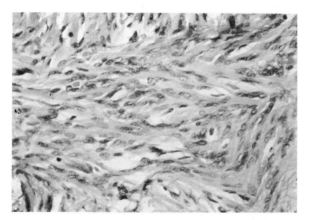

Figure 89-6. The tumor is composed of randomly arranged cytologically bland spindle cells with intervening bundles of collagen. There is minimal mitotic activity and no necrosis.

DIAGNOSIS

The final pathologic diagnosis was solitary nasal fibrous tumor.

DISCUSSION

Solitary fibrous tumor (also called fibrous mesothelioma) is a distinctive neoplasm that most often arises in the pleura. Occurrence in the nasal cavity (as in this case) has been reported. Other rare sites of occurrence include the ethmoid sinus, the peritoneal cavity, and the pericardium. Histologically, the tumors show a "patternless" arrangement of plump spindle cells in a collagenous background. Both hypercellular and hypocellular areas are often seen, along with areas containing prominent branching vessels. Although the tumor was at one time believed to arise from mesothelial cells, the current view, supported by immunohistochemical and electron microscopic findings, is that it is mesenchymal in origin.

The largest published series to date studied solitary fibrous tumors of the pleura. These tumors are often discovered as incidental findings on chest radiographs, or patients may present with cough, chest pain, or dyspnea. Associated clubbing, osteoarthropathy, and hypoglycemia have been noted. Although prognostic factors have not been completely established, large tumor size, hypercellularity, increased numbers of mitoses, pleomorphism, and necrosis are thought to be associated with a poorer prognosis. Complete resection of pleural solitary fibrous tumor is usually curative. Recurrence, however, has been reported in 13% to 20% of cases, usually locally or within the thorax. Distant metastases have also been documented.

REFERENCES

El-Naggar AK, Ro JY, Ayala AG, et al. Localized fibrous tumor of the serosal cavities. Immunohistochemical, electron-microscopic, and flow-cytometric DNA study. Am J Clin Pathol 1989; 92:561–565.

England DM, Hochholzer L, McCarthy MJ. Localized benign and malignant fibrous tumors of the pleura. Am J Surg Pathol 1989; 13:640–658.

Witkin GB, Rosai J. Solitary fibrous tumor of the mediastinum. A report of 14 cases. Am J Surg Pathol 1989; 13(7):545–557.

Young RH, Clement PB, McCaughey WTE. Solitary fibrous tumors ('fibrous mesotheliomas') of the peritoneum. A report of three cases and a review of the literature. Arch Pathol Lab Med 1990; 114:493–495.

Zukerberg LR, Rosenberg AE, Randolph G, et al. Solitary fibrous tumor of the nasal cavity and paranasal sinuses. Am J Surg Pathol 1991; 15(2):126–130.

Case 90

HISTORY

A 17-year-old male, treated successfully at age 5 years for stage IV Hodgkin's lymphoma, presented with a 1-month history of left-sided chest pain and cough.

RADIOLOGY

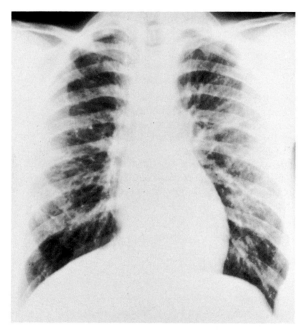

Figure 90-1. Initial chest radiograph reveals a 2- × 4-cm pleural or chest wall mass in the region of the left costophrenic angle. The patient has had a splenectomy and gastric fundoplication. Radiation changes are noted in the paramediastinal regions bilaterally.

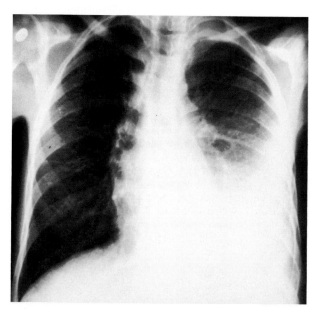

Figure 90-2. Three months later a large left pleural effusion is visible. The left 9th rib is fractured anteriorly, and this rib may be involved with the chest wall process.

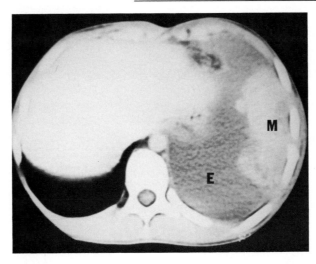

Figure 90-3. CT reveals a 4- × 11- × 9-cm left chest wall mass (M) with a large associated pleural effusion (E). The mass extends into the soft tissues, and there is associated rib destruction.

DIFFERENTIAL DIAGNOSIS

The differential diagnosis includes Ewing's sarcoma, recurrent leukemia, rhabdomyosarcoma, lymphoma, and metastatic neuroblastoma.

PATHOLOGY

The patient underwent an open biopsy and extensive left-sided chest wall resection.

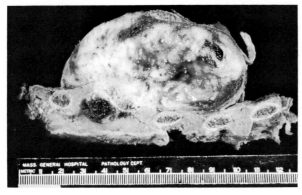

Figure 90-4. The removed segment of the chest wall shows a large soft tan hemorrhagic mass protruding from the pleural surface.

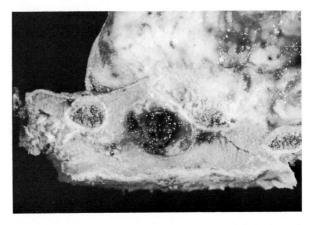

Figure 90-5. The tumor extends into adjacent rib and skeletal muscle.

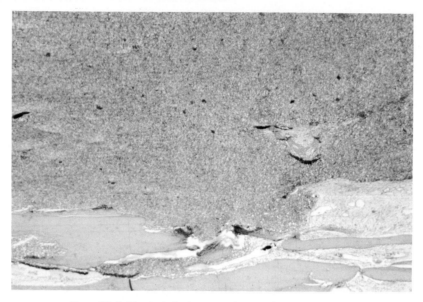

Figure 90-6. Histologically the tumor destroys the cortex of the rib.

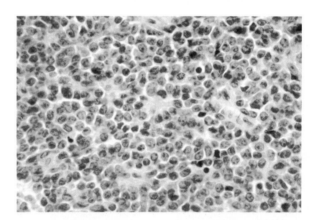

Figure 90-7. The tumor is composed of sheets of small round cells with inconspicuous cytoplasm. In some areas the tumor cells form rosettes. Immunohistochemical stains (stained specimens not shown) were positive for neuron-specific enolase. On electron-microscopic examination (not shown) the cells demonstrated neurosecretory granules and cytoplasmic projections consistent with neuroectodermal cells.

DIAGNOSIS

The final pathologic diagnosis was Askin tumor (peripheral primitive neuroectodermal tumor).

DISCUSSION

Chest wall malignancies are rare in infancy and childhood. Most of the tumors that arise in or metastasize to this area in childhood and young adulthood are small cell tumors that have a similar appearance under light microscopy: sheets of homogeneous small cells with scant cytoplasm. The pathologic differential diagnosis includes Ewing's sarcoma, metastatic neuroblastoma, rhabdomyosarcoma, leukemia, and lymphoma.

Askin and colleagues first described a set of 20 children in 1979 with a "malignant small cell tumor of the thoracopulmonary region" similar in appearance to Ewing's sarcoma. However, microscopic studies demonstrated pseudorosette formation, a relative lack of cytoplasmic glycogen, and immunohistologic staining for neuron-specific enolase. On ultrastructural examination the cells were found to possess neurosecretory granules and cytoplasmic processes with microtubules suggestive of a neuroectodermal origin. Many tumors previously diagnosed as Ewing's sarcoma may have been in fact Askin tumors. Furthermore, immunohistochemical and chromosomal similarities between Askin tumors and Ewing's sarcoma raise the possibility of a common progenitor cell.

Askin tumors typically arise during the first two decades of life. They present as a chest wall mass with or without pain. Pleural involvement and rib destruction are frequent. Despite surgical resection with adjuvant chemotherapy and radiotherapy, the rate of treatment failure is high. The tumor tends to recur locally and metastasizes to the skeleton, lungs, liver, and sympathetic chain.

Primitive neuroectodermal tumor (PNET) is a term used to describe a group of small, round cell tumors of the central nervous system, sympathetic nervous system, bones, and soft tissues (see Case 88).

REFERENCES

Askin FB, Rosai J, Sibley RK, et al. Malignant small cell tumor of the thoracopulmonary region in childhood: a distinctive clinicopathologic entity of uncertain histogenesis. Cancer 1979; 43: 2438–2451.

Boyd A. Tumors of the chest wall. *In*: Hood RM. Surgical diseases of the pleura and chest wall. Philadelphia: Saunders, 1986:239–250.

Fink IJ, Kurtz DW, Cazenav L, et al. Malignant thoracopulmonary small-cell (Askin) tumor. AJR 1985; 145:517–520.

Shamberger R. Chest wall tumors in infancy and childhood. Cancer 1989; 63:774–785.

Triche T, Askin, F. Neuroblastoma and the differential diagnosis of small-, round-, blue-cell tumors. Hum Pathol 1983; 14:569–593.

Case 91

HISTORY

A 47-year-old male presented with fever 2 years following cardiac transplantation.

RADIOLOGY

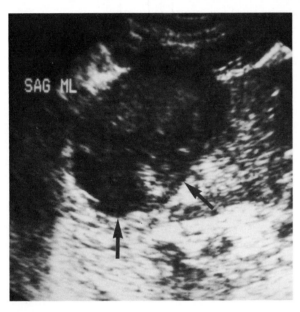

Figure 91-1. Sonography of the left hepatic lobe shows a hypoechoic mass (arrows) with enhanced through-transmission.

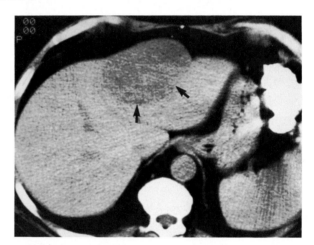

Figure 91-2. On noncontrast CT scan the sharply circumscribed mass lesion (arrows) deforms the anterior hepatic contour.

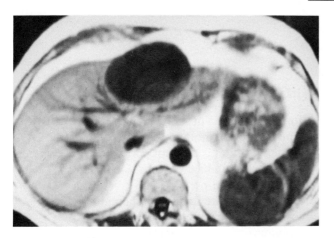

Figure 91-3. T1-weighted MR image (TR = 275, TE = 14) shows that the signal characteristics of the mass are comparable to those of spleen.

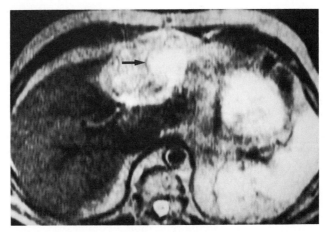

Figure 91-4. Heavily T2-weighted MR image (TR = 2350, TE = 180) demonstrates a central region of higher signal intensity (arrow) due to necrosis.

DIFFERENTIAL DIAGNOSIS

The differential diagnosis includes hepatocellular carcinoma, metastasis, abscess, and hematoma.

PATHOLOGY

An imaging-guided percutaneous needle biopsy was performed.

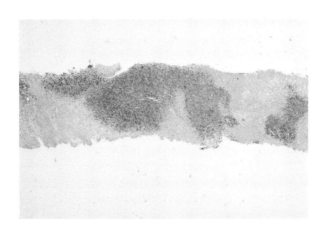

Figure 91-5. A needle biopsy shows that portions of the liver are replaced by a very cellular tumor.

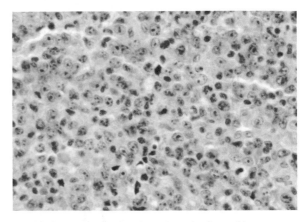

Figure 91-6. The tumor cells are moderate in size and have hyperlobulated irregular hyperchromatic nuclei with scant to moderate amounts of cytoplasm. Many of the nuclei contain prominent nucleoli.

DIAGNOSIS

The final pathologic diagnosis was primary hepatic lymphoma.

DISCUSSION

Transplant patients are at an increased risk for development of malignancies. The most common cancers to develop in transplant recipients are carcinomas of the skin and lips. Lymphomas are the second most common malignancy and account for 20% of cancers in transplant patients. The risk of developing lymphoma in these immunocompromised patients is approximately 100 times that in the general population.

In immunocompetent patients, Hodgkin's disease occurs more frequently than non-Hodgkin's disease in all age groups. In immunosuppressed patients, non-Hodgkin's lymphoma is far more frequent than Hodgkin's lymphoma and most commonly involves the central nervous system. Transplant patients who have received cyclosporine have an increased incidence of hepatic involvement. Although lymphomas arising in immuno-compromised patients typically present 4 to 5 years following transplantation, this time interval is reduced drastically, to less than 1 year, in transplantation patients who receive cyclosporine.

In immunocompetent patients, secondary hepatic lymphoma usually occurs in conjunction with widespread extrahepatic involvement and occurs as diffuse infiltration of the liver parenchyma. Primary lymphoma of the liver, which accounts for only 10% of all hepatic lymphomas, usually presents as single or multiple discrete masses. In immunocompromised patients, hepatic lymphoma may be primary or secondary, and therefore involvement may be focal or diffuse. Lymphoma arising in transplant recipients may decrease in size if the dose of immunosuppressive agents (particularly cyclosporine) is lowered. With some restrictions, chemotherapy and radiation therapy are used in immunocompromised as well as in immunocompetent patients.

Radiologic imaging includes CT, sonography, and MR imaging. On CT scan, hepatic lymphoma is usually hypodense to the surrounding liver and occasionally has a central region of lower density corresponding to necrosis. The tumor may be sharply circumscribed or infiltrative. Discrete lesions are frequently multiple. On sonography the lesions are hypoechoic and may demonstrate enhanced through transmission. MR signal characteristics are nonspecific. Indistinguishable from metastatic disease, hepatic lymphoma shows T1 and T2 signal characteristics similar to those of the spleen.

The imaging studies in this patient show a mass lesion with nonspecific findings. Central necrosis and deformity of the liver contour suggest malignancy. Figures 91–7 through 91–9 show images from the sonogram, CT, and MR imaging of a 59-year-old patient with liver lesions that were detected incidentally during pelvic sonography. Although the patient does not have a known malignancy, the multiplicity of the lesions suggests metastatic disease. However, the imaging characteristics are not typical for metastatic disease. The lesions are hyperechoic on sonography, hypodense on noncontrast-enhanced CT (NCECT) (only the contrast-enhanced study is shown), and hyperintense on MR imaging. As in the patient with primary hepatic lymphoma, the dominant lesion is anterior in location. However, unlike this patient, the liver margin is normal in contour. These findings suggest focal fatty infiltration, which was diagnosed by needle biopsy of the dominant lesion (Fig. 91–10). The pathologic specimen showed fat droplets within otherwise normal hepatocytes.

The liver may undergo diffuse or focal fatty change. Focal fatty infiltration of the liver has a variety of appearances including lobar, segmental, and nodular patterns. In these patients, radionuclide scans and angiography are normal. Sonography shows hyperechogenicity similar to that of hemangioma, NCECT shows attenuation lower than that of spleen, and MR imaging shows increased signal intensity on T1-weighted scans. There is no mass effect or heterogeneous enhancement. Vessels course through the region without encasement or displacement. Fatty infiltration is benign and requires no treatment other than that needed for the underlying condition (if reversible) such as obesity, alcohol abuse, chemotherapy, malnutrition, diabetes mellitus, or jejunoileal bypass surgery.

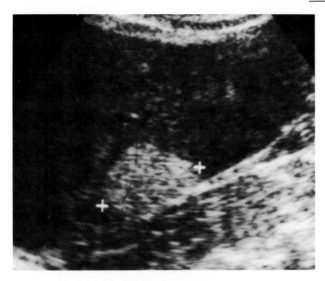

Figure 91–7. Oblique sonography of the left hepatic lobe shows a posterior region of homogeneously increased echogenicity (measuring markers). Similar hyperechoic lesions (not shown) were identified and demonstrated no enhanced through-transmission.

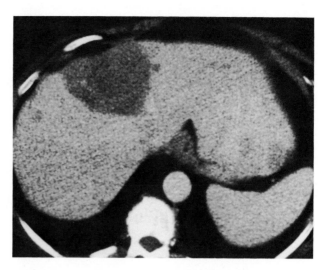

Figure 91–8. Contrast-enhanced CT scan shows multiple lesions of low attenuation. The dominant anterior lesion does not deform the hepatic contour.

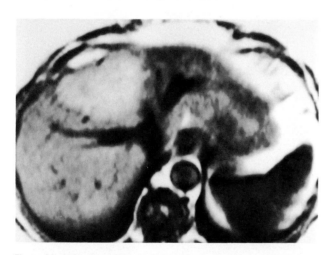

Figure 91–9. On T1-weighted MR image, the dominant anterior lesion shows increased signal intensity.

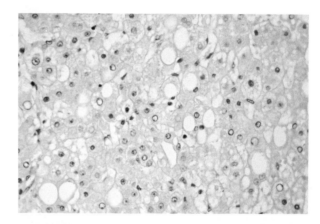

Figure 91–10. Many hepatocytes show numerous intracytoplasmic clear round vacuoles of fat.

REFERENCES

Honda H, et al. Hepatic lymphoma in cyclosporine-treated transplant recipients: sonographic and CT findings. AJR 1989; 152:501–503.

Penn I. Cancers complicating organ transplantation. N Engl J Med 1990; 323:1767–1769.

Swinnen LJ, et al. Increased incidence of lymphoproliferative disorder after immunosuppression with the monoclonal antibody OKT3 in cardiac-transplant recipients. N Engl J Med 1990; 323(25): 1723–1728.

Tubman D, et al. Lymphoma after organ transplantation: radiologic manifestations in the central nervous system, thorax, and abdomen. Radiology 1983; 149:625–631.

Yates CK, Streight RA. Focal fatty infiltration of the liver simulating metastatic disease. Radiology 1986; 159:83.

Zornoza J, et al. Computed tomography of hepatic lymphoma. Radiology 1981; 138:405–410.

Case 92

HISTORY

A 43-year-old male presented with a complaint of several months of right knee pain.

RADIOLOGY

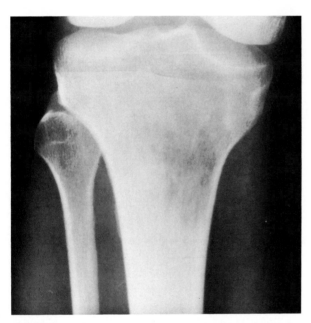

Figure 92-1. A destructive lesion of the proximal tibia has classic "moth-eaten" margins. The lesion is metaphyseal. There is no matrix mineralization, and no periosteal reaction is seen.

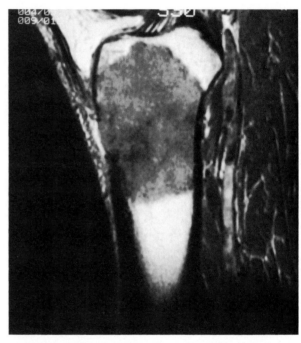

Figure 92-2. Proton-density (TR = 1000, TE = 25) sagittal MR image demonstrates penetration of the anterior cortex by the lesion.

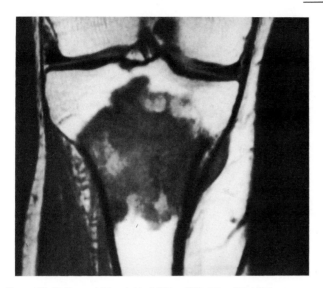

Figure 92-3. Coronal T1-weighted (TR = 600, TE = 25) MR image shows extension outside of the periosteum.

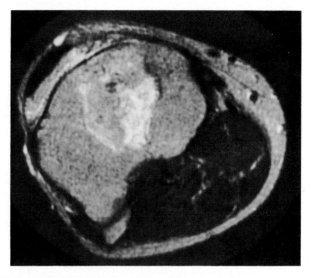

Figure 92-4. T2-weighted axial images show a markedly inhomogeneous brightening within the lesion suggesting a varying mixture of fluid and solid components.

DIFFERENTIAL DIAGNOSIS

The differential diagnosis includes metastasis, fibrosarcoma, or other high-grade sarcoma; less likely possibilities include myeloma and infection.

PATHOLOGY

The tibia was resected.

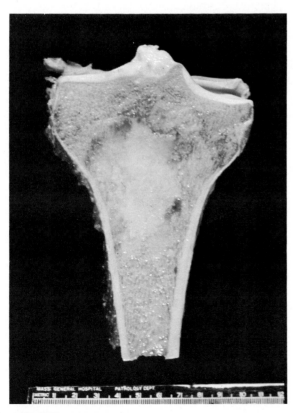

Figure 92-5. The resected tibia contains a solid tan-white mass that fills the medullary component of the metaphysis and extends into the adjacent epiphysis and diaphysis.

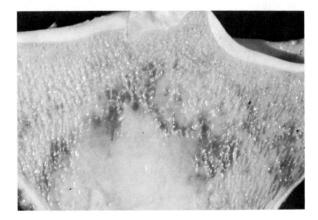

Figure 92-6. Grossly the tumor extends between preexisting bony trabeculae.

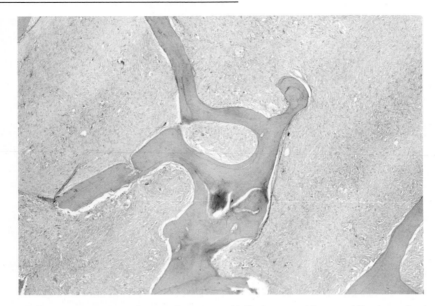

Figure 92–7. The tumor replaces the normal marrow and infiltrates around the preexisting bony structures.

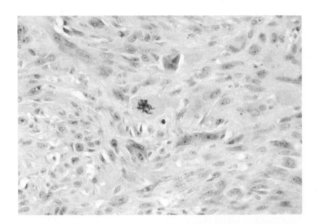

Figure 92–8. The tumor cells are very pleomorphic and range from spindle-shaped to bizarre large ovoid multinucleated giant cells. Mitotic activity is conspicuous.

DIAGNOSIS

The final pathologic diagnosis was malignant fibrous histiocytoma of bone.

DISCUSSION

Malignant fibrous histiocytoma (MFH) is a malignant tumor of mesenchymal origin. It may arise in soft tissue or (less often) bone. It has been recognized as a primary bone tumor only since 1972, previously being categorized as osteosarcoma or fibrosarcoma. MFH is the most common soft tissue sarcoma of adults; MFH of bone is rare. The male to female ratio is to 3:2. MFH most commonly occurs in the fifth to seventh decades but may occur at any age. Symptoms most commonly include a palpable mass with pain and tenderness. More acute pain can occur secondary to the common occurrence of pathologic fractures. MFH of bone can occur de novo in association with other osseous abnormalities (eg, Paget's disease or bone infarct) or following radiation treatment.

The sites of predilection are similar to those seen with osteosarcoma. The long bones are chiefly affected (75%), especially those in the lower extremity. The femur (45%), tibia (20%), and humerus (9%) are the bones most commonly involved. The metaphyseal region is most commonly involved, with frequent extension into the epiphysis or diaphysis. On plain films the lesions appear to be aggressive. Most commonly there is a poorly defined, unifocal, lytic lesion with a moth-eaten or permeated pattern. Cortical destruction almost always occurs, and the lesion extends into a soft tissue mass in 80% to 100% of cases. Periostitis is limited unless a pathologic fracture is present. Osseous expansion is unusual but may be observed in flat and irregularly shaped bones (ribs, scapula, sternum). Mottled calcifications or sclerotic margins are rarely present. On CT the lesions are predominantly of muscle density (10 to 60 HU); hypodense regions represent necrosis (55%). No fat is present. The lesions are hypervascular on angiography. MR imaging may be helpful for assessing both intraosseous and extraosseous extension. Increased uptake is seen on scans done with Tc-MDP, Tc-DTPA, and gallium.

The prognosis is poor owing to local recurrence and hematogenous metastases (most commonly lungs). Reported 5-year survival rates range from 0% to 70%, depending on the size and grade of the lesion.

REFERENCES

Enneking WF. Clinical Musculoskeletal Pathology (3rd ed). Gainesville, FL: University of Florida Press, 1990:395–397.

Hudson TM. Radiologic-Pathologic Correlation of Musculoskeletal Lesions. Baltimore: Williams & Wilkins, 1987:341–357.

Ros P, et al. Malignant fibrous histiocytoma. AJR 1984; 142:753–759.

Case 93

HISTORY

A 74-year-old female presented with an enlarging left scalp mass and gradual onset of proptosis and visual loss in the left eye.

RADIOLOGY

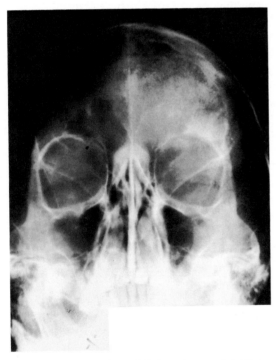

Figure 93-1. Waters' view of the skull shows increased density overlying the left frontal sinus and orbit.

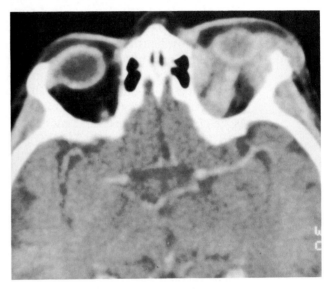

Figure 93-2. Axial contrast-enhanced CT scan shows proptosis due to abnormal soft tissue within the medial and lateral left orbit. The soft tissue lesion extends anterior to the lateral orbital wall.

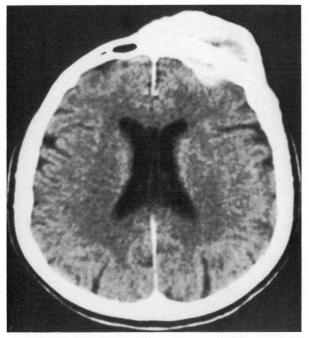

Figure 93-3. The enhancing mass is exophytic from the scalp and also extends intracranially along the inner table of the left frontal bone.

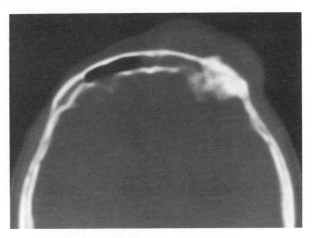

Figure 93-4. Bone windows show irregular hyperostosis involving both the outer and inner tables of the skull.

DIFFERENTIAL DIAGNOSIS

The differential diagnosis includes metastases, lymphoma, basal cell carcinoma, squamous cell carcinoma, sebaceous cell carcinoma, neurofibroma, neurofibrosarcoma, cellulitis, lacrimal duct tumors, sarcoid, meningioma, and arteriovenous malformation.

PATHOLOGY

A biopsy of the scalp lesion was obtained.

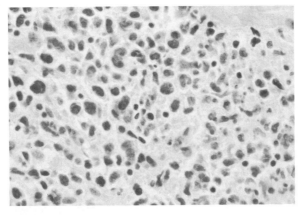

Figure 93-5. The tumor is extremely cellular and is composed of round, small to medium size cells that have very hyperchromatic nuclei, some of which have irregular contours.

DIAGNOSIS

The final pathologic diagnosis was lymphoma of the scalp.

DISCUSSION

Various types of lymphoma can involve the skin, either primarily or secondarily. The most common lymphoma of the skin is mycosis fungoides, a T cell lymphoma. In addition, diffuse large cell lymphoma of both B and T cell subtypes can occur, and a variety of nodular lymphomas of the skin have been described.

In a recent report of follicular dermal lymphomas, 9 of 15 patients had primary cutaneous lymphoma without extradermal involvement. In eight of these patients the primary site was on the scalp or forehead. The skin lesions were indurated, red or violaceous, and painless. Five small cleaved cell, seven mixed, and three large cell follicular lymphomas were found.

As this case illustrates, there is no anatomic barrier preventing scalp masses from entering the orbit by superficial extension over the bony orbital margin. Once in the orbit, proptosis can occur, and the appearance may mimic that of orbital neurofibroma, hemangioma, lymphangioma, or metastatic disease.

The CT and MR appearance of scalp lesions is nonspecific, and the differential diagnosis includes melanoma, squamous cell carcinoma, basal cell carcinoma, plexiform neurofibroma, cellulitis, and metastatic disease.

Primary follicular lymphomas of the skin respond well to radiation therapy and chemotherapy. If the disease is confined to the skin, the prognosis is generally favorable.

REFERENCES

Garcia CF, Weiss LM, Warnke RA, et al. Cutaneous follicular lymphoma. Am J Surg Pathol 1986; 10:454–463.

Ruff RJ, Osborn AG, Harnsberger HR, et al. Extracalvarial soft tissues in cranial computed tomography. Normal anatomy and pathology. Invest Radiol 1985; 20:374–380.

Willemze R, Meijer CJ, Sentis HJ, et al. Primary cutaneous large cell lymphomas of follicular center cell origin. A clinical follow-up study of nineteen patients. J Am Acad Dermatol 1987; 16:518–526.

Wood GS, Burke JS, Horning S, et al. The immunologic and clinicopathologic heterogeneity of cutaneous lymphomas other than mycosis fungoides. Blood 1983; 62:464–472.

Case 94

HISTORY

The esophagram of a 27-year-old man admitted for evaluation of epigastric pain unexpectedly showed bilateral paraspinal soft tissue masses.

RADIOLOGY

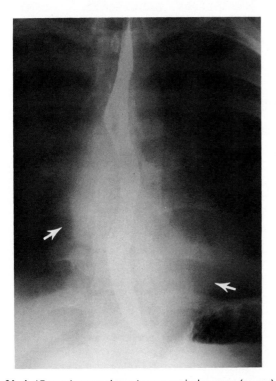

Figure 94 – 1. AP esophagram shows two paraspinal masses (arrows).

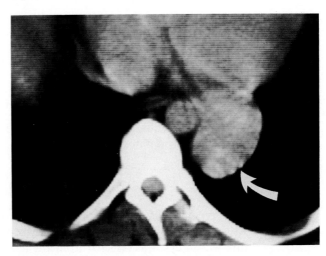

Figure 94 – 2. CT scan at the level of the left lesion shows sharp margination (arrow). The structures adjacent to the mass, including the lung, appear normal

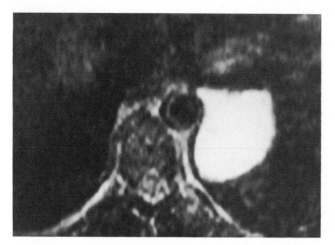

Figure 94–3. T2-weighted axial MR image demonstrates the left lesion as a bright, featureless signal with a horizontal fluid level.

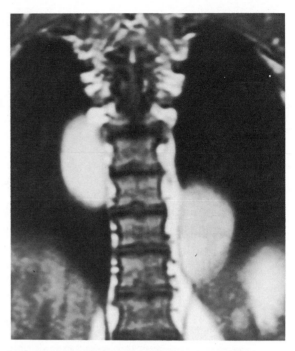

Figure 94–4. T1-weighted coronal MR image shows a bright signal in both lesions.

DIFFERENTIAL DIAGNOSIS

The differential diagnosis includes bronchogenic or respiratory cysts, enteric cysts, and lymphangiomatosis.

PATHOLOGY

Percutaneous needle aspiration of the right-sided mass produced mucoid material. At surgery the masses were completely separate from each other. A tense mucus-filled, thin-walled cyst was resected from the left side; there was no hemorrhage.

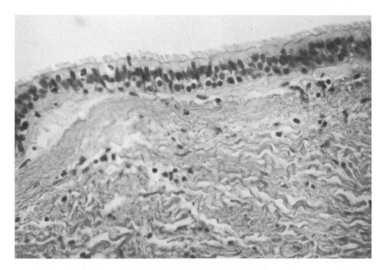

Figure 94–5. The cyst wall is lined by ciliated pseudostratified columnar respiratory epithelium and contains cartilage, smooth muscle, and glands.

DIAGNOSIS

The final pathologic diagnosis was bilateral bronchogenic cysts.

DISCUSSION

Because the walls of uncomplicated bronchogenic cysts are relatively thin and are interposed between the cyst contents and the adjacent structures, the imaging characteristics of these lesions are essentially those of the cyst contents. Radiographs show a soft tissue mass, frequently subcarinal and less frequently found in other mediastinal locations or within the lung.

CT demonstrates sharp margination and no contrast enhancement. The high protein content of the cyst fluid apparently shortens the T1 relaxation time sufficiently to result in bright signal on T1-weighted MR images. The fluid is also bright on T2-weighted images. When the cyst is complicated by infection or hemorrhage, variable attenuation values on CT scans and a range of possible signal intensities on MR may be found, sometimes with fluid-fluid levels or air-fluid levels. Bright signal on T1-weighted MR images is uncommon in mass lesions and suggests the specific tissue compositions of fat, subacute hematoma, proteinaceous material, and cellular composition with a high cytoplasm-nucleus ratio. A homogeneous appearance and concurrent bright signal on T2-weighted images eliminate fat and subacute hematoma as diagnostic possibilities. Bronchogenic cysts probably result from aberrant budding of the developing tracheobronchial tree. Adults usually present with asymptomatic masses.

REFERENCES

Barakos JA, Brown JJ, Brescia RJ, et al. High signal lesions of the chest in MR imaging. J Comput Assist Tomogr 1989; 13:797–802.

Naidich DP, Rumancik WM, Ettenger NA, et al. Congenital anomalies of the lungs in adults: MR diagnosis. AJR 1988; 151:13–19.

Nakata H, Nakayama C, Kimoto T, et al. Computed tomography of mediastinal bronchogenic cysts. J Comput Assist Tomogr 1982; 6:733–738.

Case 95

HISTORY

A 72-year-old Chinese female was admitted to the hospital because of abdominal pain, nausea, and diarrhea.

RADIOLOGY

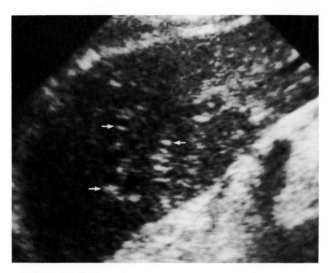

Figure 95-1. Transverse sonography of the left hepatic lobe demonstrates heterogeneity and multiple punctate, echogenic foci (arrows).

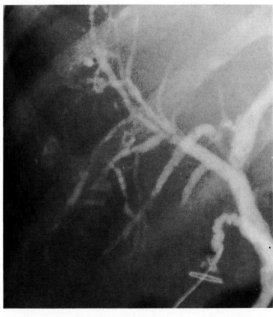

Figure 95-2. Intraoperative cholangiogram shows irregular beading of the intrahepatic biliary tree and multiple punctate collections of contrast involving the terminal branches of the intrahepatic bile ducts. The tertiary branches are pruned.

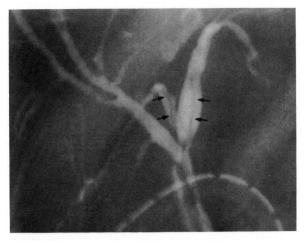

Figure 95-3. A T-tube cholangiogram demonstrates several linear filling defects (arrows) within the bile ducts.

DIFFERENTIAL DIAGNOSIS

The differential diagnosis includes ascending cholangitis with cholelithiasis, sclerosing cholangitis, *Clonorchis sinensis* cholangitis, and ascariasis.

PATHOLOGY

The patient underwent a cholecystectomy and common bile duct exploration.

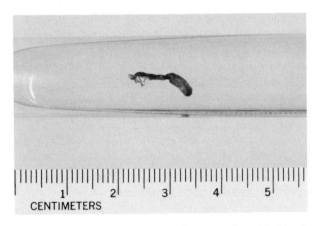

Figure 95-4. The worm has a varying diameter and a pointed head.

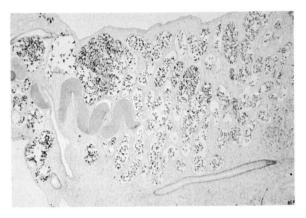

Figure 95-5. The worm has a prominent uterus.

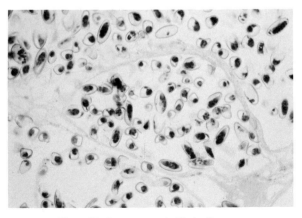

Figure 95-6. The uterus is filled with ova.

DIAGNOSIS

The final diagnosis was *Clonorchis sinensis* cholangitis.

DISCUSSION

Clonorchis sinensis, the Chinese or oriental liver fluke, is a parasite of fish-eating mammals in Japan, China, Korea, Indochina, and Taiwan. The adult fluke is a flat, elongated worm that measures between 12 and 20 mm in length. Typically, it is discolored by bile and has a deep brown color.

The life cycle of *Clonorchis* involves snails as first intermediate hosts, freshwater fish as second intermediate hosts, and mammals as definitive hosts. The ova are secreted by mature flukes into the biliary passages of the definitive host and pass out the body in the feces. Snails are infected by water contaminated with fecal discharge. The larvae grow within the snail and reenter the water as free-swimming metacercariae. The metacercariae invade the flesh of certain freshwater fish. Humans (and other mammals) are infected by eating raw or incompletely cooked fish. The metacercariae enter the duodenum and migrate into the common bile duct. The fluke matures in the distal biliary radicles and reproduces by self-fertilization. Over 2400 ova can be produced per day by an adult fluke. The fluke feeds on the mucosal secretions of the upper biliary ducts.

The movement of the flukes causes mechanical damage to the biliary epithelium. This motion induces adenomatous tissue formation and fibrosis in the periportal regions. Cirrhosis develops in severe cases. Secondary bacterial infection is a common complication. *Clonorchis* has been associated with recurrent pyogenic cholangitis (RPC, oriental cholangiohepatitis), a condition manifested by recurrent attacks of fever, chills, abdominal pain, and jaundice. RPC is thought to be secondary to repeated bacterial superinfections. In a large percentage of patients, *Escherichia coli* is cultured from the bile. Microabscesses develop in patients with significant bacterial infection.

Imaging methods include sonography and cholangiography. Sonographic findings are nonspecific. Diffuse or focal intrahepatic and extrahepatic bile duct dilatation may be present. Heterogeneous echotexture and multiple scattered echogenic foci reflect chronic liver disease, microabscesses, and possibly the presence of *Clonorchis* organisms in the biliary tree. Cholangiographic findings may suggest a specific diagnosis if the organisms are visualized as linear filling defects in the intrahepatic and extrahepatic bile. The biliary tree develops alternating segments of dilatation and stricture formation. The intrahepatic radicles become tortuous and pruned. The organisms can be seen as filling defects in the extrahepatic biliary ducts.

Praziquantel is an effective 1-day therapy that eradicates the parasite in 99% of cases. Owing to microabscess formation, however, RPC is more difficult to cure. Surgical drainage of the biliary tree is often required to prevent recurrence of symptoms.

REFERENCES

Carmona R, et al. Oriental cholangitis. Am J Surg 1984; 148:117–124.

Federle M, et al. Recurrent pyogenic cholangitis in Asian immigrants. Radiology 1982; 143:151–156.

Ho C, et al. Recurrent pyogenic cholangitis in Chinese immigrants. AJR 1974; 122(2):368–374.

Case 96

HISTORY

A 70-year-old woman presented with a 1-year history of leg pain and difficulty in walking.

RADIOLOGY

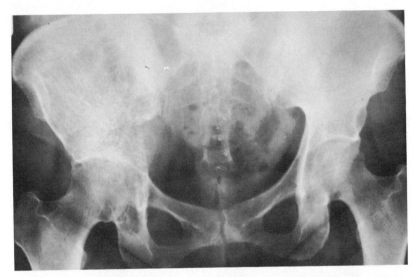

Figure 96-1. A radiating pattern of trabecular bone is present within a large, lytic, destructive lesion of the right ilium. The medial cortex is violated, resulting in a small soft tissue mass.

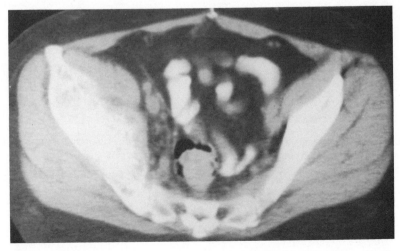

Figure 96-2. On CT scan the lesion is characterized by a radiating pattern of stellate trabecular bone.

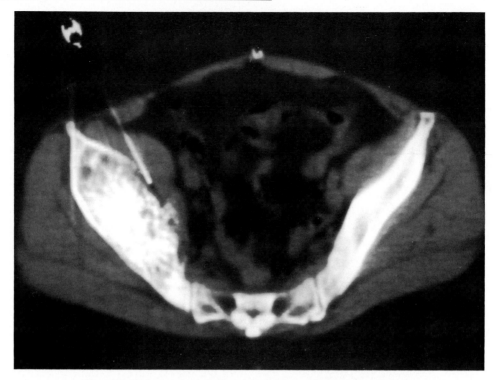

Figure 96–3. Fine-needle aspiration of the medial soft tissue mass was done.

DIFFERENTIAL DIAGNOSIS

The differential diagnosis includes hemangioma, hemangiosarcoma, angiosarcoma, lymphangioma, and Paget's disease.

PATHOLOGY

The lesion was resected.

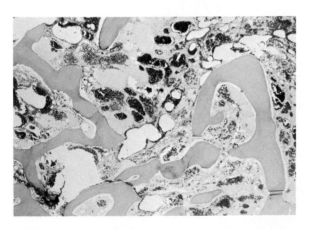

Figure 96–4. Throughout the medullary cavity are large, clear, vascular spaces, some of which are filled with red blood cells.

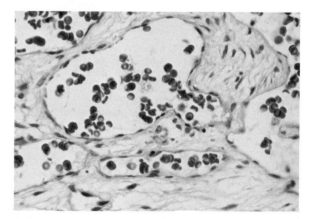

Figure 96–5. The vascular spaces are lined by uniform bland endothelial cells.

DIAGNOSIS

The final pathologic diagnosis was hemangioma of bone.

DISCUSSION

Hemangiomas of bone are uncommon lesions composed of cavernous, capillary, or venous vascular channels. They are indistinguishable histologically from hemangiomas of the soft tissues. The lesions are usually found in patients in the fourth and fifth decades of life and have a female to male predominance of 2:1. Many are silent clinically and are discovered incidentally, though some produce pain, soft tissue swelling, or pathologic fractures. Occasionally, hemangiomas in the spine cause symptoms by extension into the epidural space, narrowing of the spinal canal due to vertebral body expansion (rare), compression fractures, and epidural hemorrhage. Solitary or multiple bony lesions can lead to hemihypertrophy of an extremity. Malignant degeneration is not seen. When sectioned for biopsy, lesions can produce massive hemorrhage or exsanguination.

Any bone may be affected, including long bones, short bones, and flat bones. Most lesions are detected in the vertebrae, skull, and facial bones. Authors estimate that hemangiomas can be found in up to 10% of all spines at autopsy, most commonly in the thoracic vertebral bodies, though the lesions can extend into the posterior elements. Hemangiomas of the skull are less common but may be more clinically significant because of the mass effect they produce. Hemangiomas of the long tubular bones arise in the epiphysis or metaphysis and, although very uncommon, usually occur in the femur, humerus, or tibia. They are rarely seen in the pelvis, ribs, patella, scapula, clavicle, carpals, and tarsals; however, the largest lesions (up to 14 cm in diameter) are found in the pelvis and ribs.

Radiographically, spinal hemangiomas exhibit parallel, coarse, vertical, linear streaks representing coarsened, overlapping trabeculae, which have been likened in appearance to corduroy or a honeycomb. Usually only a segment of the vertebral body is affected. Extension into the epidural space or paraspinal soft tissues, which uncommonly occurs, can simulate malignancy. Radiographic features in extraspinal sites are less characteristic. However, the diagnosis is suggested by a lucent, expansile, well-defined osseous lesion, often containing a radiating, "sunray" spiculation or a latticelike or weblike trabecular pattern. This pattern is a frequent and somewhat specific finding. Lesions centered in the cortex or periosteum are also seen.

REFERENCES

Dahlin DC, Unni KK. Bone Tumors: General Aspects and Data on 8,542 Cases (4th ed). Springfield, IL: Thomas, 1986:167–180.

Hudson TM. Radiologic-Pathologic Correlation of Musculoskeletal Lesions. Baltimore: Williams & Wilkins, 1987:407–411.

Mirra JM. Bone Tumors: Diagnosis and Treatment. Philadelphia: Lippincott, 1980:504–509.

Resnick D, Kyriakos M, Greenway GD. Tumors and tumor-like lesions of bone: imaging and pathology of specific lesions. *In*: Resnick D, Niwayama G (eds). Diagnosis of Bone and Joint Disorders (2nd ed). Philadelphia: Saunders, 1988:3792–3798.

Case 97

HISTORY

A 14-year-old male presented with recurrent epistaxis.

RADIOLOGY

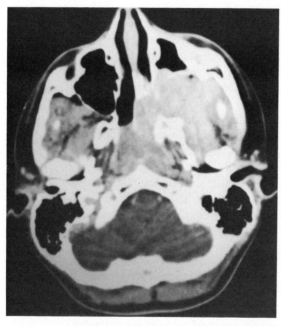

Figure 97-1. Contrast-enhanced axial CT scan shows an enhancing soft tissue mass in the left pterygopalatine fossa. The mass pushes the posterolateral wall of the left maxillary sinus anteriorly and extends posteriorly into the masticator space. There is associated obliteration of the normal fat planes around the temporalis and lateral pterygoid muscles.

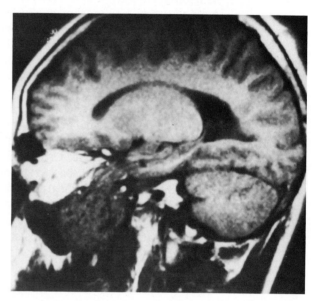

Figure 97-2. T1-weighted sagittal MR image shows numerous small signal voids in the mass that suggest flowing blood in enlarged vessels.

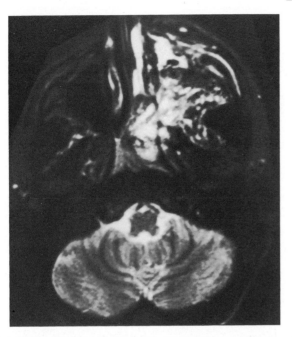

Figure 97-3. Axial late echo T2-weighted image shows heterogeneously increased signal intensity in addition to linear and punctate signal voids that are suggestive of vascular flow.

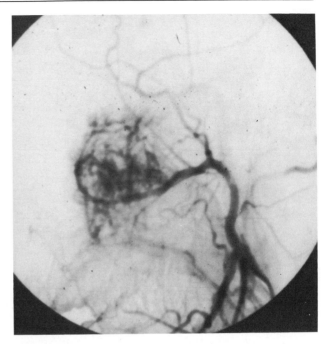

Figure 97-4. Lateral view of the head during digital subtraction left external carotid arteriography shows that feeding vessels originate from branches of the left internal maxillary artery. There is dense tumor vascularity.

DIFFERENTIAL DIAGNOSIS

The primary radiologic diagnosis is juvenile nasopharyngeal angiofibroma. Much less likely possibilities include malignant fibrous histiocytoma, rhabdomyosarcoma, and squamous cell carcinoma.

PATHOLOGY

The lesion was embolized through a catheter and then was resected.

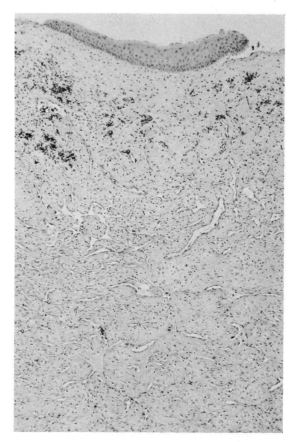

Figure 97–5. The overlying nasal mucosa, which is composed of stratified squamous epithelium, is attenuated by the underlying tumor.

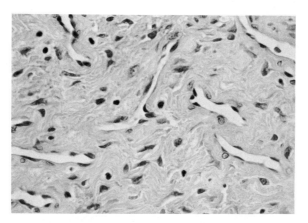

Figure 97–6. The blood vessels in the tumor branch irregularly and have the features of capillaries. Surrounding the capillaries are spindle- and stellate-shaped bland-appearing fibroblasts.

DIAGNOSIS

The final pathologic diagnosis was juvenile angiofibroma.

DISCUSSION

Juvenile nasopharyngeal angiofibroma is a benign but locally aggressive neoplasm that originates near the sphenopalatine foramen within the pterygopalatine fossa. It occurs almost exclusively in adolescent males, presenting with recurrent epistaxis, nasal obstruction, and nasal discharge. Grossly, the tumor appears as a pink-blue nodular nasopharyngeal mass. Microscopically, it consists of thin-walled vessels of varied caliber surrounded by a moderately cellular fibroblastic stroma.

Juvenile angiofibromas tend to spread locally along fissures and foramina. Initially, the tumor enlarges the sphenopalatine foramen and grows medially into the nose and nasopharynx. Characteristic extension into the pterygopalatine fossa causes anterior deviation of the posterior maxillary sinus and posterior deviation or erosion of the pterygoid plates. These findings are visible on lateral skull films or on CT in the great majority of patients. Spread into the sphenoid, ethmoid, or maxillary sinuses is not uncommon. More aggressive tumors may spread into the orbit through the inferior orbital fissure or intracranially through the superior orbital fissure or through the sphenoid roof. Spread into the infratemporal soft tissues is also seen.

CT shows the extent of the tumor mass and best evaluates the underlying bony structures. The tumor enhances homogeneously with contrast. On MR imaging, a soft tissue mass of intermediate T1 signal intensity is demonstrated. Both T1- and T2-weighted images may show punctate or serpiginous flow voids within the mass similar to those seen in highly vascular tumors such as paragangliomas.

Angiography has traditionally played a major role in the evaluation of juvenile nasopharyngeal angiofibromas. The tumor receives the majority of its blood supply from the internal maxillary artery. Collateral supply can also be seen from the ascending pharyngeal and ascending palatine arteries. In the arterial phase, multiple tortuous vessels are seen, followed by a dense homogeneous blush during the capillary phase. Early draining veins are not present.

The treatment of juvenile nasopharyngeal angiofibroma remains controversial. Cases of spontaneous involution of tumor mass have been documented. Angiographic preoperative embolization is increasingly performed to reduce blood loss at surgery. This combined technique results in a low rate of complications and few recurrences. Radiation therapy is generally reserved for unresectable tumor or cases of recurrence.

REFERENCES

Davis KR. Embolization of epistaxis and juvenile nasopharyngeal angiofibromas. AJR 1987; 148: 209–218.

Grybauskas V, Parker J, Friedman M. Juvenile nasopharyngeal angiofibroma. Otolaryngol Clin North Am 1986; 19(4):647–657.

Lloyd GA, Phelps PD. Juvenile angiofibroma: imaging by MRI, CT and conventional techniques. Clin Otolaryngol 1986; 11:247–259.

Jacobsson M, Petruson B, Svendsen P, et al. Juvenile nasopharyngeal angiofibroma. A report of eighteen cases. Acta Otolaryngol (Stockh) 1989; 105: 132–139.

Case 98

HISTORY

The chest radiograph of a 49-year-old woman admitted for wrist surgery was found incidentally to be abnormal.

RADIOLOGY

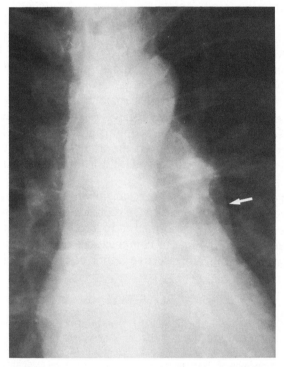

Figure 98-1. PA chest film shows a broad mediastinal contour. An abnormal density is projected over the left pulmonary artery (arrow). The lateral chest film (not shown) was normal and demonstrated in particular that there was no mass in the anterior mediastinum.

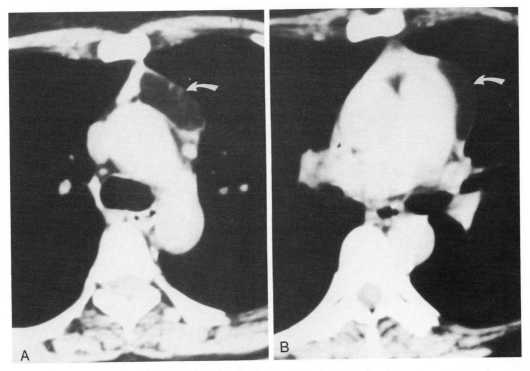

Figure 98-2. *A-B.* CT scan shows an anterior fatty mass (arrows) adjacent to the thymus. The mass extends caudad 6 cm along the ascending aorta and the left cardiac margin.

DIFFERENTIAL DIAGNOSIS

The differential diagnosis includes lipoma, liposarcoma, and thymolipoma.

PATHOLOGY

Surgical resection was performed.

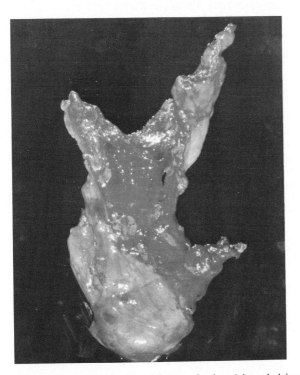

Figure 98-4. The mass abuts the residual thymic parenchyma and is composed of fat.

Figure 98-3. The removed enlarged thymus gland contains a bulging mass in the inferior portion of the gland.

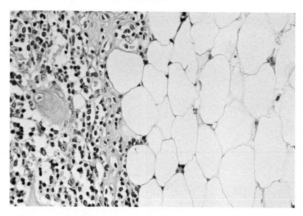

Figure 98-5. Present within the thymic parenchyma are Hassall's corpuscles. The adipocytes of the tumor are mature.

DIAGNOSIS

The final pathologic diagnosis was thymolipoma.

DISCUSSION

Thymolipomas are unusual benign mediastinal tumors composed of thymic and adipose tissue. The imaging characteristics are simply those of fat, although the thymic tissue may appear as islands of soft tissue density within the fat. Arising in the anterior mediastinum at the level of the thymus gland, these soft and pliable tumors droop inferiorly as they enlarge and are said to slump onto the diaphragms, accommodating themselves to the potential spaces between the lungs and the heart, diaphragms, or anterior mediastinum. Their pendulous, elongated, teardrop shape leaves the anterior clear space unencumbered on the lateral chest film. They may simulate cardiomegaly on the frontal chest film. Because they are asymptomatic until marked mass effect occurs, thymolipomas often reach a large size, sometimes weighing several kilograms at the time of excision.

Thymolipomas are uncommon, comprising approximately 5% of all thymic tumors. Most are discovered incidentally. In a very few cases, myasthenia gravis is a concurrent condition, but the strength of the association is weak and is probably coincidental.

When they are treated, the treatment is surgical resection. The tumors do not recur.

REFERENCES

Faerber EN, Balsara RK, Shidlow DV, et al. Thymolipoma: computed tomographic appearances. Pediatr Radiol 1990; 20:196–197.

Pan CH, Chiang CY, Chen SS. Thymolipoma in patients with myasthenia gravis: report of two cases and a review. Acta Neurol Scand 1988; 78:16–21.

Shirkhoda A, Chasen MH, Eftekhari F, et al. MR imaging of mediastinal thymolipoma. J Comput Assist Tomogr 1987; 11:364–365.

Teplick JG, Nedwich A, Haskin ME. Roentgenographic features of thymolipoma. Am J Roentgenol 1973; 117:873–877.

Case 99

HISTORY

A 44-year-old man stated that he had had left thigh pain and swelling, fevers and night sweats, and anorexia for 2 months and had lost 10 pounds. These symptoms began after he was kicked by a horse.

RADIOLOGY

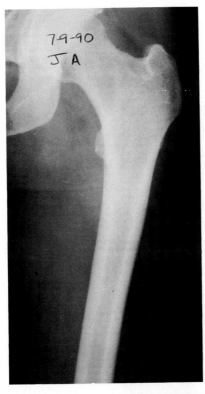

Figure 99-1. At the time of presentation radiographs of the femur were normal.

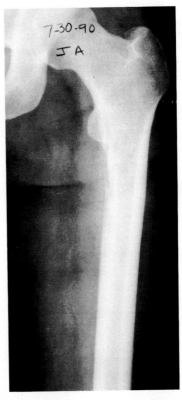

Figure 99-2. Three weeks later there is permeated destruction of the subtrochanteric part of the femur.

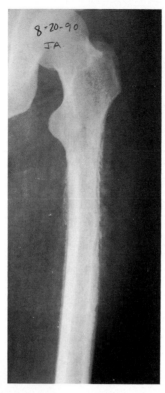

Figure 99–3. After an additional month, the area of bone destruction has extended down the shaft of the femur. There is a mixture of spiculated and layered periosteal reaction.

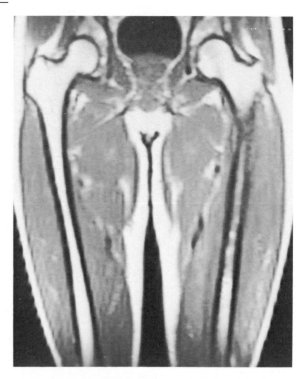

Figure 99–4. A coronal T1-weighted (TR = 480, TE = 20) MR image demonstrates replacement of the fatty signal from the bone marrow by low signal intensity.

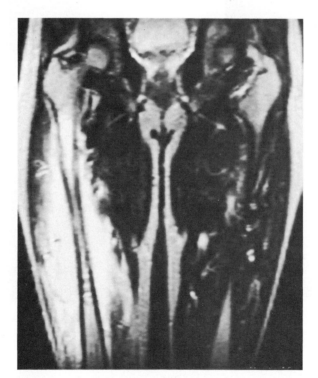

Figure 99–5. A coronal T2-weighted (TR = 2010, TE = 20) MR image demonstrates an extensive area of bright signal abnormality involving the bone marrow and the contiguous muscle.

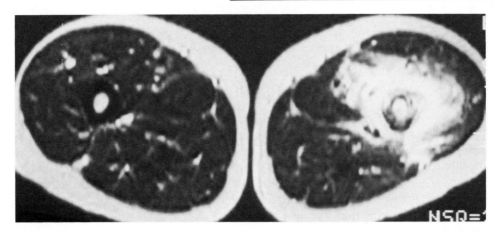

Figure 99-6. Axial T2-weighted (TR = 2196, TE = 100) MR images demonstrate a bright signal within the medullary canal, permeating the cortex and extending out into the soft tissues. The area of signal abnormality is very poorly marginated.

DIFFERENTIAL DIAGNOSIS

The differential diagnosis includes round cell tumor (lymphoma, Ewing's sarcoma, primitive neuroectodermal tumor), fibrosarcoma, osteosarcoma, and metastasis, but the rapid progression argues in favor of osteomyelitis.

PATHOLOGY

A biopsy of the lesion was performed.

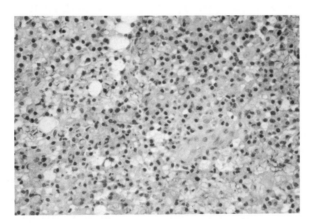

Figure 99-7. The specimen consists of an aggregate of plasma cells, lymphocytes, and scattered macrophages.

DIAGNOSIS

The final pathologic diagnosis was acute osteomyelitis.

DISCUSSION

Osteomyelitis continues to present a difficult diagnostic problem because its clinical, laboratory, and radiographic signs may mimic those of a variety of other conditions. Radiographic findings usually are delayed after the onset of clinical signs of infection, with 90% of findings remaining invisible for up to 1 month after clinical signs have appeared. Thus, extensive destruction of bone may occur before accurate identification and therapy take place. Before the era of antibiotics, osteomyelitis had a 25% mortality. The morbidity resulting from chronic infection was high owing to deformity and growth abnormalities.

The overall incidence of osteomyelitis has decreased severalfold since the advent of antibiotics in the early 1940s, but cases resulting from contiguous spread have increased. Acute and chronic forms of the disease are seen. Chronic cases are often subclinical but are punctuated by recurrent exacerbation. Spontaneous drainage through an osteocutaneous sinus tract may occur.

Responsible organisms include pyogenic bacteria (especially *Staphylococcus aureus*), mycobacteria, fungi, and viruses. Nonpyogenic opportunistic infection is especially prevalent among immunosuppressed patients. Fungal infection involving the spine, hands, and feet is usually confined to endemic areas. *Pseudomonas aeruginosa* is particularly common in penetrating wounds of the feet and among intravenous drug abusers. Patients with sickle cell disease, because of autosplenectomy, have an increased risk of infection with encapsulated organisms. In this group of patients *Pneumococcus* and *Salmonella* are the most frequent causes of bacteremia, with *Salmonella* responsible for 60% of cases of osteomyelitis. Many bones may be affected. Radiographically, the condition can be very difficult to differentiate from bone infarcts (for which this patient group is also at increased risk).

Hematogenous osteomyelitis commonly occurs after a transient bacteremia. In up to one third of cases a history of adjacent blunt trauma is recorded. Blood culture is positive in 60% of patients. This disease is especially well known among children, who typically present with toxic symptoms and local inflammation. Cases in infants are less dramatic and usually result from infected umbilical catheters or delivery complicated with group B streptococcal infection. Adults often have a more insidious course. Long bone infection is seen in all age groups, but the spine is commonly involved in adults. Neonatal cases typically involve multiple bones.

The location of infection in the long bones is a direct reflection of the vascular anatomy at different ages. All bones are penetrated by one or two diaphyseal nutrient canals, which contain both an artery and a vein, both of which split into ascending and descending branches. These connect with the capillaries of the haversian systems and continue as cortical capillaries, which anastomose with periosteal capillary plexuses. The capillaries drain into venous sinuses. In children, capillary growth is blocked by the cartilaginous physis; the terminal capillaries on the metaphyseal side turn back in acute loops to join the sinusoidal veins. It is here that flow is slow and turbulent, and capillaries are incomplete and fenestrated, creating increased opportunities for organisms to lodge. In adults the cartilaginous growth plate is not present, allowing vessels to penetrate to the epiphysis, and in infants up to 1 year of age the growth plate is incomplete, allowing penetrating epiphyseal vessels to persist. Because of these variations in anatomy, childhood osteomyelitis is commonly metaphyseal, whereas infantile and adult osteomyelitis can be epiphyseal.

The pathophysiology of hematogenous osteomyelitis is well documented in avian models. When blood-borne organisms lodge in the metaphyseal blood vessels the result is a focal area of thrombophlebitis. The infecting organisms colonize and grow in the areas of infarction, isolated from the usual host defenses. Infection spreads along the paths of least resistance, namely the haversian systems, toward the cortex. Vascular engorgement, edema, and cellular exudate increase intramedullary pressure. This, in addition to the thrombophlebitis spreading toward the periosteal vessels, leads to more widespread areas of bone infarction (sequestra) and abscess formation (Brodie's abscess), increasing the risk of chronic osteomyelitis.

As the inflammatory exudate spreads to the cortical surface, periosteal elevation occurs (particularly in infants and children, whose periosteum is loosely apposed), and extensive periosteal new bone formation results (involucrum). Increased internal pressure may result in penetration of the periosteum and involucrum in places (cloaca) with subsequent formation of sinus tracts to the skin surface through which pus and sequestra can escape.

In children the shoulders and hip joints are at special risk of contiguous involvement from an infected joint because these joint capsules attach beyond the growth plates. Infants and adults are at risk of contiguous joint involvement in any bone because subcortical epiphyseal infection is the rule. Infants are at particular risk of damage to the epiphyseal side of the growth plate, which can result in severe growth disturbances.

Nonhematogenous osteomyelitis is more common among patients more than 50 years old. The disease may occur in patients with peripheral vascular disease and long-standing skin ulceration (diabetics), overlying infection (decubitus ulcers, dental abscess), previous orthopedic manipulation (total hip replacement, allograft), or direct implantation of organisms (open fracture). Special cases of contiguous osteomyelitis are worth noting. *Pseudomonas* foot infection due to penetrating trauma has already been mentioned. Other examples include *Pasteurella multocida* infection complicating animal bites, anaerobic infection complicating human bites, the sacrum becoming infected from decubitus ulcers, the feet of diabetics developing osteomyelitis owing to vascular ulcers, and the frontal bone becoming infected owing to longstanding sinus infection (Pott's puffy tumor).

Treatment necessitates immediate and appropriate antibiotic therapy. Diagnosis usually requires a positive blood culture or open bone biopsy. If clinical improvement does not occur within 48 to 72 hours, chronic infection with sequestra or abscess can be assumed, and surgical debridement may be required. Antibiotic therapy must be extended over many weeks, and the course can be complicated by pathologic fracture, nonunion, spread of infection to the joint, or hematogenous dissemination. Promising results have been documented with soft tissue reconstruction with flaps and hyperbaric oxygen to induce revascularization, and recently subcutaneous antibiotic pumps have become available. Chronic osteomyelitis is complicated at times by the development of amyloidosis as well as by late squamous cell carcinoma arising in chronically draining and epithelialized sinus tracts. The incidence of this complication is low, and it is rarely seen in the absence of a history of chronic osteomyelitis for 20 to 30 years. The cancers are generally low grade but may metastasize.

REFERENCES

Emslie KR, et al. Acute haematogenous osteomyelitis: an experimental model. Pathology 1983; 141:157–167.

Emslie KR, Nade S. Acute hematogenous staphylococcal osteomyelitis: an avian model. Am J Pathol 1983; 110:333–345.

Enneking WF. Clinical Musculoskeletal Pathology (3rd rev ed). Gainesville, FL: University of Florida Press, 1990:105–123.

Hudson TM. Radiologic-Pathologic Correlation of Musculoskeletal Lesions. Baltimore: Williams & Wilkins, 1987:441–489.

Modic T, et al. MRI of musculoskeletal infection. Radiol Clin North Am 1986; 24:247–258.

Sankaran-Kutty M, et al. Squamous cell carcinoma in chronic osteomyelitis. Clin Orthop 1985; 198: 264–267.

Smith DJ Jr, Colyer RA. An aggressive therapeutic approach for adult osteomyelitis. Am Surg 1985; 51:363–366.

Case 100

HISTORY

A 74-year-old man with a history of chronic lymphocytic leukemia and 4 months of left-sided headache presented with progressive visual loss.

RADIOLOGY

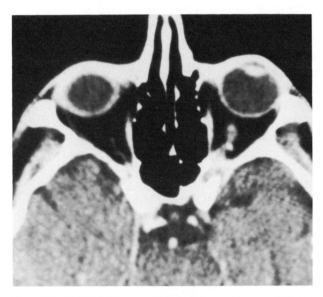

Figure 100–1. Orbital CT scan demonstrates an enhancing soft tissue mass at the left orbital apex. Bone windows (not shown) demonstrate adjacent erosion at the anterior wall of the left middle cranial fossa.

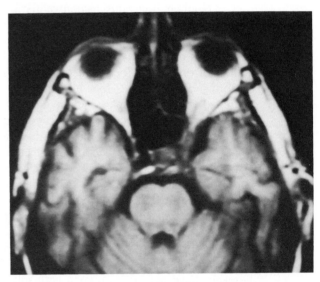

Figure 100–2. An axial T1-weighted MR image shows intermediate signal soft tissue mass occupying the left orbital apex and extending into the left cavernous sinus.

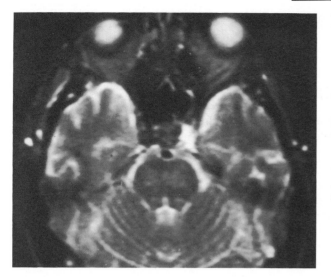

Figure 100-3. The soft tissue mass is hyperintense on late echo T2-weighted images.

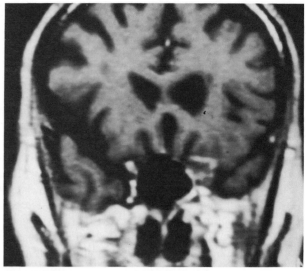

Figure 100-4. Coronal T1-weighted MR images after gadolinium injection show inhomogeneous enhancement along the left optic canal and superior orbital fissure.

DIFFERENTIAL DIAGNOSIS

The differential diagnosis includes lymphomatous infiltrate, meningioma, granulomatous disease (sarcoid, Wegener's granuloma), and fungal or granulomatous infection.

PATHOLOGY

Resection of the tumor and dura adjacent to the optic nerve was performed.

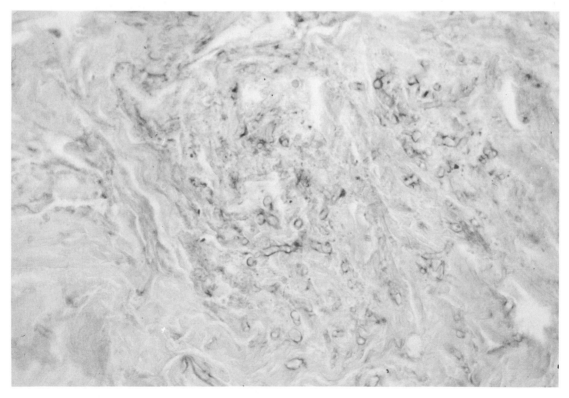

Figure 100-5. Numerous branching hyphae are seen infiltrating necrotic fibrous tissue.

DIAGNOSIS

The final diagnosis was aspergilloma involving the orbit.

DISCUSSION

Generally, aspergillous fungal infections of the orbit begin in the nasal cavity or paranasal sinuses and extend secondarily into the orbit, usually the apex. The *Aspergillus flavus* species is responsible for many cases of this type of infection. Pathologically, the lesions of invasive aspergillosis demonstrate a fungal mycelial mass with narrow septate hyphae and acutely angled branching. Blood vessel invasion with thrombosis is common.

Paranasal sinus infections with *Aspergillus* have a range of severity. The most benign infection is a low-grade, noninvasive colonization of an abnormal sinus, analogous to colonization of lung cavities by aspergilloma. A condition analogous to allergic broncho-pulmonary aspergillosis, called allergic aspergillous sinusitis, may also be seen. Involvement of the orbit occurs only in the two most aggressive forms of infection: subacute or chronic invasive aspergillous sinusitis (usually seen in mildly immunocompromised patients such as diabetics) and fulminant aspergillous sinusitis (usually seen in severely neutropenic patients, such as patients with leukemia undergoing chemotherapy or steroid treatment). In both these aggressive forms, erosion of the bony sinus wall can result in extension of infection into the intracranial space, orbit, or cavernous sinus. Patients with orbital involvement may present with decreasing visual acuity, unilateral proptosis, or retro-orbital pain.

CT and MR imaging are important techniques for defining the extent of disease and determining the best approach for possible diagnostic or therapeutic surgery. The modalities are complementary, with MR imaging best demonstrating soft tissue extension outside of the paranasal sinuses, and CT best evaluating the bony orbital walls. On CT, aspergillosis involving the paranasal sinus can appear as intrasinus soft tissue masses of relatively high density, sometimes containing frank calcifications or a linear interlacing network of high attenuation, and sometimes surrounded by a relatively radiolucent rim. On T2-weighted MR images, the intrasinus mass can appear rather hypointense relative to typical mucosal disease.

Treatment of sino-orbital aspergillosis frequently consists of surgical orbital exenteration and use of the antifungal agent amphotericin B. Rifampin and 5-fluorouracil are sometimes used as adjunctive therapy.

REFERENCES

Dyken ME, Biller J, Yuh WT, et al. Carotid-cavernous sinus thrombosis caused by *Aspergillus fumigatus*: magnetic resonance imaging with pathologic correlation—a case report. Angiology 1991; 41(8):652–657.

Patel PJ, Kolawole TM, Malabarey TM, et al. CT findings in paranasal aspergillosis. Clin Radiol 1992; 45(5):319–321.

Sacho H, Stead KJ, Klugman KP, et al. Infection of the human orbit by *Aspergillus stromatoides*. Case report. Mycopathologia 1987; 97(2):97–99.

Talbot GH, Huang A, Provencher M. Invasive aspergillus rhinosinusitis in patients with acute leukemia. Rev Infect Dis 1991; 13(2):219–232.

Yumoto E, Kitan S, Okamura H, et al. Sino-orbital aspergillosis associated with total ophthalmoplegia. Laryngoscope 1985; 95:190–192.

Case 101

HISTORY

A 69-year-old male presented with dysphagia, weight loss, and an upper abdominal mass.

RADIOLOGY

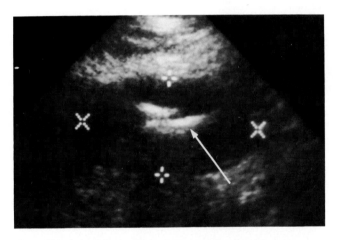

Figure 101-1. A midline sagittal sonogram of the stomach demonstrates a markedly thickened, hypoechoic gastric wall (measuring marks) with echogenic gastric lumen (arrow).

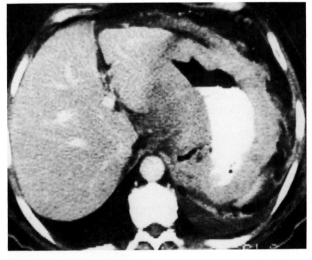

Figure 101-2. Contrast-enhanced CT scan shows circumferential, irregular gastric wall thickening.

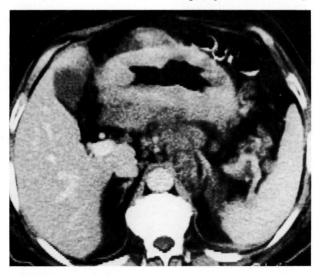

Figure 101-3. At a more caudal level, the gastric mucosal surface is nodular and polypoid.

DIFFERENTIAL DIAGNOSIS

The differential diagnosis includes linitis plastica (scirrhous metastatic disease or primary gastric adenocarcinoma), lymphoma, and Menetrier's disease.

PATHOLOGY

Gastrectomy was performed.

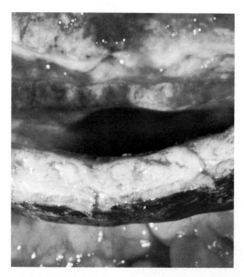

Figure 101-4. The removed stomach shows a markedly thickened tan-white wall. All layers of the wall are involved.

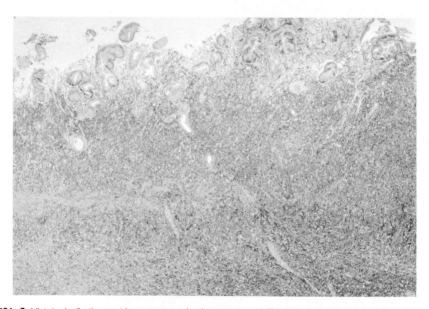

Figure 101-5. Histologically the gastric mucosa and submucosa are infiltrated by a dense population of tumor cells.

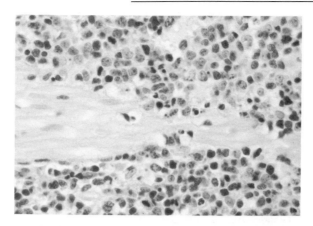

Figure 101-6. The tumor cells are small to intermediate in size. They are cytologically malignant and have hyperchromatic nuclei and scant cytoplasm. The tumor cells can also be seen infiltrating throughout the muscularis propria.

DIAGNOSIS

The final pathologic diagnosis was primary gastric lymphoma.

DISCUSSION

Lymphoma may arise as a primary neoplasm of the gastrointestinal tract or may involve the bowel during systemic dissemination. The gastrointestinal tract is the most common extranodal site involved by primary non-Hodgkin's lymphoma. Primary lymphoma usually is limited to one segment of the gastrointestinal tract, such as the stomach, ileum, large intestine, or appendix. Lymphoma arising from mesenteric or retroperitoneal nodes typically involves multiple contiguous bowel segments.

Primary gastric lymphoma occurs in middle-aged patients and has an equal sex distribution. Presenting symptoms usually are related to ulcer formation. Lymphoma of the stomach accounts for 3% to 5% of all malignant gastric neoplasms and 50% of all primary gastrointestinal lymphomas. Primary lymphoma of the stomach usually is isolated to its lower and middle thirds, although diffuse infiltration also occurs. Involvement may be classified as polypoid or infiltrative. Polypoid growth shows irregular nodules projecting into the gastric lumen. Polypoid lesions vary in size and may be single or multiple. Although this entity may resemble multiple polyposis of the stomach, the intervening mucosa is thickened and rigid in lymphoma but atrophic and distensible in polyposis. Lymphomatous nodules are usually irregular and ulcerated, whereas benign polyps have a smooth contour.

Infiltrative growth shows diffuse or segmental giant rugae with or without tiny tumor nodules. Wild, bizarre gastric folds are similar to those seen in Menetrier's disease or scirrhous carcinoma. Infiltrative lymphoma commonly ulcerates. This ulcer may become deep and develop an aneurysmal configuration resembling leiomyosarcoma in appearance. Extensive ulceration results in perforation. Gastric lymphoma rarely presents as an isolated ulcerated mass but can appear identical to gastric carcinoma.

Barium examination usually is the first radiologic study undertaken in patients with symptoms referable to the stomach. Common findings include narrowing and rigidity of the antrum and body of the stomach. Segmental and diffuse gastric involvement is demonstrated as well as nodularity and ulceration. Peristalsis is decreased or absent. A double-contrast upper gastrointestinal series shows subtle mucosal nodularity that may not be detected by endoscopy because the tumor can spread along the submucosa and muscularis mucosa without involving the mucosal lining. CT scans show irregular mural thickening even when luminal distention can be achieved. On CT gastric lymphoma is staged by defining its direct extension into adjacent structures as well as by showing the presence of enlarged mesenteric and retroperitoneal lymph nodes. If the diagnosis cannot be made by endoscopy, CT-guided biopsy of the stomach or peritoneal metastases can be performed.

Gastric lymphoma may be identical in appearance to linitis plastica caused by either primary adenocarcinoma or metastatic spread from adenocarcinoma of the breast, gallbladder, or prostate. Primary lymphoma isolated to the stomach is surgically resected for cure. Chemotherapy, radiation therapy, and combination therapy can induce long-term remissions in nonresectable cases. The prognosis is much better than for adenocarcinoma.

REFERENCES

Levine MS, Kong V, Rubesin SE, et al. Scirrhous carcinoma of the stomach: radiologic and endoscopic diagnosis. Radiology 1990; 175:151–154.

Makepeace AR, et al. Gastrointestinal non-Hodgkin's lymphoma. Clin Radiol 1987; 38:609–614.

Sato T, et al. Radiologic manifestations of early gastric lymphoma. AJR 1986; 146:513–517.

Case **102**

HISTORY

A 67-year-old Portuguese man presented with a several-month history of intermittent bloating, midepigastric pain, and a 25-pound weight loss. An upper abdominal mass was palpated.

RADIOLOGY

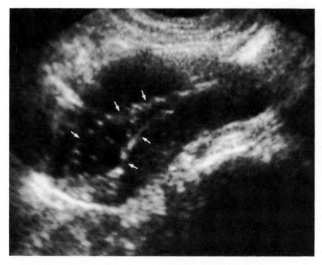

Figure 102-1. A transverse, midline sonogram of the duodenum demonstrates a markedly thickened, relatively hypoechoic wall with through-transmission. The central heterogeneous region (arrows) represents the duodenal lumen and produces the "pseudokidney sign."

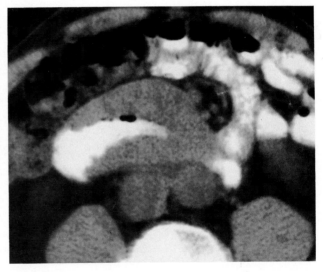

Figure 102-2. At a comparable level, a CT scan following oral contrast administration demonstrates circumferential thickening of the duodenal wall with irregularity and nodularity of the mucosa.

DIFFERENTIAL DIAGNOSIS

The differential diagnosis includes adenocarcinoma of the duodenum, metastases, lymphoma, leiomyosarcoma, intramural hematoma, and Crohn's disease.

PATHOLOGY

Pancreaticoduodenectomy was performed. A 9-cm segment of enlarged, rigid duodenum demonstrated serosal adhesions. The wall was markedly thickened (more than 1.5 cm) and nodular.

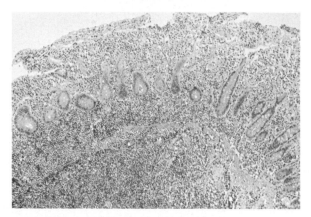

Figure 102-3. A dense cellular infiltrate involves the duodenal submucosa and mucosa.

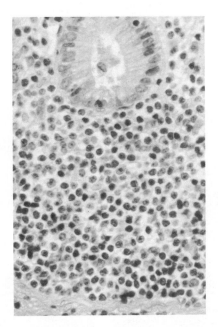

Figure 102-4. Intestinal gland with adjacent cellular infiltrate is composed of sheets of small lymphoid cells.

DIAGNOSIS

The final pathologic diagnosis was primary duodenal lymphoma.

DISCUSSION

This case provides radiographic comparison with Case 101.

Tumors of the small bowel are relatively uncommon, representing less than 5% of gastrointestinal malignancies. Because presenting symptoms are nonspecific and radiographic examination of the small bowel is difficult, diagnosis is often delayed until local or distant metastases have occurred. Clinical signs and symptoms are insidious and include bleeding, obstruction, poorly localized abdominal pain, and palpable mass.

Adenocarcinoma is the most common small bowel malignancy and frequently occurs in the duodenum and proximal jejunum. Malignant carcinoid, the second most common small bowel malignancy, usually arises in the ileum or appendix. Leiomyosarcomas usually arise distal to the duodenum. Primary lymphoma of the duodenum is uncommon. Like primary gastric lymphoma, tumor spreads in the submucosal or muscularis mucosal layers and causes circumferential infiltration. Less commonly, a focal, exophytic lymphomatous mass ulcerates into the bowel lumen and cavitates in a fashion similar to leiomyosarcoma. Intramural duodenal hematoma is a benign lesion that also results in circumferential bowel wall thickening.

Although upper gastrointestinal series with small bowel follow-through (UGI/SBFT) and CT remain the primary imaging modalities, ultrasound may also identify bowel pathology. The "pseudokidney sign," described in 1979, consists of a central hyperechoic focus surrounded by a hypoechoic periphery corresponding to the intraluminal bowel contents and bowel wall, respectively. When the bowel is imaged in the longitudinal axis, the appearance of a kidney is produced. In the transverse plane, a doughnut or sandwich appearance is produced. The sign is considered positive when bowel wall thickening is greater than 10 mm. Although the sign indicates pathology, both benign and malignant causes are possible. In the present case, for example, both the sonographic and CT appearances are identical to those in intramural duodenal hematoma, although, if acute, hemorrhage can be high in attenuation.

REFERENCE

Bluth EI, et al. Ultrasound evaluation of the stomach, small bowel, and colon. Radiology 1979; 133: 677–680.

Case 103

HISTORY

A 36-year-old female had a 10-year history of unresectable cardiac tumor. Coronary artery bypass surgery had been performed at age 28.

RADIOLOGY

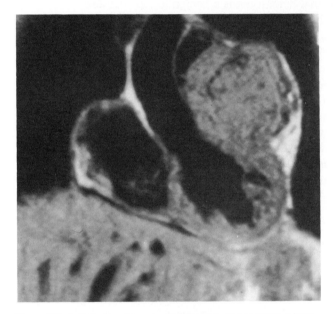

Figure 103-1. Gated cardiac coronal MR image demonstrates a large mass compressing the left atrium and infiltrating between the cardiac chambers. The tumor appears to be a myocardial tumor.

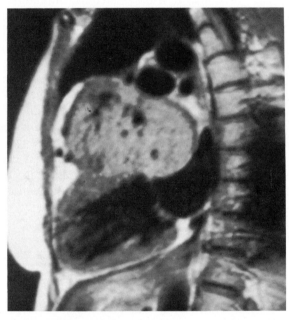

Figure 103-2. Gated cardiac sagittal MR image also shows the mass and its relationships.

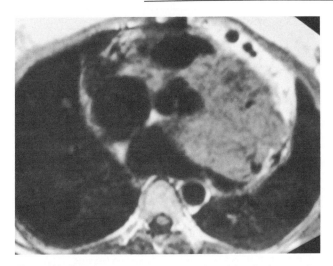

Figure 103-3. Gradient echo technique in the axial projection reveals the hypervascularity of the lesion.

DIFFERENTIAL DIAGNOSIS

The differential diagnosis includes lymphoma and angiosarcoma.

PATHOLOGY

The patient had undergone biopsy of the mass during a previous hospitalization.

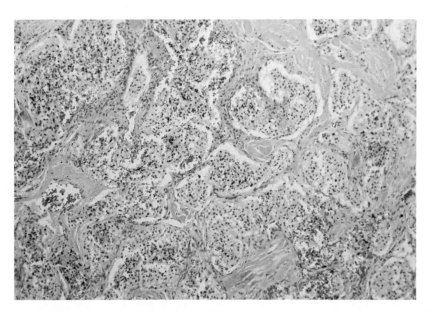

Figure 103-4. Histologically the tumor cells are arranged in round nests, which are compartmentalized by fibrous septa and numerous capillaries.

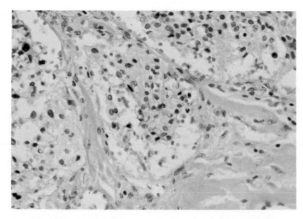

Figure 103–5. The tumor cells are polyhedral and have a moderate amount of eosinophilic cytoplasm. Although there is some pleomorphism, there is little mitotic activity and no necrosis.

DIAGNOSIS

The final pathologic diagnosis was cardiac paraganglioma.

DISCUSSION

Paragangliomas are tumors of the paraganglia. The adrenal medulla and the extra-adrenal paraganglia constitute the paraganglion system, a component of the autonomic nervous system. The parenchymal (chief) cells of the paraganglia are derived from the neural crest and migrate during development throughout the autonomic system. All paraganglia, including the nonsecretory chemoreceptors, contain dense core granules within the chief cells. The distribution of paraganglia in the fetus and neonate is much more extensive than that in the adult. Most paragangliomas arise within the paraganglion system; those few that are found in atypical locations probably arise in rests of cells that failed to involute.

There are four types of extra-adrenal paraganglia: (1) branchiomeric, associated with arteries and cranial nerves of the branchial arches, including the carotid and aortic body chemoreceptors (intercarotid and aorticopulmonary paraganglia), jugulotympanic (glomus jugulare), coronary (between the ascending aorta and pulmonary trunk), and pulmonary; (2) intravagal, located along the peripheral distribution of the vagus nerve; (3) aorticosympathetic, associated with segmental sympathetic ganglia and retroperitoneal ganglia in the neck, thorax, and abdomen (including the organ of Zuckerkandl); and (4) visceral-autonomic, associated with blood vessels and visceral organs and found in the atria and interatrial septum, urinary bladder and gallbladder, and liver hilum.

Ninety percent of paragangliomas are functioning adrenal pheochromocytomas. Extra-adrenal paragangliomas may be functional or nonfunctional. Patients with functional tumors often present with hypertension. Well-described paragangliomas include those of the carotid body (most common), jugulotympanic types (glomus jugulare tumor), anterosuperior mediastinum (aorticopulmonic), posterior mediastinum (aortico-sympathetic), and retroperitoneum (including the organ of Zuckerkandl near the angle of the anterior aorta and the origin of the inferior mesenteric artery). Multicentric tumors have been noted in sporadic cases and in certain families.

Paragangliomas are highly vascular tumors composed of nests of cuboidal cells (zellballen) separated by vascular fibrous septa. Sustentacular cells are found in addition to chief cells. Bizarre nuclei and vascular invasion occur but do not indicate malignancy. Mitoses are rare. As a group, 10% of paragangliomas are malignant. Metastases occur most commonly to lung (also brain, liver, heart, and lymph nodes). Cardiac paragangliomas are rare tumors that may be intrapericardial or myocardial and can reside within any of the chambers, most often the left atrium. Paraganglion tissue has been identified in the pericardium, interatrial septum, and posterior walls of both atria. In two recent literature reviews a total of 19 cases were reported with an age range of 18 to 76 years (mean 44) and a male to female ratio of 2:3. Tumors were both functional and nonfunctional. One patient had lung metastases. Frequent symptoms included chest pain and, in functional tumors, hypertension. The tumors were vascular and adherent to adjacent structures.

Gated cardiac MR imaging is the modality of choice for evaluation of cardiac paragangliomas. Paragangliomas, including cardiac tumors, exhibit prolonged T1 and T2 times relative to the surrounding tissue. Some noncardiac tumors have been reported to exhibit characteristic serpiginous areas of signal void on T2-weighted images secondary to high vascular flow. Preoperative coronary angiography can define the vascular supply of the tumor and determine its resectability. Cardiac echocardiography can reliably detect intracardiac but not intrapericardial tumors. CT features of paragangliomas in all locations include a mass of soft tissue density, which is best visualized by bolus intravenous contrast administration owing to its extensive vascularity. Radionuclide scanning with ^{131}I-meta-iodobenzylguanidine (MIBG) can localize functional and nonfunctional paragangliomas.

Cardiac paragangliomas are very difficult to resect because they are highly vascular and adherent to adjacent structures. Cardiopulmonary bypass and coronary artery reconstruction are often required. Excision of the left atrial wall may be necessary. Many tumors are judged to be unresectable.

REFERENCES

Conti VR, Saydjari R, Amparo EG. Paraganglioma of the heart: the value of magnetic resonance imaging in the preoperative evaluation. Chest 1986; 90:604–606.

Glenner GG, Grimley PM. Tumors of the extra-adrenal paraganglion system (including chemoreceptors). Atlas of Tumor Pathology (2nd Series, Fascicle 9). Washington, DC: Armed Forces Institute of Pathology, 1974.

Hui G, McAllister HA, Angelini P. Left atrial paraganglioma: report of a case and review of the literature. Am Heart J 1987; 113:1230–1234.

Johnson TL, Shapiro B, Beierwaltes WH, et al. Cardiac paragangliomas: a clinicopathologic and immunohistochemical study of four cases. Am J Surg Pathol 1985; 9:827–834.

Case 104

HISTORY

An 18-year-old male presented with worsening left hip pain of several months duration.

RADIOLOGY

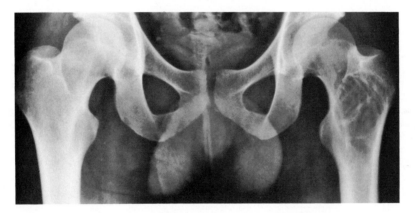

Figure 104-1. There is a lytic lesion of the intertrochanteric part of the femur. Note the prominent ridges of bone surrounding the lesion.

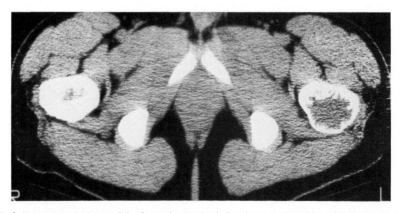

Figure 104-2. The trabecular bone of the femoral metaphysis has been replaced by a lytic lesion that has soft tissue attenuation values. The prominent bony ridges observed on the plain film are seen at the periphery of the lesion.

DIFFERENTIAL DIAGNOSIS

The differential diagnosis includes fibrous dysplasia, aneurysmal bone cyst, giant cell tumor, nonossifying fibroma, simple bone cyst, chondromyxoid fibroma, plasmacytoma, brown tumor, hydatid cyst, metastases, and low-grade sarcomas, including fibrosarcoma and chondrosarcoma.

PATHOLOGY

The lesion was resected.

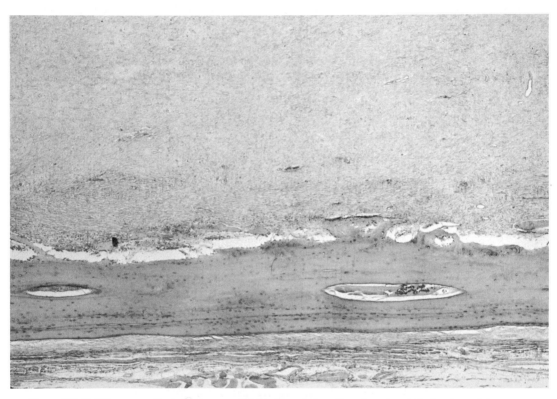

Figure 104–3. At low power the lesion has a well-defined margin from the adjacent endosteal surface of the cortex. Arising from the endosteum are small spicules of reactive bone, which form the bony ridges seen on x-ray.

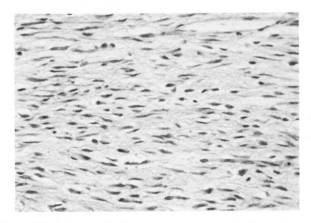

Figure 104–4. Microscopically the tumor appears moderately cellular and is composed of a uniform population of spindle cells with intervening collagen fibers.

DIAGNOSIS

The final pathologic diagnosis was desmoplastic fibroma.

DISCUSSION

Desmoplastic fibroma is an uncommon benign lesion of bone composed of fibroblasts and large amounts of collagen. The cells are relatively well differentiated and do not show nuclear atypia. It occurs most commonly in the second and third decades of life. Seventy-five percent of reported patients are less than 30 years old, and gender incidence is equal. At the time of presentation swelling and pain have typically been present for months. Pathologic fractures occur in a small percentage (10%) of cases. The lesion has been most commonly described in the mandible, femur, humerus, tibia, radius, and ilium but has been observed in many locations. The location is characteristically metaphyseal when the lesion occurs in tubular bones and centrally situated within the bone (in distinction to lesions such as nonossifying fibroma and chondromyxoid fibroma). Involvement of the epiphysis is rare.

Radiographically, an expanded metaphyseal lesion with well-demarcated borders is seen in the majority of cases. The characteristic appearance of coarse trabeculation is due to prominent ridges of bone at the margins of the lesion. A cortical defect may be present, but a prominent soft tissue mass is unusual. Periosteal reaction is not prominent, and an internal calcific matrix is not present. CT may be better for demonstrating the extension of the lesion within the medullary cavity and is more sensitive for delineating cortical erosion and associated soft tissue abnormalities. MR imaging of desmoplastic fibroma shows nonspecific decreased signal on T1-weighted images and increased signal on T2-weighted studies.

Microscopically, the tumor is composed of spindle-shaped fibroblasts of uniform size and appearance, separated by abundant collagen. The nuclei do not demonstrate pleomorphism or hyperchromasia, and mitoses are rare. Fibrosarcoma typically shows larger, more atypical cells with a less prominent collagenous stroma and more numerous mitoses.

Surgical resection of the tumor is considered curative. Recurrence of lesions of similar histology and location has been reported with conservative resection; however, malignant transformation is not typical.

REFERENCES

Dahlin DC, Unni KK. Bone Tumors: General Aspects and Data on 8,542 cases (4th ed). Springfield, IL: Thomas, 1986:366–378.

Enneking WF. Clinical Musculoskeletal Pathology (3rd rev ed). Gainesville, FL: University of Florida Press, 1990:347–349.

Gebhart MC, et al. Desmoplastic fibroma of bone. A report of eight cases and review of the literature. J Bone Joint Surg 1985; 67:732.

Hardy R, Lehrer H. Desmoplastic fibroma vs. desmoid tumor of bone. Radiology 1967; 88:899.

Hudson TM. Radiologic-Pathologic Correlation of Musculoskeletal Lesions. Baltimore: Williams & Wilkins, 1987:305–345.

Lichtman EA, Klein MJ. Case report 302. Skel Radiol 1985; 13:160–163.

Resnick D, Kyriakos M, Greenway GD. Tumors and tumor-like lesions of bone: imaging and pathology of specific lesions. *In*: Resnick D, Niwayama G (eds). Diagnosis of Bone and Joint Disorders (2nd ed). Philadelphia: Saunders, 1988:3746–3752.

Case 105

HISTORY

A 26-year-old woman complained of back pain.

RADIOLOGY

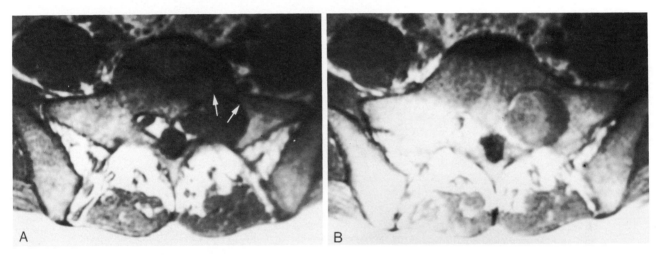

Figure 105-1. T1-weighted MR image (*A*) shows a mass of intermediate signal intensity involving the left S1 nerve root and enlarging the neural foramen (arrows). The mass was hyperintense on T2-weighted images (not shown). There is mild enhancement after intravenous gadolinium infusion (*B*). Other images (not shown) demonstrated extradural extension into the presacral soft tissues.

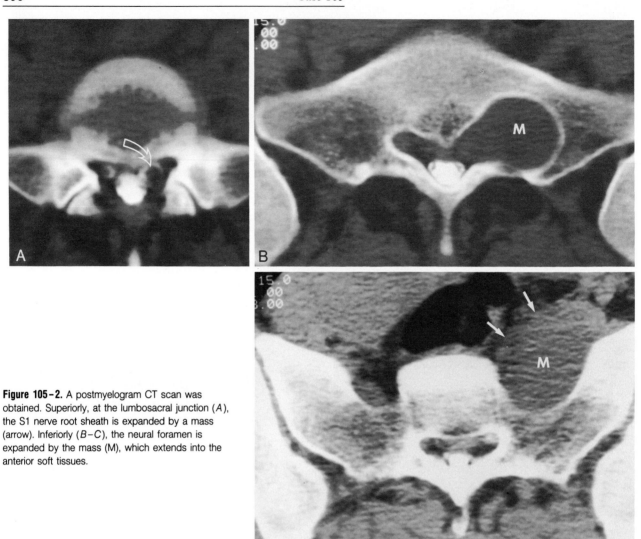

Figure 105-2. A postmyelogram CT scan was obtained. Superiorly, at the lumbosacral junction (*A*), the S1 nerve root sheath is expanded by a mass (arrow). Inferiorly (*B-C*), the neural foramen is expanded by the mass (M), which extends into the anterior soft tissues.

DIFFERENTIAL DIAGNOSIS

The differential diagnosis includes neurofibroma, schwannoma, and meningioma.

PATHOLOGY

The lesion was resected.

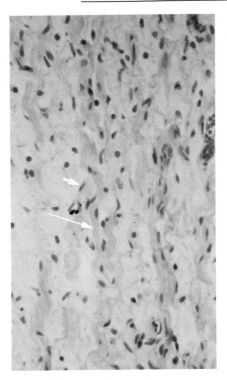

Figure 105-3. Photomicrograph shows wirelike bundles of collagen (long arrow) and spindle cells (short arrow) with abundant intercellular myxoid matrix.

DIAGNOSIS

The final pathologic diagnosis was sacral neurofibroma. The patient did not have other known stigmata of neurofibromatosis.

DISCUSSION

Neurofibromas are benign fibroblastic neoplasms of peripheral nerves whose consistency and histologic appearance vary from myxoid to fibrous according to the differentiation of the neoplastic elements. The bulk of the tumor consists of intercellular collagen fibrils in a nonorganized myxoid matrix. The imaging characteristics depend on the relative amounts of fibrous and myxoid material. Unlike schwannomas, neurofibromas contain neural fibers scattered within the tumor.

Nerve sheath tumors are generally tumors of midlife, with female patients slightly more common than males. They are the most common masses of the spinal canal, accounting for 16% to 30% of such tumors, and are typically intradural and extramedullary. The most common symptoms are pain and radiculopathy due to compression of the affected nerve root. Neurofibromas are slow growing, noninvasive, soft, and elastic tumors that may expand bony foramina and erode pedicles but do not cause bone destruction. They can appear as a single well-circumscribed lesion or as plexiform or multiple lesions in neurofibromatosis. Unlike meningiomas, which in the spine also commonly present as intradural extramedullary masses, they rarely calcify and much more frequently have a bilobed "dumbbell" appearance. On MR imaging, neurofibromas tend to be isointense to muscle on T1-weighted images and show marked brightening on T2-weighted images. A central area of low T2 signal is not unusual.

The primary treatment for neurofibromas is surgical resection. Neurologic outcome is related to the tumor bulk and to whether the adjacent nerve root can be spared. Malignant degeneration to neurofibrosarcoma occurs in 4% to 11% of patients with neurofibromatosis but is otherwise rare.

REFERENCES

Barboriak DP, Rivitz SM, Chew FS. Sacral neurofibroma. AJR 1992; 159:600.

Benzel EC, Morris DM, Fowler MR. Nerve sheath tumors of the sciatic nerve and sacral plexus. J Surg Oncol 1988; 39(1):8–16.

Breidahl WH, Khangure MS. MRI of lumbar and sacral plexus nerve sheath tumours. Australas Radiol 1991; 35:140–144.

Feldenzer JA, McGauley JL, McGillicuddy JE. Sacral and presacral tumors: problems in diagnosis and management. Neurosurgery 1989; 25:884–891.

Harkin JC, Reed RJ. Tumors of the peripheral nervous system. Washington DC: Armed Forces Institute of Pathology, 1969:51–97.

Zimmerman RA, Bilaniuk LT. Imaging of tumors of the spinal canal and cord. Radiol Clin North Am 1988; 26(5):965–1007.

Case 106

HISTORY

A 25-year-old previously healthy male with a weight loss of 25 pounds over 2 months developed progressive facial and bilateral arm swelling and dyspnea.

RADIOLOGY

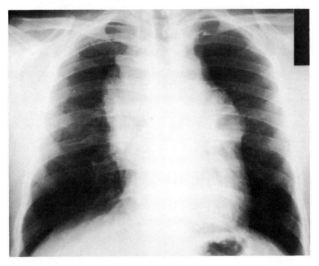

Figure 106-1. Chest radiograph demonstrates the presence of a large, noncalcified anterior mediastinal mass. No pulmonary parenchymal lesions are seen.

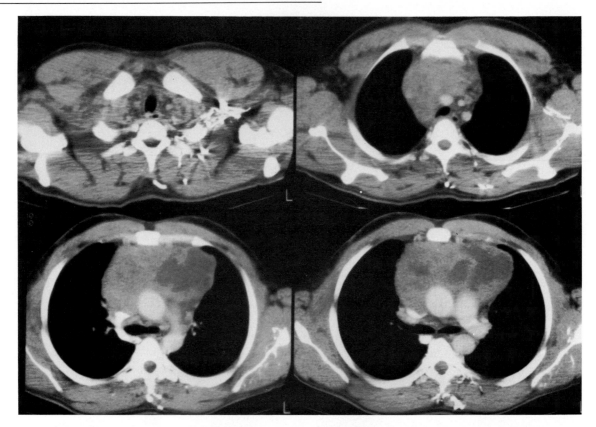

Figure 106-2. CT performed after contrast infusion into the left antecubital vein demonstrates a patent subclavian vein but shows nonfilling of the superior vena cava (SVC) above the azygous arch. The mediastinal mass has large areas of low attenuation that suggest necrosis. Extensive venous collaterals are opacified, including dilated azygos (1.7 cm), hemiazygous, internal mammary, lateral thoracic, anterior subcutaneous, and perivertebral veins. The compressed contrast-filled SVC is seen below the level of the azygous arch, and the trachea is eccentrically compressed by the mass.

DIFFERENTIAL DIAGNOSIS

The differential diagnosis includes lymphoma, teratoma, metastases, inflammatory adenopathy, thymoma, thymic cyst, neuroenteric cysts, sarcoidosis, substernal thyroid, and pericardial cyst.

PATHOLOGY

Surgical biopsy was performed. The lesion was largely necrotic.

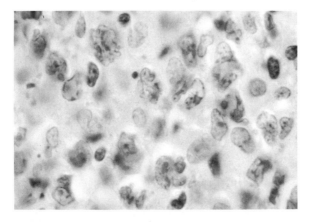

Figure 106-3. The tumor cells are small to medium size and have round nuclei, some of which have irregular contours. The cytoplasm is scant and eosinophilic.

DIAGNOSIS

The final diagnosis was non-Hodgkin's lymphoma causing superior vena cava syndrome.

DISCUSSION

The first description of the superior vena cava syndrome is William Hunter's 1757 description of a patient with an ascending aortic aneurysm. The clinical syndrome consists of plethora and edema of the face and upper body, dyspnea, cough, conjunctival edema with or without proptosis, headache, visual difficulty, pain, and dilation of collateral vessels of the neck and upper torso. Males are affected more frequently (2 : 1), and the median age at presentation has been reported as 50 to 60 years, but there is wide variation.

In approximately 80% of cases of superior vena cava obstruction, the source is a malignant neoplasm. Primary lung carcinoma accounts for most cases, followed by lymphoma, metastases, and other primary mediastinal neoplasms. Rapid development of symptoms is more commonly noted in patients with malignant causes. Among benign causes, ascending aortic aneurysms were most common in early series; however, inflammatory nodal enlargement (due to tuberculosis, histoplasmosis, and other pathogens), postirradiation change, fibrosing mediastinitis, and catheter-induced thrombosis are now more commonly described. Superior vena caval obstruction may also be associated with central venous monitors, hyperalimentation lines, transvenous pacemakers, and leVeen shunts. Finally, superior vena cava syndrome has been described in an aortocaval fistula without obstruction.

With superior vena cava occlusion, collateral venous flow is achieved primarily through the azygous-hemiazygous, internal mammary, lateral thoracic, and vertebral venous systems. If the superior vena cava obstruction occurs below the azygous arch, flow through collateral veins will reach the azygos vein and flow caudally to the ascending lumbar veins and ultimately to the inferior vena cava. Symptoms in this situation tend to be more prominent.

Plain chest radiographs may show mediastinal widening, pleural effusion, or hilar mass on the right more often than on the left. The chest film may be normal. Although venography demonstrates the degree of obstruction, the thrombus, and collateral channels, CT with contrast is more likely to reveal the obstructing lesion itself. The CT diagnosis of superior vena cava obstruction requires demonstration not only of absent or decreased opacification of the superior vena cava but also opacification of the collateral vessels. Using these criteria, CT findings of obstruction were seen in over 80% of patients with documented superior vena cava syndrome in a retrospective study. Contrast enhancement should be performed with bilateral antecubital injection to reduce nonenhanced flow artifacts.

Malignant lesions causing superior vena cava syndrome are often treated by radiation therapy, although there may be medical (chemotherapy, steroids, and diuretics) or surgical options. Overall, the mean survival of patients with superior vena cava syndrome due to malignant lesions is brief—8 months in one series. Thrombolysis or anticoagulation (with line removal) is performed for catheter-related events.

REFERENCES

Brown RC, Nelson CM, Lerona PT. Angiographic demonstration of collateral circulation in a patient with the superior vena caval syndrome. Am J Roentgenol 1973; 119:543–546.

Engel IA, Auh YH, Rubenstein WA, et al. CT diagnosis of mediastinal and thoracic inlet venous obstruction. AJR 1983; 141:521–526.

Moncada R, Cardella R, Demos TC, et al. Evaluation of superior vena cava syndrome by axial CT and CT phlebography. AJR 1984; 143:731–736.

Parish JM, Marschke RF Jr, Dines DE, et al. Etiologic considerations in superior vena cava syndrome. Mayo Clin Proc 1981; 56:407–413.

Yedlicka JW Jr, Cormier MG, Gray R, et al. Computed tomography of superior vena cava obstruction. J Thorac Imag 1987; 2:72–78.

Case 107

HISTORY

A 73-year-old man presented with progressive bilateral lower extremity weakness (left greater than right), paresthesias, and bowel and bladder incontinence.

RADIOLOGY

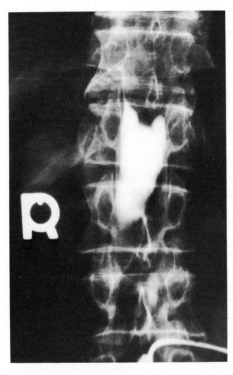

Figure 107-1. Single AP film from a lumbar myelogram obtained with the patient in the Trendelenburg position shows a complete block of myelographic contrast at the level of T11. The inferior margin of the block is lobular.

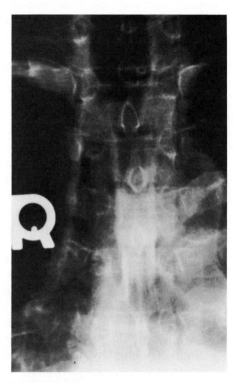

Figure 107-2. AP film from a cervical myelogram with the patient upright shows a complete block at the T5-T6 level.

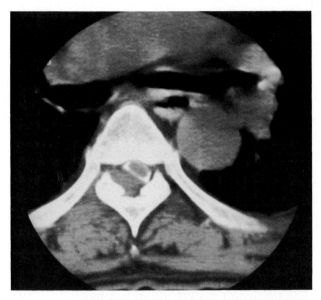

Figure 107-3. Postmyelogram CT scan of the thoracic spine taken at the level of the 6th rib shows a right posterolateral extradural mass that displaces the thoracic spinal cord and thecal sac.

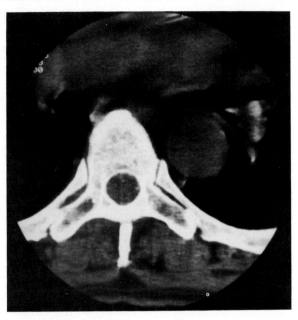

Figure 107-4. At the level of the T6 vertebral body the extradural mass causes complete myelographic block and cord compression. No bony abnormality is seen.

DIFFERENTIAL DIAGNOSIS

The differential diagnosis includes metastasis, lymphoma, extradural schwannoma or neurofibroma, epidural abscess, epidural hemorrhage, sarcoma, multiple myeloma, and extramedullary plasmacytoma.

PATHOLOGY

The lesion was resected.

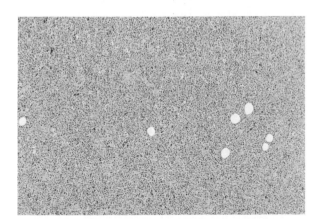

Figure 107-5. Histologically, this section shows a very cellular neoplasm infiltrating around preexisting adipocytes.

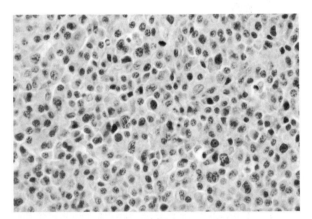

Figure 107-6. The tumor cells have eccentrically placed nuclei and a moderate amount of eosinophilic to slightly basophilic cytoplasm. Adjacent to the nucleus is a crescent-shaped area of cytoplasmic clearing known as a perinuclear huff.

DIAGNOSIS

The final pathologic diagnosis was extramedullary plasmacytoma.

DISCUSSION

Extradural lesions of the spinal canal account for about 85% of cases of spinal cord compression. The great majority of these extradural lesions are due to masses extending from primary and metastatic tumors of the adjacent vertebrae. When no evidence of adjacent bony involvement is seen, entities that present as isolated epidural masses must be considered. These include metastatic disease (particularly prostate or ovarian carcinoma spreading via the epidural venous plexus), lymphoma, sarcoma, epidural abscess, and epidural hematoma. Purely extradural schwannomas and neurofibromas are rare.

Plasma cell malignancies occur in several forms that can involve the spinal canal. Multiple myeloma is a widespread process that can involve multiple vertebral bodies, particularly in the thoracic spine. Skeletal involvement at a single site is seen in solitary osseous plasmacytoma, which accounts for about 10% of extradural tumors and is an uncommon cause of spinal cord compression. Extramedullary plasmacytoma is a rare lesion that is particularly unlikely to occur in the epidural space. Although any nonskeletal body part can be involved by extramedullary plasmacytoma, more than 80% of reported cases occur in the nasal cavity, paranasal sinuses, or upper airway. A single case report of extramedullary plasmacytoma of the epidural space appeared in 1987.

The diagnosis of extramedullary plasmacytoma is made by the histologic demonstration of abnormal aggregates of plasma cells in the extraskeletal soft tissues. Unlike multiple myeloma, urinalysis findings for Bence Jones protein and serum protein electrophoresis are normal in the great majority of patients with extramedullary plasmacytoma. Although subsequent development of multiple myeloma has been documented, this is more commonly seen in solitary osseous plasmacytoma than in extramedullary plasmacytoma.

Early recognition of spinal cord compression is critical for the institution of appropriate therapy. Back pain, weakness in the extremity, bladder and bowel dysfunction, and sensory loss are the most common presenting symptoms. Emergency MR imaging, if available, or myelography followed by CT are the diagnostic methods of choice. Sagittal T1-weighted images are frequently sufficient to rule out high-grade spinal cord compression, and axial imaging by either postmyelographic CT or MR best localizes the mass relative to the spinal cord and thecal sac while evaluating the adjacent bony structures. In cases of complete block, myelography should be performed using small volumes of dense water-soluble contrast because collected intrathecal contrast may be neurotoxic.

Spinal cord compression is a neurologic emergency, and treatment depends on the cause. Radiosensitive tumors such as extramedullary plasmacytoma can be treated with high-dose steroids and radiation therapy. Decompressive laminectomy is generally reserved for patients with nonradiosensitive tumors or for those who relapse and cannot be treated with additional radiation.

REFERENCES

Brinch L, Hannisdal E, Abrahamsen AF, et al. Extramedullary plasmacytomas and solitary plasma cell tumours of bone. Eur J Haematol 1990; 44: 132–135.

Colak A, Cataltepe O, Ozgen T, et al. Spinal cord compression caused by plasmocytomas. A retrospective review of 14 cases. Neurosurg Rev 1989; 12:305–308.

Jungreis CA, Rothfus WE, Latchaw RE. Tumors and infections of the spine and spinal cord. *In:* Latchaw RE (ed). MR and CT Imaging of the Head, Neck and Spine. St. Louis: Mosby-Year Book, 1991.

Kato T, Nakagawa Y, Sawamura Y, et al. Extramedullary plasmacytoma forming a mass in the epidural space of the spinal cord: report of a case. No Shinkei Geka 1987; 15:213–218.

Meis JM, Butler JJ, Osborne BM, et al. Solitary plasmacytomas of bone and extramedullary plasmacytomas. A clinico-pathologic and immunohistochemical study. Cancer 1987; 59:1475–1485.

Schabel SI, Roger CI, Rittenberg GM, et al. Extramedullary plasmacytomas. Radiology 1978; 128:625–628.

Wiltshaw E. The natural history of extramedullary plasmacytoma and its relation to solitary myeloma of bone and myelomatosis. Medicine 1976; 217–238.

Case 108

HISTORY

A 56-year-old Jamaican woman presented with fever, chills, cough, and pleuritic pain of rapid onset.

RADIOLOGY

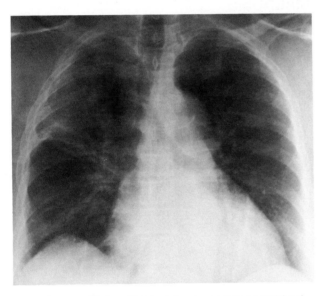

Figure 108-1. Initial AP upright chest film demonstrates a peripheral, sharply marginated right upper lobe consolidation. The lateral film (not shown) localized the abnormality to the apical and posterior segments.

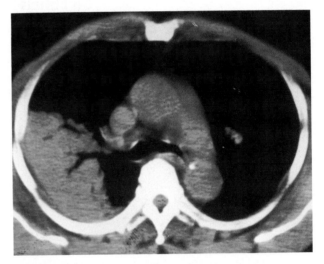

Figure 108-2. Nonenhanced CT scan demonstrates homogeneous soft tissue density of the mass with central air bronchograms. Focal, bilateral pleural disease is present.

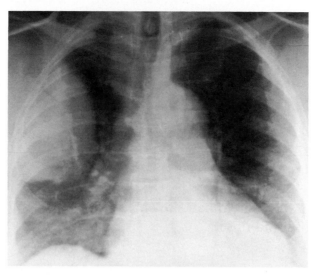

Figure 108-3. Following 6 days of medical therapy, the chest film reveals partial resolution of the consolidation and volume loss.

DIFFERENTIAL DIAGNOSIS

The differential diagnosis includes pneumonia, lymphoma, bronchioloalveolar cell carcinoma, and pseudolymphoma.

PATHOLOGY

Sputum culture was positive for *Streptococcus pneumoniae.*

DIAGNOSIS

The final diagnosis was pneumococcal pneumonia.

DISCUSSION

In the United States, community-acquired pneumonias affect more than 3 million people per year and account for 500,000 hospital admissions. Mortality is approximately 10% to 15% but can exceed 30% in the elderly. *Streptococcus* pneumococci were responsible for 95% of cases in the preantibiotic era. In multiple series between 1971 and 1985, *Streptococcus* was identified as the cause in about 76% of cases and thus remains the most common etiologic agent. The next most common agents are viruses and mycoplasmas. Often the cause cannot be identified, sometimes because of partial antibiotic treatment and sometimes because of less than fastidious culture techniques. An increasing incidence of gram-negative pneumonias in the elderly has been observed, with mortality rates exceeding 70% in some series. *Legionella* and *Haemophilus influenzae* are becoming increasingly common causes of community-acquired pneumonias.

Pneumococci are gram-positive diplococci that possess polysaccharide capsules. The capsular polysaccharide antigen has been used to identify more than 85 serotypes. Generally, the serotypes that cause pneumonia in adults are different from those that affect children, and these in turn are different from those that affect the elderly. Pneumococci remain common because of their high prevalence of colonization in the oropharynx and nasopharynx (40% to 70% of cases), the susceptibility of patients in all age ranges, and the organism's ability to infect secondarily following a viral respiratory illness.

Predisposing factors that interfere with normal host defense mechanisms are important in the development of pneumonia. These include previous viral infection, alcoholism, diabetes, decreased splenic function, chronic obstructive pulmonary disease, congestive heart failure, and advanced age. Classic signs and symptoms include sudden onset of fever and chills, cough productive of rusty sputum, and pleuritic pain. Leukocytosis with a left shift is common. The complications of empyema, endocarditis, pericarditis, and meningitis are rare. The route of infection in pneumococcal pneumonia is aspiration. Organisms penetrate to the periphery where they elicit an outpouring of fibrinous edema and where they can multiply rapidly. Spread of edema, bacteria, red cells, and leukocytes occurs through the canals of Lambert and the pores of Kohn and results in homogeneous consolidation in an initially nonsegmental distribution. Involvement of contiguous alveoli may result in a masslike pneumonia, but fully developed lobar consolidation is uncommon.

The infection usually abuts a pleural surface, and air bronchograms are almost invariable. Atelectasis may be seen during resolution. Involvement of more than one lobe is uncommon and carries a worse prognosis. Pleural effusion is not common. Bronchopneumonia-type inhomogeneous segmental density may be seen in infants, the elderly, and the immunocompromised. Treatment with antibiotics should elicit rapid cessation of the consolidation process, but complete radiologic clearing takes 8 to 10 weeks and lags far behind clinical improvement.

REFERENCES

Jawetz E. Medical Microbiology (18th ed). Norwalk, CT: Appleton & Lang, 1989.

Pare JAP, Fraser RG. Synopsis of Diseases of the Chest. Philadelphia: Saunders, 1983:267–269.

Reed JC. Chest Radiology: Plain Film Patterns and Differential Diagnoses (2nd ed). Chicago: Year Book, 1987:149–160.

Wollschlager CM, Khan FA, Khan A. Utility of radiography and clinical features in the diagnosis of community-acquired pneumonia. Clin Chest Med 1987; 8:393–404.

Case **109**

HISTORY

A 10-year-old boy complained of right knee pain.

RADIOLOGY

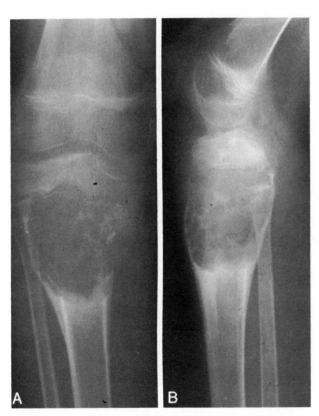

Figure 109-1. *A–B.* There is a destructive lesion of the proximal tibial metaphysis. The lesion is lytic and contains no internal calcification. There is endosteal scalloping, cortical expansion, and a pathologic fracture. Solid periosteal new bone is seen at the lesion margins (Codman triangle).

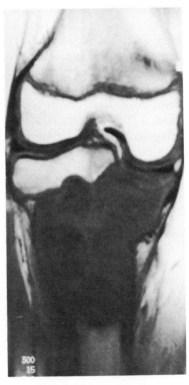

Figure 109-2. Coronal T1-weighted MR image (TR = 300, TE = 15) shows that the mass is centered in the metaphysis but has crossed the open growth plate to involve the subarticular bone of the medial tibia.

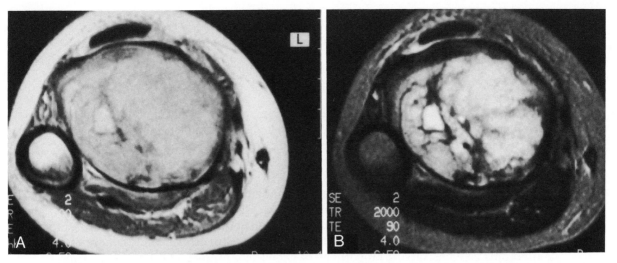

Figure 109-3. Axial proton-density (TR = 2000, TE = 25) (*A*) and T2-weighted (TR = 2000, TE = 90) (*B*) MR images reveal that the lesion is heterogeneous and has hyperintense areas.

DIFFERENTIAL DIAGNOSIS

The differential diagnosis includes giant cell tumor, aneurysmal bone cyst, desmoplastic fibroma, osteoblastoma, brown tumor of hyperparathyroidism, chondroblastoma, and fibrous dysplasia.

PATHOLOGY

The lesion was resected.

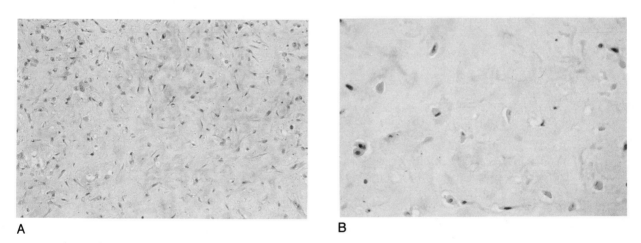

Figure 109-4. Photomicrograph of the more cellular myxoid component (*A*) of the tumor shows scattered neoplastic cells surrounded by an acellular myxoid matrix. The cartilaginous component (*B*) of the tumor has round and elongated chondrocytes residing in lacunar spaces and surrounded by hyaline-type matrix.

DIAGNOSIS

The final pathologic diagnosis was chondromyxoid fibroma.

DISCUSSION

Chondromyxoid fibroma is the least common benign cartilaginous neoplasm of bone, comprising less than 1% of all bone tumors and 2% of benign neoplasms. It is most common in the second and third decades and has a male to female ratio of 1.5:1. The most common symptoms are pain and swelling. Pathologic fracture is uncommon, and the joint is rarely involved.

Chondromyxoid fibroma has a metaphyseal origin but may extend to the epiphysis. The lesion probably arises from the growth plate. The most common location is the proximal tibia followed by the distal femur and less often the fibula, bones of the feet, and the hand. It is rare in bones formed entirely by membranous ossification. Chondromyxoid fibroma contains varying proportions of chondroid, myxoid, and fibrous elements, with occasional hemorrhage and cystic degeneration. The lesions may resemble aneurysmal bone cyst, chondroblastoma, and chondrosarcoma. The lobular growth pattern simulates trabeculation, but true bony trabeculae are not present. On radiographic studies, chondromyxoid fibroma is metaphyseal, eccentric, lucent, and elongated along the long axis of long bones. Cortical expansion, endosteal sclerosis and scalloping, and pseudotrabeculation are characteristic. Pathologic fracture, periosteal reaction, and calcification are uncommon. An intracortical location has been reported but is rare.

Surgical resection is the treatment of choice. Because these lesions are locally aggressive, wide resection and bone grafting with either homograft or allograft is usually required. If simply curetted or incompletely excised, the recurrence rate is high, varying from 10% to 80% in different studies. Radiation and chemotherapy are not used. Malignant transformation has been documented very rarely.

REFERENCES

Begg IG, Staker DJ. Chondromyxoid fibroma of bone. Clin Radiol 1982; 33:671.

Cherlinzoni F, Rock M, Picci P. Chondromyxoid fibroma. J Bone Joint Surg 1983; 65(A):198.

Enneking WF. Clinical Musculoskeletal Pathology (3rd rev ed). Gainesville, FL: University of Florida Press, 1990:337–341.

Hudson TM. Radiologic-Pathologic Correlation of Musculoskeletal Lesions. Baltimore: Williams & Wilkins, 1987:147–152.

McFarland GB, Morden ML. Benign cartilaginous lesion. Orthop Clin North Am 1977; 8:737.

Resnick D. Bone and Joint Imaging. Philadelphia: Saunders, 1989:1131–1132.

Schajowicz F. Chondromyxoid fibroma. Report of 3 cases with predominant cortical involvement. Radiology 1987; 164:783.

Case 110

HISTORY

A 34-year-old Cambodian male presented with a left neck mass that had been progressively enlarging for 2 years.

RADIOLOGY

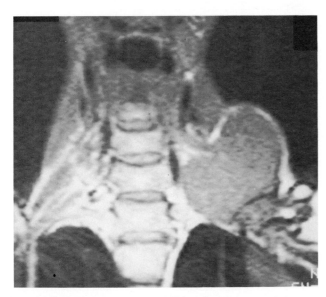

Figure 110-1. T1-weighted coronal MR image shows a rounded mass of intermediate signal at the base of the left neck. The mass is continuous with the left brachial plexus.

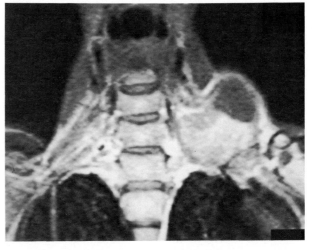

Figure 110-2. On postgadolinium images the inferior solid portion of the mass enhances heterogeneously whereas the superior portion of the mass does not enhance.

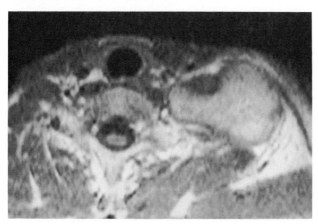

Figure 110-3. Postgadolinium T1-weighted axial image shows that the tail of the comet-shaped enhancing solid component approaches but does not extend into the lower cervical neural foramen.

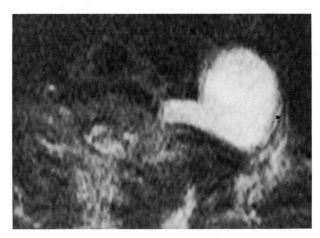

Figure 110-4. The solid component shows a markedly increased signal on the late echo T2-weighted MR sequence.

DIFFERENTIAL DIAGNOSIS

The differential diagnosis includes cystic neurofibroma, schwannoma, cystic gang-lioneuroma, paraganglioma (glomus vagale tumor), and malignant or necrotic ade-nopathy.

PATHOLOGY

An incisional biopsy was performed, followed by resection of the mass. The mass was lobulated and compartmentalized by layers of fibrous tissue. Morphologically, the mass was typified by areas of increased cellularity (Antoni A areas) alternating with less cellular regions (Antoni B).

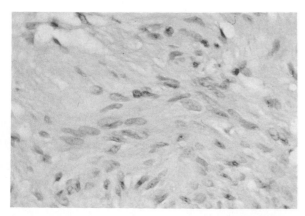

Figure 110–5. In the cellular Antoni A regions the neoplastic spindle cells are arranged in parallel array forming Verocay bodies.

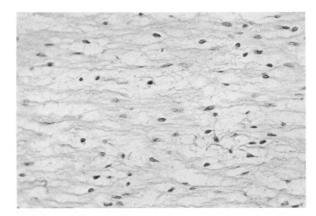

Figure 110–6. In the less cellular Antoni B regions the spindle cells tend to be haphazardly arranged and are separated by myxoid stroma and thin wirelike collagen fibers.

DIAGNOSIS

The final pathologic diagnosis was schwannoma of the brachial plexus.

DISCUSSION

Schwannomas consist of proliferating Schwann cells and fibroblasts. Microscopically, areas of both high and low cellularity (Antoni A and Antoni B tissue) are seen. Typically, schwannomas arise eccentrically along nerve roots. Unlike neurofibromas, they do not contain nerve fibers scattered in the tumor. Grossly, the lesion is well circumscribed, solitary, and usually lobulated. Although hemorrhage within the tumor is unusual, cyst formation is common.

In a large series, nerve sheath tumors were the most common neoplasms of the brachial plexus, with neurofibromas accounting for 46% and benign schwannomas for 14%. The benign schwannomas tended to occur at the C5 or C6 root on the upper trunk. The tumors displace rather than envelop adjacent neural structures. The most common presentation in the neck is a palpable mass. If the tumor reaches sufficient size, pain and paresthesias may radiate along the course of the compressed nerve. Muscles supplied by the involved nerve may atrophy.

Plain films may demonstrate a soft tissue mass that may be associated with bony erosion and, rarely, with punctate calcifications. CT appearance depends upon the relative proportion of soft tissue and cystic degeneration. Varying degrees of contrast enhancement occur. On MR imaging, the T1-weighted signal intensity of the tumor is similar to that of spinal cord and muscle, and there is marked brightening on T2-weighted images. On postgadolinium images, enhancement of schwannomas is marked and, in the absence of cystic degeneration or necrosis, homogeneous. No vascular encasement is seen. Angiography demonstrates a hypervascular lesion.

Sarcomatous degeneration of a schwannoma into neurofibrosarcoma rarely occurs. With complete resection, recurrence is unusual.

REFERENCES

Harkins JC, Reed RJ. Tumors of the Peripheral Nervous System. Atlas of Tumor Pathology (2nd series, Fascicle 3). Washington DC: Armed Forces Institute of Pathology, 1969.

Horowitz J, Kline DG, Keller SM. Schwannoma of the brachial plexus mimicking an apical lung tumor. Ann Thorac Surg 1991; 52:555–556.

Lusk MD, Kline DG, Garcia CA. Tumors of the brachial plexus. Neurosurgery 1987; 21:439–453.

Reed JC, Hallett KK, Feigin DS. Neural tumors of the thorax: subject review from the AFIP. Radiology 1978; 126:9–17.

Shields TW, Reynolds M. Neurogenic tumors of the thorax. Surg Clin North Am 1988; 68(3):645–668.

Case 111

HISTORY

A 31-year-old woman presented with a 3-month history of pleuritic chest pain, mild shortness of breath, night sweats, and low grade fever. The initial chest radiograph was clear.

RADIOLOGY

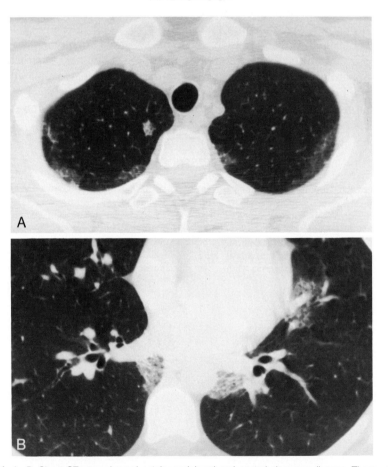

Figure 111-1. *A–B*. Chest CT scan showed patchy peripheral and central air-space disease. There was no cavitation, effusion, or adenopathy.

DIFFERENTIAL DIAGNOSIS

The differential diagnosis includes pneumonia, hemorrhage, lymphoma, bronchioloalveolar cell carcinoma, pulmonary alveolar proteinosis, and opportunistic infections in patients with acquired immune deficiency syndrome (AIDS).

PATHOLOGY

Open lung biopsy was performed.

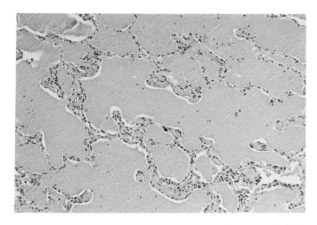

Figure 111-2. Low power view of the lung demonstrates alveolar filling with homogeneous eosinophilic material.

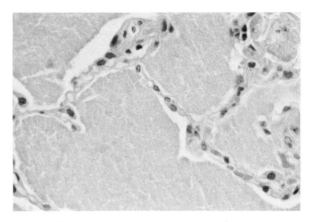

Figure 111-3. No inflammatory or fibrotic reaction is seen in the alveolar walls or interstitium.

DIAGNOSIS

The final pathologic diagnosis was pulmonary alveolar proteinosis.

DISCUSSION

Pulmonary alveolar proteinosis is a rare disease of unknown etiology. The classic radiologic finding is bilateral, symmetric, perihilar air space disease in a "bat-wing" distribution simulating severe acute pulmonary edema but with normal heart size. However, studies with CT have shown that peripheral or central ill-defined nodular opacities or patchy consolidation are more common appearances. This pattern of abnormality results from large groups of otherwise normal alveoli filling with material that is mostly phospholipid and protein constituents of both surfactant and degenerated cell membranes. Occasionally, superimposed septal edema, infiltration, or fibrosis results in an interstitial pattern of abnormality. Involvement is occasionally asymmetric or unilateral.

Pulmonary alveolar proteinosis is a nonspecific tissue response to a variety of injuries to alveolar macrophages, type II pneumocytes, or both. It is associated with altered immunity and exposure to dusts or fumes. Proposed pathogenetic mechanisms include unbalanced turnover and defective production or clearance of surfactant.

Insidious onset of mild dyspnea and cough are the most common symptoms, but hemoptysis, intermittent low-grade fevers, pleuritic chest pain, weight loss, clubbing, and cyanosis have been associated. Pulmonary function testing typically shows restrictive dysfunction with decreased diffusing capacity and compliance. Due to its rarity, initial misdiagnosis is not uncommon. Opportunistic superinfection, particularly with *Nocardia*, and pulmonary fibrosis are possible complications.

The diagnosis of pulmonary alveolar proteinosis is made by biopsy, but detection of surfactant apoprotein A in sputum could allow a less invasive diagnosis. Bronchoalveolar lavage to remove the alveolar material usually improves pulmonary function, sometimes dramatically. Although the disease in some patients resolves spontaneously or after a single lavage, most require chronic treatment for months or years.

REFERENCES

Dail DH. Metabolic and other disease. *In*: Dail DH, Hammar SP (eds). Pulmonary Pathology. New York: Springer-Verlag, 1988:561–567.

Godwin JD, Muller NL, Takasugi JE. Pulmonary alveolar proteinosis: CT findings. Radiology 1988; 169:609–613.

Masuda T, Shimura S, Sasaki H, et al. Surfactant apoprotein-A concentration in sputum for diagnosis of pulmonary alveolar proteinosis. Lancet 1991; 337:580–582.

Case 112

HISTORY

A 69-year-old woman presented with fever, bloody diarrhea, and abdominal pain 7 days following surgical repair of an abdominal hernia.

RADIOLOGY

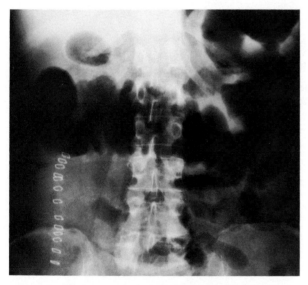

Figure 112-1. Kidney, ureter, bladder (KUB) film shows haustral thickening of the transverse colon.

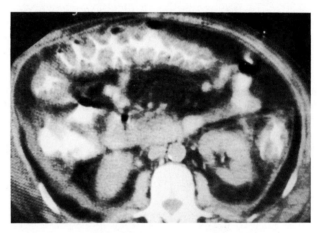

Figure 112-2. Following oral Gastrografin administration, noncontrast CT scan demonstrates nodular wall thickening involving the transverse colon.

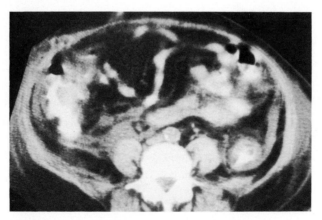

Figure 112-3. The cecum and descending colon show symmetric nodular wall thickening with adjacent inflammatory changes.

DIFFERENTIAL DIAGNOSIS

The differential diagnosis includes infectious colitis, inflammatory bowel disease, ischemic bowel, and pseudomembranous colitis.

PATHOLOGY

The patient had been treated with clindamycin postoperatively. *Clostridium difficile* was isolated from the bowel. The *C. difficile* toxin titer measured 1:6000. Because the patient did not respond to conservative therapy, partial colectomy was performed.

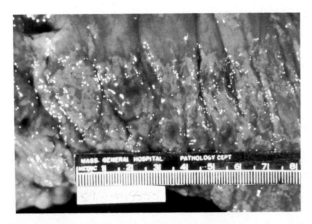

Figure 112-4. The segment of removed bowel shows a very hyperemic mucosa in which pale pink regions are covered by a pseudomembrane.

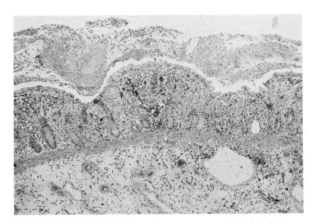

Figure 112-5. The focally necrotic bowel mucosa is covered by a pseudomembrane (lumen at top of figure).

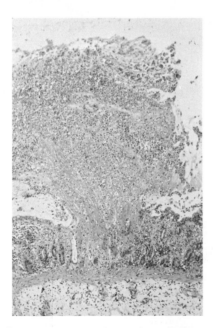

Figure 112-6. In the early stages the membrane begins as a mushroomlike aggregate of inflammation admixed with fibrin.

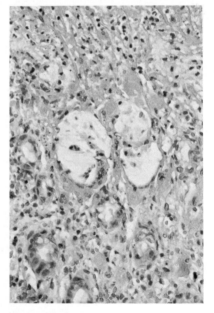

Figure 112-7. Some of the underlying obstructed necrotic glands become filled with mucin.

DIAGNOSIS

The final diagnosis was pseudomembranous colitis.

DISCUSSION

Enterocolitis in the elderly encompasses a broad spectrum of disorders. The differential diagnosis includes infectious colitis, antibiotic-associated colitis, ischemic colitis, ulcerative colitis, Crohn's disease, radiation colitis, or infiltrative tumors such as lymphoma. The differentiation between infectious, ischemic, and inflammatory bowel disease may be difficult.

Ischemic enterocolitis results in a segmental distribution with infrequent involvement of the rectum. The most common clinical presentation is bloody diarrhea associated with mild to moderate lower abdominal pain. In the first 48 to 72 hours, radiographs may show thumbprinting from submucosal hemorrhage. If the acute edema and hemorrhage resolve, the healing process may be complicated by submucosal fibrosis, stricture formation, and obstruction. Without resolution, the bowel wall becomes necrotic, perforates, and requires surgical resection. Ominous radiographic signs include gas in the bowel wall and portal venous system.

Like ischemic enterocolitis, infectious enterocolitis is common in the elderly. Acute inflammation of the terminal ileum and colon is caused by numerous infectious agents, including viruses, bacteria, and parasites. Specific organisms include *Campylobacter*, *Yersinia*, *Escherichia coli*, *Mycobacterium tuberculosis*, *Shigella*, and *Entamoeba histolytica*. Infection due to these agents typically occurs in a segmental distribution.

Pseudomembranous colitis is a common cause of infectious pancolitis. This disease often involves the small bowel as well. Clinically, it can follow a course ranging from mild, watery diarrhea to the development of toxic megacolon. Inflammation of the colonic and rectal mucosa is characterized histologically and pathologically by the formation of elevated yellowish-white plaques. The plaques, or pseudomembranes, are composed of necrotic debris that adheres to the ulcerated mucosa. *Clostridium difficile* is the predominant causative agent and usually superinfects patients taking antibiotics. Although all antibiotics inhibit the normal intestinal flora and permit overgrowth of a resistant enteric pathogen, clindamycin is most commonly associated with pseudomembranous colitis. *C. difficile* also occurs as an opportunistic infection in patients with leukemia or cancer and in those receiving chemotherapy. Treatment with oral vancomycin or metronidazole is usually effective. The offending antibiotic must be stopped.

Plain radiographs of the abdomen may show a dynamic ileus pattern and nodular thickening or thumbprinting of the transverse colon. A segmental distribution simulates the appearance of ischemic colitis. A dilated colon with irregular wall thickening contraindicates barium enema examination. Barium enema, which increases the intraluminal pressure and can perforate the bowel wall in patients with toxic megacolon, shows numerous nodular plaques that are most predominant in the transverse colon. The contour of the colon wall is irregular and polypoid owing to pseudomembranous and submucosal hemorrhage. Ulcerations are not seen because they are covered by pseudomembranes. The haustra are blunted or thickened, and the inflamed mucosa is poorly coated by barium. CT scan shows marked, low attenuation edema of the bowel wall, which is thick and nodular. Although the entire colon is involved, the distribution may be markedly asymmetric or segmental. Inflammatory stranding involves the mesentery and adjacent fat. In contrast, ulcerative colitis produces thickening of the colonic wall without significant surrounding inflammatory changes.

Figures 112–8 and 112–9 show images from the CT scan of a 52-year-old patient with pseudomembranous colitis. In this case, the ascending, transverse, and descending colon are diffusely involved. Although the transverse colon is diffusely involved with nodular transmural edema, there is asymmetric thickening of the ascending colon compared with the descending colon. In patients with asymmetric distribution, the left colon is typically affected to a greater degree. This patient developed pseudomembranous colitis during antibiotic treatment of pyelonephritis.

Bowel wall thickening of the colon is nonspecific and may have a vascular, infectious, inflammatory, or neoplastic causes. Figure 112–10 shows images from the CT scan of a 40-year-old patient who had AIDS. This patient also had thickening of the wall of the ascending and transverse colon with relative sparing of the descending colon. He under-

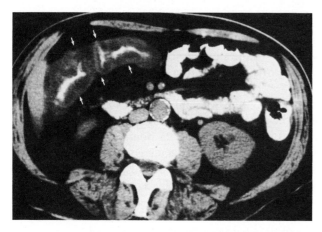

Figure 112–8. Noncontrast-enhanced CT scan demonstrates a low attenuation, nodular, thickened wall (arrows) of the transverse colon.

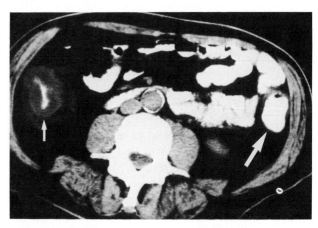

Figure 112–9. Nodular wall thickening and surrounding inflammatory changes involve the ascending colon (small arrow), but there is relative sparing of the descending colon (large arrow).

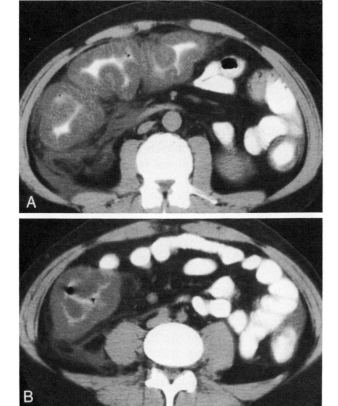

Figure 112–10. *A–B.* Noncontrast CT scan shows marked wall thickening of the ascending and transverse colon with relative sparing of the descending colon. Inflammatory changes involve the adjacent retroperitoneal fat.

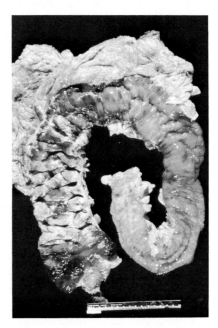

Figure 112–11. Resected colon with hyperemic mucosa is focally covered by a pale tan-yellow pseudomembrane.

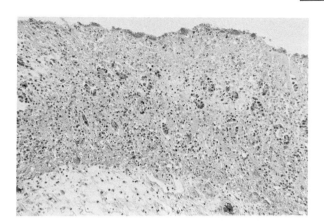

Figure 112–12. The mucosa is largely necrotic with scattered residual portions of colonic glands.

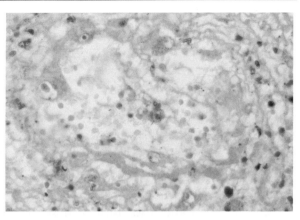

Figure 112–13. Many of the vessels within the submucosa are partially occluded by fibrin and are lined by enlarged endothelial cells that have prominent nuclear viral inclusions.

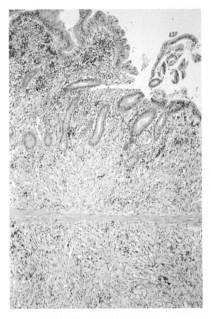

Figure 112–14. Elsewhere in the small bowel are well-circumscribed red-purple nodules that are composed histologically of a proliferation of spindle cells that infiltrate throughout the mucosa and submucosa.

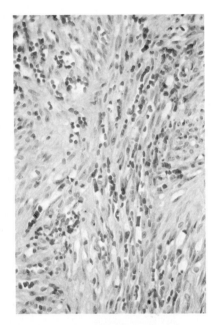

Figure 112–15. These spindle cells are arranged in interlacing fascicles with numerous red blood cells filling subtle slitlike vascular spaces. They indicate the presence of Kaposi's sarcoma.

went colectomy, which revealed cytomegalovirus colitis as well as Kaposi's sarcoma of the bowel wall (Figs. 112–11 through 112–15).

REFERENCES

Scully R, Mark E, McNeely W, et al. Case records of the MGH. N Engl J Med 1990; 323:113.

Stanley R, Melson G, Tedesco F. The spectrum of radiographic findings in antibiotic-related pseudo-membranous colitis. Radiology 1974; 111:519.

Talbot RW, Walker RC, Beart RW Jr. Diagnosis and treatment of *Clostridium difficile* toxin-associated colitis. Br J Surg 1986; 73:457.

Wittenberg J, Athanasoulis C, Shapiro J, et al. A radiological approach to the patient with acute, extensive bowel ischemia. Radiology 1973; 106:13.

Wittenberg J, Athanasoulis C, Williams L, et al. Ischemic colitis. AJR 1975; 123:287.

Case 113

HISTORY

A 75-year-old man presented with vague left knee pain.

RADIOLOGY

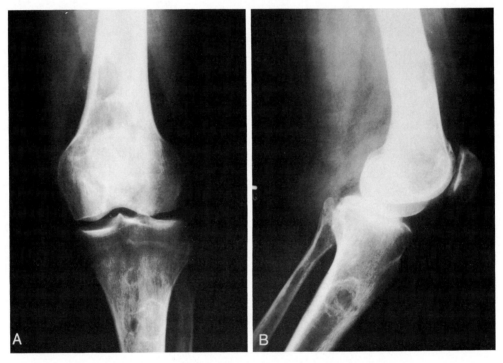

Figure 113-1. AP radiograph (*A*) of the knee shows multiple lytic lesions affecting the femur, tibia, and fibula. The lesions are well circumscribed and appear round, ovoid, or lobulated. Lateral radiograph (*B*) shows a cortically based lesion in the distal femur with a soft tissue component.

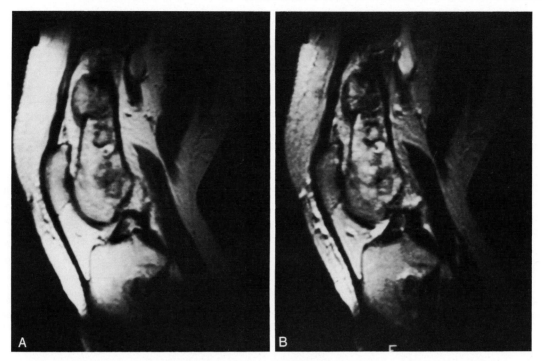

Figure 113-2. Proton-density (TR = 2500, TE = 30) weighted MR image (*A*) shows a diffusely inhomogeneous, mottled, abnormal signal in the distal femoral marrow. T2-weighted (TR = 2500, TE = 80) MR image (*B*) demonstrates cortical destruction and extension into the soft tissues anterior to the femur. There is relatively little increase in signal intensity.

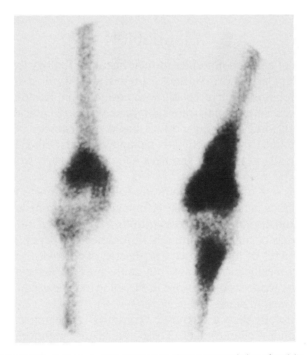

Figure 113-3. Radionuclide bone scan shows accumulation of activity in the lesions.

DIFFERENTIAL DIAGNOSIS

The differential diagnosis includes hemangiomas, cystic angiomatosis, lymphangi-omatosis, hemangioendotheliomas, histiocytoses, and infection by unusual organism.

PATHOLOGY

An incisional biopsy was done of one of the lesions.

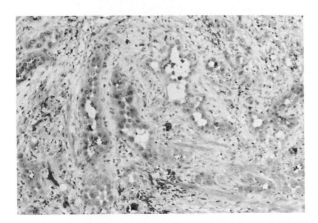

Figure 113-4. The lesion is composed of a conglomerate of capillaries lined by plump endothelial cells.

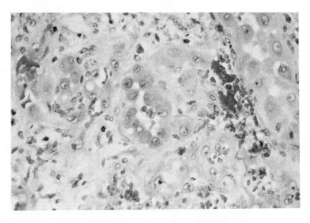

Figure 113-5. The endothelial cells are large, round, and have abundant eosinophilic cytoplasm. These features are typical of "epithelioid" endothelial cells.

DIAGNOSIS

The final pathologic diagnosis was epithelioid hemangioma involving bone.

DISCUSSION

Hemangiomas of bone do not differ in their histomorphology from those in the skin and soft tissues. Capillary and cavernous varieties are the most frequent. Epithelioid hemangiomas (angiolymphoid hyperplasia with eosinophilia, Kimura's disease, histiocytoid hemangioma) are an extremely rare subtype that radiographically appears identical to cavernous hemangioma. The diagnosis is based on histology because many of the vessels appear to be lined by distinct epithelial-appearing endothelial cells. Most lesions are situated superficially in the head and neck and occur in early to mid adult life (20 to 40 years).

Hemangioma is one of the most common soft tissue tumors and is the most common tumor in infancy and childhood. Hemangiomas of bone are significantly less frequent but not uncommon lesions constituting about 1% of primary bone tumors. Osseous hemangiomas occur predominantly in middle-aged patients, particularly in the fourth and fifth decades of life. Women are affected about twice as frequently as men. Most lesions are clinically insignificant, but some may be associated with soft tissue swelling or pain. On rare occasions, lesions in the spine may be accompanied by signs and symptoms of cord compression.

Spinal lesions usually show a diagnostic "corduroy" appearance. In extraspinal sites, the findings are often less characteristic. These lesions are radiolucent, slightly expansile, and intraosseous, possessing a radiating, latticelike or weblike trabecular pattern. Cortical thinning may be seen, but extensive periostitis or soft tissue mass is rare. A distinctive trabecular pattern comprising retained trabeculae within the lesion is most helpful though not always seen. Multiple skeletal hemangiomas appear as roundish or ovoid lucencies. Sharply marginated and often with thin, reactive sclerotic rims, the appearance is sometimes multiloculated or honeycombed. On MR images there is a mottled, increased signal in T1- and T2-weighted images from the osseous portions. Increased signal on T1 is secondary to the adipose content. In one study, the extraosseous component of the tumor contained little fat and therefore had a long T1 signal.

Solitary lesions predominate. The most common sites of involvement are the skull or facial bones and the vertebrae. Hemangiomas in the long tubular bones are uncommon and are usually found in the epiphysis or metaphysis, especially in the femur, tibia, and humerus. A subtype known as intracortical predominates in the diaphysis of long bones. Multiple skeletal hemangiomas occur rarely, often in association with more or less extensive soft tissue involvement. These are benign lesions that may progress slowly in size. Clinical manifestations, when present, are related to local effects such as osseous expansion or soft tissue extension. Malignant degeneration is not encountered.

Rare lesions have been noted to regress spontaneously, but in general, surgical excision is required if the lesions are symptomatic. Up to one third may recur following resection. Eighty percent show at least a partial response to superficial radiotherapy.

REFERENCES

Enzinger FM, Weiss SW. Soft Tissue Tumors (2nd ed). St. Louis: Mosby, 1988:502–508.

Hudson TM. Radiologic-Pathologic Correlation of Musculoskeletal Lesions. Baltimore: Williams & Wilkins, 1987:407–411.

Resnick D, Kyriakos M, Greenway GD. Tumors and tumor-like lesions of bone: imaging and pathology of specific lesions. *In*: Resnick D, Niwayama G (eds). Diagnosis of Bone and Joint Disorders (2nd ed). Philadelphia, Saunders, 1988:3792–3798.

Ross JS, Masaryk TJ, Modic MT, et al. Vertebral hemangiomas: MR imaging. Radiology 1987; 165:165–169.

Case 114

HISTORY

A 19-year-old male presented with progressive facial and skull deformities.

RADIOLOGY

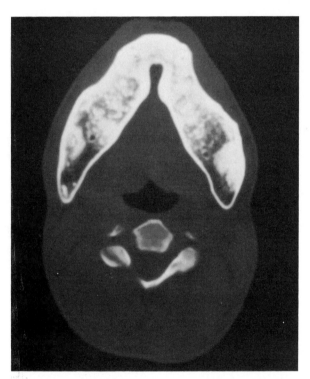

Figure 114–1. An axial CT image through the mandible reveals massively enlarged dysplastic bone with areas of lucency, sclerosis, and a ground-glass appearance. The overlying cortex is intact.

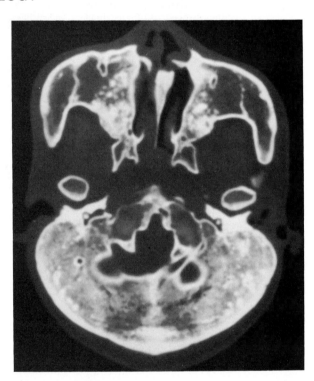

Figure 114–2. Axial image through the maxilla and base of the skull reveals similar findings.

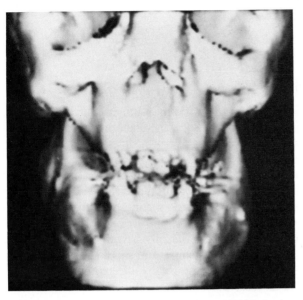

Figure 114-3. AP view of the 3-dimensional CT reconstruction displayed for bones demonstrates the very marked hypertrophy of the mandible, particularly on the right side. Severe dental malalignment, hypertelorism, and low-set ears are also present.

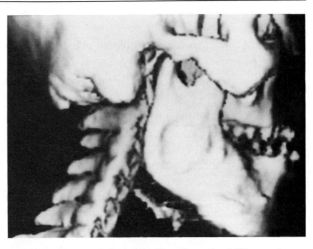

Figure 114-4. A lateral view of the three-dimensional CT scan shows the lumpy and irregular contour of the mandible. The occiput displays a similar appearance, suggesting its involvement.

DIFFERENTIAL DIAGNOSIS

The differential diagnosis includes fibrous dysplasia and the mixed phase of Paget's disease.

PATHOLOGY

A biopsy was performed.

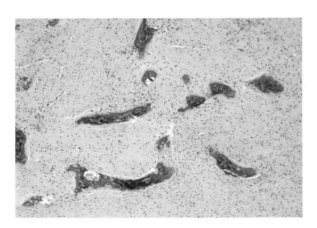

Figure 114-5. The specimen contains round and curvilinear trabeculae of woven bone surrounded by a moderately cellular spindle cell proliferation.

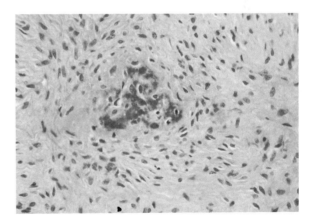

Figure 114-6. The woven bone is focally mineralized and is not rimmed by conspicuous osteoblasts. The spindle cell component contains uniform bland spindle cells with no mitotic activity.

DIAGNOSIS

The final pathologic diagnosis was fibrous dysplasia.

DISCUSSION

Fibrous dysplasia is a benign nonhereditary developmental bone lesion in which failure of osteoblastic differentiation and maturation is associated with replacement of normal bone by fibrous connective tissue showing varying degrees of osseous metaplasia. It affects males and females equally.

The monostotic form accounts for 70% to 80% of cases and tends to involve (in decreasing order of frequency) the ribs, femur, tibia, mandible, calvarium, and humerus, although any bone may be affected. Most cases are diagnosed in the second and third decades (range 10 to 70 years).

The polyostotic form may be unilateral or bilateral (but is usually asymmetric). Craniofacial involvement is common, as are lesions of the pelvis, spine, and shoulder. In comparison with the monostotic form, larger segments of bone are usually affected, and gross deformities are more frequent. Two thirds of cases present before the age of 10 years. A small number of cases of fibrous dysplasia are associated with an endocrine abnormality. The best known lesions (although they comprise only a small percentage of the total) are the McCune-Albright syndrome of female sexual precocity, polyostotic fibrous dysplasia, and pigmented cutaneous lesions.

Craniofacial fibrous dysplasia occurs in 10% to 25% of patients with monostotic and 50% of patients with polyostotic disease. Most often affected are the frontal, sphenoid, maxillary, and ethmoid bones; involvement of the mandible and the occipital and temporal bones is less common. Craniofacial fibrous dysplasia most often presents with asymmetric deformity and occasionally with pathologic fracture. Orbital involvement can result in hypertelorism, proptosis, and optic nerve compromise. Hearing and vestibular dysfunction can result from involvement of the temporal and sphenoid bones, and anosmia can occur if the cribriform plate is affected. Occasionally, hypertrophic changes in the base of the skull affect the neural foramina.

Fibrous dysplasia is characterized by a fibrocellular matrix with haphazardly embedded, irregular ossicles of woven bone with varying degrees of mineralization. Cartilaginous nodules and cystic changes are occasionally found. A variety of radiographic appearances may be seen depending on the location and histology. Extensive sclerosis of the sphenoid wing and base of the skull is a common finding (as in Paget's disease, craniometaphyseal dysplasia, Engelmann's disease, meningioma, osteopetrosis, and some other diseases). Mandibular and maxillary involvement is characterized by expansion (focal or diffuse) with mixed lucent and sclerotic regions (similar to the mixed phase of Paget's disease), malocclusion, displacement of teeth and obliteration of the paranasal sinuses. Focal areas of mandibular expansion may resemble adamantinoma or dentigerous cyst. Lucent lesions of the calvarium or facial bones are associated with widening of the diploic space and focal or extensive outward expansion.

CT may help to define lesions in the face and skull including those with osseous and the rare extraosseous involvement. It may help to narrow the differential diagnosis in equivocal cases by defining the character and attenuation values of the matrix and may be useful for evaluation of malignant change. The three-dimensional reformations are particularly useful for surgical planning. Although it may be reactivated by estrogen therapy or pregnancy, fibrous dysplasia most often becomes quiescent after puberty. Extensive, early, and deforming disease may continue to progress after puberty.

The risk of malignant change is said to be 0.4% to 1%, most often to osteosarcoma or fibrosarcoma and occasionally to chondrosarcoma. Excision or curettage is used to correct functional and cosmetic deformities and to provide relief of neurologic compromise. It is best to postpone surgery until the lesion stabilizes. Radiation therapy is seldom used because of the hazard of secondary malignancy.

REFERENCES

Feldman F. Tuberous sclerosis, neurofibromatosis, and fibrous dysplasia. *In*: Resnick D, Niwayama G (eds). Diagnosis of Bone and Joint Disorders (2nd ed). Philadelphia: Saunders, 1988:4057–4070.

Leeds N, Seaman WB. Fibrous dysplasia of the skull: a clinical and roentgenographic study of 46 cases. Radiology 1962; 78:570–581.

Mendelsohn DB, et al. Computed tomography of craniofacial fibrous dysplasia. J Comput Assist Tomogr 1984; 8:1062–1065.

Sherman NH, et al. Fibrous dysplasia of the facial bones and mandible. Skel Radiol 1982; 8:141–143.

Index

Note: Page numbers in *italics* refer to illustrations.